USMLE STEP 2 SECRETS

SECRETS

USMLE STEP 2 SECRETS

Third Edition

Theodore X. O'Connell, MD
Program Director
Family Medicine Residency Program
Kaiser Permanente Woodland Hills, Woodland Hills, California;
Assistant Clinical Professor
Department of Family Medicine
David Geffen School of Medicine at UCLA, Los Angeles, California;
Partner Physician
Southern California Permanente Medical Group, Woodland Hills, California

Adam Brochert, MD
Staff Radiologist
Eisenhower Medical Center
Rancho Mirage, California

MOSBY

ELSEVIER

MOSBY
ELSEVIER

1600 John F. Kennedy Blvd.
Ste 1800
Philadelphia, PA 19103-2899

USMLE STEP 2 SECRETS   ISBN: 978-0-323-05713-4

Notice

Knowledge and best practice in this field are constantly changing. As new research and experience broaden our knowledge, changes in practice, treatment and drug therapy may become necessary or appropriate. Readers are advised to check the most current information provided (i) on procedures featured or (ii) by the manufacturer of each product to be administered, to verify the recommended dose or formula, the method and duration of administration, and contraindications. It is the responsibility of the practitioner, relying on his or her own experience and knowledge of the patient, to make diagnoses, to determine dosages and the best treatment for each individual patient, and to take all appropriate safety precautions. To the fullest extent of the law, neither the Publisher nor the Editors assume any liability for any injury and/or damage to persons or property arising out of or related to any use of the material contained in this book.

The Publisher

Library of Congress Cataloging-in-Publication Data
O'Connell, Theodore X.
    USMLE step 2 secrets / Theodore X. O'Connell, Adam Brochert. – 3rd ed.
        p. ; cm. – (Secrets series)
    Rev. ed. of: USMLE step 2 secrets / Adam Brochert. 2nd ed. c2004.
    Includes bibliographical references and index.
    ISBN 978-0-323-05713-4
    1. Clinical medicine–Examinations, questions, etc. I. Brochert, Adam. II. Brochert, Adam,
    - USMLE step 2 secrets. III. Title. IV. Title: USMLE step two secrets. V. Series: Secrets series.
    [DNLM: 1. Clinical Medicine–Examination Questions. WB 18.2 O18u 2010]
    RC58.B76 2010
    616.0076–dc22

                                                                    2009039617

Acquisitions Editor: James Merritt
Developmental Editor: Christine Abshire
Publishing Services Manager: Hemamalini Rajendrababu
Project Manager: Sukanthi Sukumar
Marketing Manager: Jason Oberacker

Printed in the United States of America

Last digit is the print number: 9 8 7 6 5 4 3

Working together to grow
libraries in developing countries

www.elsevier.com | www.bookaid.org | www.sabre.org

ELSEVIER   BOOK AID International   Sabre Foundation

DEDICATION

For Claire.
Welcome to the world, little one.

CONTENTS

100 TOP SECRETS

These secrets are 100 of the top board alerts. They summarize the concepts, principles, and most salient details that you should review before you take the Step 3 exam. Understanding of these Top Secrets will serve you well in your final review.

1. **Smoking** is the number-one cause of preventable morbidity and mortality in the United States (e.g., atherosclerosis, cancer, chronic obstructive pulmonary disease).

2. **Alcohol** is the number-two cause of preventable morbidity and mortality in the United States. More than half of accidental and intentional (e.g., murder and suicide) deaths involve alcohol. Alcohol is the number-one cause of preventable mental retardation (fetal alcohol syndrome); it also causes cancer and cirrhosis and is potentially fatal in withdrawal.

3. In **alcoholic hepatitis** the classic ratio of aspartate aminotransferase (AST) to alanine aminotransferase (ALT) is greater than or equal to 2:1, although both may be elevated.

4. **Vitamins:** Give folate to reproductive-age women to prevent neural tube defects. Watch for pernicious anemia, and treat with vitamin B12 to prevent permanent neurologic deficits. Isoniazid causes pyridoxine (vitamin B6) deficiency. Watch for Wernicke encephalopathy in alcoholics, and treat with thiamine to prevent Korsakoff dementia.

5. **Minerals:** Iron-deficiency anemia is the most common cause of anemia. Think of menstrual loss in reproductive-age women and of cancer in men and older women if no other cause is obvious.

6. **Vitamin A** is a known teratogen. Counsel and treat reproductive-age women appropriately (e.g., take care in treating acne with the vitamin A analog isotretinoin).

7. Complications of **atherosclerosis** (e.g., myocardial infarction, heart failure, stroke, gangrene) are involved in roughly one half of deaths in the United States. The primary risk factors for atherosclerosis are age/sex, family history, cigarette smoking, hypertension, diabetes mellitus, high LDL cholesterol, and low HDL cholesterol.

8. **Diabetes** leads to atherosclerosis and its complications, retinopathy (a leading cause of blindness), nephropathy (a leading cause of end-stage renal failure), peripheral vascular disease (a leading cause of limb amputation), peripheral neuropathy (sensory and autonomic), and an increased incidence of infections.

9. Although hypertension is most often mild or moderate and clinically silent, **severe hypertension** can lead to acute problems (known as a hypertensive emergency): headaches, dizziness, blurry vision, papilledema, cerebral edema, altered mental status, seizures, intracerebral hemorrhage (classically in the basal ganglia), renal failure/azotemia, angina, myocardial infarction, and/or heart failure.

10. In **milder cases,** lifestyle modifications (e.g., diet, exercise, weight loss, cessation of alcohol/tobacco use, elevation of head of bed) may be able to treat the following disorders without the use of medications: hypertension, hyperlipidemia, diabetes, gastroesophageal reflux disease (GERD), insomnia, obesity, and sleep apnea.

11. **Arterial blood gas analysis:** In general, pH tells you the primary event (acidosis vs. alkalosis), whereas carbon dioxide and bicarbonate values give you the cause (same direction as pH) and suggest any compensation present (opposite of pH).

12. **Exogenous causes of hyponatremia** to keep in mind: oxytocin, surgery, narcotics, inappropriate IV fluid administration, diuretics, and antiepileptic medications.

13. **EKG findings in electrolyte disturbances:** tall, tented T waves in hyperkalemia; loss of T waves/T-wave flattening and U waves in hypokalemia; QT prolongation in hypocalcemia; QT shortening in hypercalcemia.

14. **Shock:** First give the patient oxygen, start an IV line, and set up monitoring (pulse oximetry, EKG, frequent vital signs). Then give a fluid bolus (1 L normal saline or lactated Ringer solution) if no signs of congestive heart failure (e.g., bibasilar rales) are present while you try to figure out the cause if it is not known.

15. **Virchow triad** of deep venous thrombosis: endothelial damage (e.g., surgery, trauma), venous stasis (e.g., immobilization, surgery, severe heart failure), and hypercoagulable state (e.g., malignancy, birth control pills, pregnancy, lupus anticoagulant, inherited deficiencies).

16. **Therapy for congestive heart failure:** diuretics (e.g., furosemide), ACE inhibitors, and beta blockers (for stable patients) are the mainstays of pharmacologic treatment. Be sure to screen for and address underlying atherosclerosis risk factors (e.g., smoking, hyperlipidemia).

17. **Cor pulmonale:** right-sided heart enlargement, hypertrophy, or failure due to primary lung disease (usually chronic obstructive pulmonary disease). The most common cause of right heart failure, however, is left heart failure (not cor pulmonale).

18. In patients with **atrial fibrillation,** the main issues are ventricular rate (if needed, slow the rate with medications) and atrial clot formation/embolic disease (consider anticoagulation with warfarin).

19. **Ventricular fibrillation** requires immediate defibrillation pulseless ventricular tachycardia is treated with defibrillation followed by epinephrine, vasopressin, amiodarone, and lidocaine. If a pulse is present, treat with amiodarone and synchronized cardioversion.

20. **Obstructive vs. restrictive lung disease:** the FEV1/FEV ratio is the most important parameter on pulmonary function testing to distinguish the two (FEV1 may be the same). In obstructive lung disease, the FEV1/FEV ratio is less than normal. In restrictive disease the FEV1/FEV ratio is often normal.

21. The **most common cause of esophageal cancer:** reflux disease → Barrett metaplasia → adenocarcinoma. Smoking and alcohol abuse are the second most common causes (squamous cell carcinoma).

22. All **gastric ulcers** must be biopsied or followed to resolution to exclude malignancy.

23. Testing a nasogastric tube aspirate for blood is the best initial test **to distinguish an upper from a lower GI bleed,** although bright red blood via mouth or anus is a fairly reliable sign of a nearby bleeding source.

24. **Irritable bowel syndrome** is one of the most common causes of GI complaints. Physical exam and basic tests are by definition negative; this is a diagnosis of exclusion. The classic patient is a young adult female with a chronic history of alternating constipation and diarrhea.

25. **Crohn disease vs. ulcerative colitis**

	Crohn Disease	Ulcerative Colitis
Place of origin	Distal ileum, proximal colon	Rectum
Thickness of pathology	Transmural	Mucosa/submucosa only
Progression	Irregular (skip-lesions)	Proximal, continuous from rectum; no skipped areas
Location	From mouth to anus	Involves only colon, rarely extends to ileum
Bowel habit changes	Obstruction, abdominal pain	Bloody diarrhea
Classic lesions	Fistulas/abscesses, cobblestoning, string sign on barium x-ray	Pseudopolyps, lead-pipe colon on barium x-ray, toxic megacolon
Colon cancer risk	Slightly increased	Markedly increased
Surgery	No (may make worse)	Yes (proctocolectomy with ileoanal anastomosis)

26. All forms of **viral hepatitis** can present similarly in the acute stage; serology testing and history are needed to distinguish them. Hepatitis B, C, and D are transmitted parenterally and can lead to chronic infection, cirrhosis, and hepatocellular carcinoma.

27. **Hereditary hemochromatosis** is currently the most common known genetic disease in white people. The initial symptoms (fatigue, impotence) are nonspecific, but patients often have hepatomegaly. Screen with transferrin saturation test (serum iron/total iron binding capacity) and ferritin level. Treat with phlebotomy after confirming the diagnosis with genetic testing and liver biopsy.

28. **Sequelae of liver failure:** coagulopathy (that cannot be fixed with vitamin K), jaundice/hyperbilirubinemia, hypoalbuminemia, ascites, portal hypertension, hyperammonemia/encephalopathy, hypoglycemia, and disseminated intravascular coagulation.

29. **Pancreatitis** is usually due to alcohol or gallstones. Patients present with abdominal pain, nausea/vomiting, and elevated amylase and lipase. Treat supportively and provide pain control. Complications include pseudocyst formation, infection/abscess, and adult respiratory distress syndrome.

30. **Jaundice/hyperbilirubinemia in neonates** is usually physiologic (only monitoring and follow-up lab tests are needed), but jaundice present at birth is always pathologic.

31. **Primary vs. secondary endocrine disturbances.** In primary disorders (e.g., Graves, Hashimoto, or Addison disease), the gland malfunctions, but the pituitary or another gland and the central nervous system respond appropriately (e.g., TSH, TRH, or ACTH elevate or depress as expected in the setting of a malfunctioning gland). In secondary disorders (e.g., ACTH-secreting lung carcinoma, heart failure-induced hyperreninemia, renal failure-induced hyperparathyroidism), the gland itself is doing what it is told to do by other controlling forces (e.g., pituitary gland, hypothalamus, tumor, disease); they are the problem, not the gland itself.

32. **Corticosteroid side effects:** weight gain, easy bruising, acne, hirsutism, emotional lability, depression, psychosis, menstrual changes, sexual dysfunction, insomnia, memory loss, buffalo hump, truncal and central obesity with wasting of extremities, round plethoric facies, purplish skin striae, weakness (especially of the proximal muscles), hypertension, peripheral edema, poor wound healing, glucose intolerance or diabetes, osteoporosis, and hypokalemic metabolic alkalosis (due to mineralocorticoid effects of certain corticosteroids). Growth can also be stunted in children.

33. **Osteoarthritis** is by far the most common cause of arthritis ($\geq$ 75% of cases) and usually does not have hot, swollen joints or significant findings if arthrocentesis is performed.

34. Cancer incidence and mortality in the United States.

Overall Highest Incidence		Overall Highest Mortality Rate	
Male	Female	Male	Female
1. Prostate	1. Breast	1. Lung	1. Lung
2. Lung	2. Lung	2. Prostate	2. Breast
3. Colon	3. Colon	3. Colon	3. Colon

35. **Sequelae of lung cancer:** hemoptysis, Horner syndrome, superior vena cava syndrome, phrenic nerve involvement/diaphragmatic paralysis, hoarseness from recurrent laryngeal nerve involvement, and paraneoplastic syndromes (Cushing, SIADH, hypercalcemia, Eaton-Lambert syndrome).

36. **Bitemporal hemianopsia** (loss of peripheral vision in both eyes) is due to a space-occupying lesion pushing on the optic chiasm (classically a pituitary tumor) until proven otherwise. Order a CT or MRI of the brain.

37. **Potential risks and side effects of estrogen therapy** (e.g., contraception, postmenopausal hormone replacement): endometrial cancer, hepatic adenomas, glucose intolerance/diabetes, deep venous thrombosis, stroke, cholelithiasis, hypertension, endometrial bleeding, depression, weight gain, nausea/vomiting, headache, weight gain, drug-drug interactions, teratogenesis, and aggravation of preexisting uterine leiomyomas (fibroids), breast fibroadenomas, migraines, and epilepsy. The risks of coronary artery disease and breast cancer are increased with combined estrogen and progesterone therapy.

38. **ABCD characteristics of a mole** that should make you suspicious of malignant transformation: asymmetry, borders (irregular), color (change in color or multiple colors), and diameter (the bigger the lesion, the more likely that it is malignant). Do an excisional biopsy of such moles and/or if a mole starts to itch or bleed.

39. **Bronchiolitis vs. croup vs. epiglottitis**

	Bronchiolitis	Croup (Acute Laryngotracheitis)	Epiglottitis
Child's age	0–18 months	1–2 years	2–5 years
Common	Yes	Yes	No
Common cause(s)	Repiratory syncytial virus (≥ 75%), Parainfluenza, Influenza	Parainfluenza virus (50–75% of cases), Influenza	*Haemophilus influenzae*, *Staphylococcus spp.*, *Streptococcus spp.*
Symptoms/ signs	Initial viral URI symptoms followed by tachypnea and expiratory wheezing	Initial viral URI symptoms followed by "barking" cough, hoarseness, and inspiratory stridor	Rapid progression to high fever, toxicity, drooling, and respiratory distress
X-ray findings	Hyperinflation	Subglottic tracheal narrowing on frontal x-ray (steeple sign)	Swollen epiglottis on lateral neck x-ray (thumb sign)
Treatment	Humidified oxygen, bronchodilators (controversial), Ribavarin used for severe RSV infection or high risk for RSV infection.	Humidified oxygen, bronchodilators	Prepare to establish an airway, antibiotics (e.g., third-generation cephalosporin)

40. **Sequelae of streptococcal infection:** rheumatic fever, scarlet fever, and poststreptococcal glomerulonephritis. Only the first two can be prevented by treatment with antibiotics.

41. **Multiple sclerosis** should be suspected in any young adult with recurrent, varied neurologic symptoms/signs when no other causes are evident. Best diagnostic tests: MRI (most sensitive), lumbar puncture (elevated IgG oligoclonal bands and myelin basic protein levels, mild elevation in lymphocytes and protein), and evoked potentials (slowed conduction through areas with damaged myelin).

42. For the **unconscious or delirious patient** in the emergency department with no history or signs of trauma: consider empiric treatment for hypoglycemia (glucose), opioid overdose (naloxone), and thiamine deficiency (thiamine should be given before glucose in a suspected alcoholic). Other commonly tested causes are alcohol, illicit or prescription drugs, diabetic ketoacidosis, stroke, epilepsy or postictal state, and subarachnoid hemorrhage (e.g., aneurysm rupture).

43. **Delirium vs. dementia**

	Delirium	Dementia
Onset	Acute and dramatic	Chronic and insidious
Common causes	Illness, toxin, withdrawal	Alzheimer disease, multi-infarct dementia, HIV/AIDS
Reversible	Usually	Usually not
Attention	Poor	Usually unaffected
Arousal level	Fluctuates	Normal

44. **Always consider the possibility of pregnancy** (and order a pregnancy test to rule it out, unless pregnancy is an impossibility) in reproductive-age women before advising potentially teratogenic therapies or tests (e.g., antiepileptic drugs, x-ray, CT scan). Pregnancy is in the differential diagnosis of both primary and secondary amenorrhea.

45. **Anaphylaxis** is commonly caused by bee stings, food allergy (especially peanuts and shellfish), medications (especially penicillins and sulfa drugs), or rubber glove allergy. Patients become agitated and flushed and shortly after exposure develop itching (urticaria), facial swelling (angioedema), and difficulty in breathing. Symptoms develop rapidly and dramatically in true anaphylaxis. Treat immediately by securing the airway (laryngeal edema may prevent intubation, in which case do a cricothyroidotomy, if needed), and give subcutaneous or IV epinephrine. Antihistamines and corticosteroids are not useful for immediate, severe reactions that involve the airway.

46. **Cancer screening in asymptomatic adults**

Cancer	Procedure	Age	Frequency
Colorectal	Colonoscopy or	> 50 yr for all studies	Every 10 years
	Flexible sigmoidoscopy or		Every 5 years
	Double contrast barium enema or		Every 5 years
	CT colonography or		Every 5 years
	Fecal occult blood test or		Annually
	Fecal immunochemical test or		Annually
	Stool DNA test		Interval uncertain
Colon, prostate	Digital rectal exam	> 40 yr	Annually
Prostate	Prostate specific antigen test	> 50 yr*	Controversial, but offer annually

(continued)

Cancer	Procedure	Age	Frequency
Cervical	Pap smear	Within 3 years of onset of sexual activity or age 21, whichever comes first	If conventional Pap test is used → test annually; every 2-3 years for women ≥ 30 who have had three negative cytology tests. If Pap and HPV testing are used → every 3 years if HPV negative and cytology negative.
Gynecologic	Pelvic examination	21–64 yr	Annually. Every 2–3 years after 3 normal tests.
		> 65	Annually. When to stop is not clearly established.
Endometrial	Endometrial biopsy	Menopause	No recommendation for routine screening.
Breast	Breast self-examination	> 20 yr	Benefits and limitations should be discussed, but breast self examination is no longer recommended by the American Cancer Society.
Breast	Physical exam by doctor	20–40 yr	Every 3 yrs
		> 40 yr	Annually
Breast	Mammography	> 40 yr	Annually
Lung	Sputum, chest x-ray, CT scan		Testing is not recommended for asymptomatic individuals, even if they are high-risk.

*Start at age 45 in African Americans and at age 40 for patients with a first degree relative diagnosed at an early age.

47. **Biostatistics calculations using a 2 × 2 table**

		Disease		Test Name	Formula
		(+)	(−)	Sensitivity	A/(A + C)
				Specificity	D/(B + D)
Test	(+)	A	B	PPV	A/(A + B)
or				NPV	D/(C + D)
Exposure	(−)	C	D	Odds ratio	(A × D)/(B × C)
				Relative risk	[A/(A + B)]/[C/(C + D)]
				Attributable risk	[A/(A + B)]−[C/(C + D)]

48. The **p-value** reflects the likelihood of making a type I error, or claiming an effect or difference where none existed (i.e., results were obtained by chance). When we reject the null hypothesis (i.e., the hypothesis of no difference) in a trial testing a new treatment, we are saying that the new treatment works. We use the p-value to express our confidence in the data.

49. **Side effects of antipsychotics:** acute dystonia (treat with antihistamines or anticholinergics), akathisia (beta blocker may help), tardive dyskinesia (switching to newer agent may have benefit), parkinsonism (treat with antihistamines or anticholinergics), neuroleptic malignant syndrome, hyperprolactinemia (may cause breast discharge, menstrual dysfunction and/or sexual dysfunction), and autonomic nervous system-related effects (e.g., anticholinergic, antihistamine and alpha$_1$ receptor blockade).

50. Asking about **depression and suicidal thoughts**/intent is important in the right setting and does not cause people to commit suicide. Hospitalize psychiatric patients against their will if they are a danger to self or others.

51. **Drugs of abuse:** potentially fatal in withdrawal include alcohol, barbiturates, and benzodiazepines. Alcohol, cocaine, opiates, barbiturates, benzodiazepines, phencyclidine (PCP), and inhalants are potentially fatal in overdose.

52. **Pelvic inflammatory disease** is the most common preventable cause of infertility in the United States and the most likely cause of infertility in younger, normally menstruating women.

53. **Polycystic ovarian syndrome** is classically associated with women who are "heavy, hirsute, and [h]amenorrheic". It is the most common cause of dysfunctional uterine bleeding. Remember the increased risk of endometrial cancer due to unopposed estrogen.

54. **Fetal/neonatal macrosomia** is due to maternal diabetes until proven otherwise. Use diet and insulin (not oral agents) to treat maternal diabetes.

55. **Low maternal serum alpha-fetoprotein** causes: Down syndrome, inaccurate dates (most common), and fetal demise. **High maternal serum alpha-fetoprotein causes:** neural tube defects, ventral wall defects (e.g., omphalocele, gastroschisis), inaccurate dates (most common), and multiple gestation. Measurement generally is obtained between 16 and 20 weeks gestation.

56. Hypertension plus proteinuria in pregnancy equals **preeclampsia** until proven otherwise.

57. Positive pregnancy test (i.e., not a clinically apparent pregnancy) plus vaginal bleeding and abdominal pain equals **ectopic pregnancy** until proven otherwise. Order an ultrasound test if the patient is stable.

58. **Decelerations during maternofetal monitoring:** *early* decelerations are normal and due to head compression. *Variable* decelerations are common and usually due to cord compression (turn the mother on her side, give oxygen and fluids, and stop oxytocin). *Late* decelerations are due to uteroplacental insufficiency and are the most worrisome pattern (turn the mother on her side, give oxygen and IV fluids, stop oxytocin, and measure fetal oxygen saturation or scalp pH). Prepare for prompt delivery.

59. Always perform ultrasound before pelvic exam in the setting of **third-trimester bleeding** (in case placenta previa is present).

60. **Uterine atony** is the most common cause of postpartum bleeding and is typically due to uterine overdistension (e.g., twins, polyhydramnios), prolonged labor, and/or oxytocin usage.

61. **Acute abdomen pathology localization by physical exam**

Area	Organ (Conditions)
Right upper quadrant	Gallbladder/biliary (cholecystitis, cholangitis) or liver (abscess)
Left upper quadrant	Spleen (rupture with blunt trauma)
Right lower quadrant	Appendix (appendicitis), pelvic inflammatory disease (PID)
Left lower quadrant	Sigmoid colon (diverticulitis), pelvic inflammatory disease (PID)
Epigastric area	Stomach (peptic ulcer) or pancreas (pancreatitis)

62. The **"6 Ws" of postoperative fever:** water, wind, walk, wound, "wawa," and weird drugs. Water stands for urinary tract infection, wind for atelectasis or pneumonia, walk for deep venous thrombosis, wound for surgical wound infection, "wawa" for breast (usually relevant only in the postpartum state), and weird drugs for drug fever. In patients with daily fever spikes that do not respond to antibiotics, think about a postsurgical abscess. Order a CT scan to locate, then drain the abscess if one is present.

63. **ABCDEs of trauma** (follow in order if you are asked to choose): **a**irway, **b**reathing, **c**irculation, **d**isability, and **e**xposure.

64. **Six rapidly fatal thoracic injuries** that must be recognized and treated immediately:
    1. Airway obstruction (establish airway)
    2. Open pneumothorax (intubate and close defect on three sides)
    3. Tension pneumothorax (perform needle thoracentesis followed by chest tube)
    4. Cardiac tamponade (perform pericardiocentesis)

5. Massive hemothorax (place chest tube to drain; thoracotomy if bleeding doesn't stop)
6. Flail chest (consider intubation and positive pressure ventilation if oxygenation inadequate)

65. **Neonatal conjunctivitis** may be caused by chemical reaction (in first 12 to 24 hours of giving drops for prophylaxis), gonorrhea (2 to 5 days after birth; usually prevented by prophylactic drops), and chlamydial infection (5 to 14 days after birth; often not prevented by prophylactic drops).

66. **Glaucoma** is usually (90%) due to the open-angle form, which is painless (no "attacks") and asymptomatic until irreversible vision loss (that starts in the periphery) occurs. Screening is thus important. Open-angle glaucoma is the most common cause of blindness in African Americans.

67. **Uveitis** is often a marker for systemic conditions: juvenile rheumatoid arthritis, sarcoidosis, inflammatory bowel disease, ankylosing spondylitis, Reiter syndrome, multiple sclerosis, psoriasis, or lupus. Photophobia, blurry vision, and eye pain are common complaints.

68. **Bilateral (though often asymmetric) painless gradual loss of vision** in older adults is usually due to cataracts, macular degeneration, or glaucoma, which can be distinguished on physical exam. Presbyopia is a normal part of aging and affects only near vision (i.e., accommodation).

69. **Compartment syndrome,** usually in the lower extremity after trauma or surgery, causes the "6 Ps":
    1. Pain (present on passive movement and often out of proportion to injury)
    2. Paresthesias (numbness, tingling, decreased sensation)
    3. Pallor (or cyanosis)
    4. Pressure (firm feeling muscle compartment, elevated pressure reading)
    5. Paralysis (late, ominous sign)
    6. Pulselessness (very late, ominous sign)
    Treat with fasciotomy to relieve compartment pressure and prevent permanent neurologic damage.

70. **Peripheral nerve evaluation**

Nerve	Motor Function	Sensory Function	Clinical Scenario
Radial	Wrist extension (watch for wrist drop)	Back of forearm, back of hand (first 3 digits)	Humeral fracture
Ulnar	Finger abduction (watch for "claw hand")	Front and back of last 2 digits	Elbow dislocation
Median	Pronation, thumb opposition	Palmar surface of hand (first 3 digits)	Carpal tunnel syndrome, humeral fracture
Axillary	Abduction, lateral rotation	Lateral shoulder	Upper humeral dislocation or fracture
Peroneal	Dorsiflexion, eversion (watch for foot drop)	Dorsal foot and lateral leg	Knee dislocation

71. **Pediatric hip disorders**

Name	Age	Epidemiology	Symptoms/signs	Treatment
CHD	At birth	Female, first-borns, breech delivery	Barlow and Ortolani signs	Harness
LCPD	4–10 yr	Short male with delayed bone age	Knee, thigh, groin pain, limp	Orthoses
SCFE	9–13 yr	Overweight male adolescent	Knee, thigh, groin pain, limp	Surgical pinning

CHD = congenital hip dysplasia; LCPD = Legg-Calvé-Perthes disease; SCFE = slipped capital femoral epiphysis.

Note: All of these conditions may present in an adult as arthritis of the hip.

72. **Avoid lumbar puncture** in a patient with head trauma or signs of increased intracranial pressure. Perform CT scan without contrast instead.

73. In children, 75% of **neck masses** are benign (e.g., lymphadenitis, thyroglossal duct cyst), but 75% of neck masses in adults are malignant (e.g., squamous cell carcinoma and/or metastases, lymphoma).

74. Manage **carotid artery stenosis** 70% to 99% with carotid endarterectomy for symptomatic patients; less than 50% with medical management (e.g., aspirin and/or clopidogrel) and treatment of atherosclerosis risk factors. For stenosis between 50% and 69%, management is controversial.

75. Pulsatile abdominal mass plus hypotension equals ruptured **abdominal aortic aneurysm** until proven otherwise. Perform an immediate laparotomy (90% mortality rate).

76. Conditions best viewed as **anginal equivalents:** transient ischemic attacks, claudication, and chronic mesenteric ischemia. Arterial work-up and imaging are indicated.

77. **Cryptorchidism** is the main identifiable risk factor for testicular cancer and can also cause infertility. Treat with surgical retrieval and orchiopexy (or removal).

78. **Benign prostatic hypertrophy/hyperplasia** can present as acute renal failure. Patients have a distended bladder and bilateral hydronephrosis on ultrasound (neither is present with "medical" renal disease). Drain the bladder first (catheterize), then perform transurethral resection of the prostate (TURP).

79. **Impotence** may be physical (e.g., vascular, nervous system, drugs) or, less commonly, psychogenic (patients have normal nocturnal erections and a history of dysfunction only in certain settings).

80. The **overall pattern of growth** in a child is more important than any one measurement. Consider close follow-up and remeasurement of growth parameters if you do not have enough data. A stable pattern is less worrisome and less likely to be correctable than a sudden change in previously stable growth. For example, the most common cause of delayed puberty is constitutional delay, a normal variant.

81. **Findings suspicious for child abuse,** assuming that other explanation are not provided: failure to thrive, multiple injuries in different stages of healing, retinal hemorrhages plus subdural hematoma(s) ("shaken baby" syndrome), sexually transmitted diseases, caretaker story that does not fit child's injury or complaint, childhood behavioral or emotional problems, and multiple personality disorder as an adult.

82. The **APGAR score** (commonly performed at 1 and 5 minutes after birth; maximum score is 10):

Category	Number of Points Given		
	0	1	2
Heart rate	Absent	< 100 beats/min	> 100 beats/min
Respiratory effort	None	Slow, weak cry	Good, strong cry
Muscle tone	Limp	Some flexion of extremities	Active motion
Reflex irritability*	None	Grimace	Grimace and strong cry, cough, and sneeze
Color	Pale, blue	Body pink, extremities blue	Completely pink

*Reflex irritability usually is measured by the infant's response to stimulation of the sole of the foot or a catheter put into the nose.

83. **Diuretics** are a common cause of metabolic derangement. *Thiazide diuretics* cause calcium retention, hyperglycemia, hyperuricemia, hyperlipidemia, hyponatremia, hypokalemic metabolic alkalosis, and hypovolemia; because they are sulfa drugs, watch out for sulfa allergy. *Loop diuretics* cause hypokalemic metabolic alkalosis, hypovolemia (more potent than thiazides), ototoxicity, and calcium excretion; with the exception of ethacrynic acid, they also are sulfa drugs. *Carbonic anhydrase inhibitors* cause metabolic acidosis, and *potassium-sparing diuretics* (e.g., spironolactone) may cause hyperkalemia.

84. **Overdoses and antidotes**

Poison or Medication	Antidote
Acetaminophen	Acetylcysteine
Cholinesterase inhibitors	Atropine, pralidoxime
Quinidine or tricyclic anti-depressants	Sodium bicarbonate (cardioprotective)
Iron	Deferoxamine
Digoxin	Normalize potassium and other electrolytes; digoxin antibodies
Methanol/ethylene glycol	Ethanol
Benzodiazepines	Flumazenil
Beta blockers	Glucagon
Lead	Edetate (EDTA); use succimer in children
Copper or gold	Penicillamine

(continued)

Poison or Medication	Antidote
Opioids	Naloxone
Carbon monoxide	Oxygen (hyperbaric in cases of severe poisoning)
Muscarinic blockers	Physostigmine

85. **Aspirin/NSAID side effects:** GI bleeding, gastric ulcers, renal damage (e.g., interstitial nephritis, papillary necrosis), allergic reactions, platelet dysfunction (life of platelet for aspirin, reversible dysfunction with NSAIDs), and Reye syndrome (aspirin given to child with viral infection). Aspirin overdose can be fatal and classically leads to both metabolic acidosis and respiratory alkalosis.

86. **Central pontine myelinolysis** (brainstem damage and possibly death) may result from overly rapid correction of hyponatremia.

87. Due to cellular shifts, **alkalosis and acidosis** can cause symptoms of potassium and/or calcium derangement (e.g., alkalosis can lead to symptoms of hypokalemia or hypocalcemia). In this setting, pH correction is needed (rather than direct treatment of the calcium or potassium levels). Magnesium depletion can also make hypocalcemia and hypokalemia unresponsive to replacement therapy (until magnesium is corrected).

88. Adult patients of sound mind are allowed to **refuse any form of treatment.** Watch for depression as a cause of "incompetence." Treat depression before wishes for death are respected.

89. **If a patient is incompetent** (including younger minors who lack adequate decision-making capacity) and an emergency treatment is needed, seek family member or court-appointed guardian to make health care decisions. If no one available, treat as you see fit in an emergency, or contact the courts in a nonemergency setting.

90. **Respect patient wishes and living wills** (assuming that they are appropriate) even in the face of dissenting family members, but take time to listen to family members' concerns.

91. **Always be a patient advocate** and treat patients with respect and dignity, even if they refuse your proposed treatment or are noncompliant. If patients' actions puzzle you, do not be afraid to ask them why they are doing or saying what they are.

92. **Break doctor-patient confidentiality only in the following situations:**
    - The patient asks you to do so.
    - Child abuse is suspected.
    - The courts mandate you to do so.
    - You must fulfill the duty to warn or protect (if a patient says that he is going to kill someone or himself, you have to tell the someone, the authorities, or both).
    - The patient has a reportable disease.
    - The patient is a danger to others (e.g., if a patient is blind or has seizures, let the proper authorities know so that they can revoke the patient's license to drive; if the patient is an airplane pilot and is a paranoid, hallucinating schizophrenic, then authorities need to know).

93. **Causes of "false" lab disturbances:** hemolysis (hyperkalemia), pregnancy (elevated sedimentation rate and alkaline phosphatase), hypoalbuminemia (hypocalcemia), and hyperglycemia (hyponatremia).

94. **EKG findings of myocardial infarction:** flipped or flattened T waves, ST-segment elevation (depression means ischemia; elevation means injury), and/or Q waves in a segmental distribution (e.g., leads II, III, and AVF for an inferior infarct). ST depression may also be seen in "reciprocal"/opposite leads.

95. Drugs that may be useful in the setting of **acute coronary syndrome:** aspirin, morphine, nitroglycerin, beta blocker, ACE inhibitor, clopidogrel, HMG-CoA reductase inhibitor, glycoprotein IIb/IIIa receptor inhibitors, heparin (unfractionated or low molecular weight heparin), and tissue-plasminogen activator (t-PA; strict criteria for use).

96. **Cholesterol management guidelines** (numbers in the chart represent mg/dL)

No CHD Risk Factors	$\geq$2 CHD Risk Factors*	Known CAD/ Equivalent[†]	Very High Risk[‡]	Intervention
LDL < 160	LDL < 100	LDL < 100	LDL < 70	None (meets goal)
LDL 160–189	LDL 100–129		LDL 70–99	Diet $\pm$ medications[§]
LDL $\geq$ 190	LDL $\geq$ 130	LDL $\geq$ 100	LDL $\geq$ 100	Medications (+ diet)

*CHD = coronary heart disease. Risk factors for CHD are listed in question 4.
[†]CAD = coronary artery disease. CHD equivalents include diabetes mellitus, peripheral arterial atherosclerotic disease, symptomatic carotid artery disease, and abdominal aortic aneurysm.
[‡]"Very" high-risk patients are those with CAD who have a heart attach, diabetes or other severe and poorly controlled risk factors (e.g., metabolic syndrome, heavy smoking).
[§]"Diet" includes general lifestyle modifications such as eating less and healthier, decreasing alcohol intake, exercising, etc. The trend is toward more aggressive intervention, so you will not be faulted for initiating medications at these "gray area" LDL levels, particularly in higher risk people.

97. **Type 1 vs. type 2 diabetes**

	Type 1 (10% of Cases)	Type 2 (90% of Cases)
Age at onset	Most commonly < 30 yr	Most commonly > 30 yr
Associated body habitus	Thin	Obese
Development of ketoacidosis	Yes	No
Development of hyperosmolar state	No	Yes
Level of endogenous insulin	Low to none	Normal to high (insulin resistance)

(continued)

	Type 1 (10% of Cases)	Type 2 (90% of Cases)
Twin concurrence	< 50%	> 50%
HLA association	Yes	No
Response to oral hypoglycemics	No	Yes
Antibodies to insulin	Yes (at diagnosis)	No
Risk for diabetic complications	Yes	Yes
Islet-cell pathology	Insulitis (loss of most B cells)	Normal number, but with amyloid deposits

Remember, however, that these findings may overlap.

98. **Hypertension classification**

Systolic BP* (mm Hg)	Diastolic BP* (mm Hg)	Classification
< 120	< 80	Normal
120–139	80–89	Prehypertension
140–159	90–99	Stage I hypertension
≥ 160	≥ 100	Stage II hypertension

*Classification is based on the worst number (e.g., 168/60 mm Hg considered stage II hypertension even though diastolic pressure is normal).

99. Word associations (not 100%, but they can help when you have to guess):

Buzz Phrase or Scenario	Condition
Friction rub	Pericarditis
Kussmaul breathing (deep, rapid breathing)	Diabetic ketoacidosis
Kayser-Fleischer ring in the eye	Wilson disease
Bitot spots	Vitamin A deficiency
Dendritic corneal ulcers on fluorescein stain of the eye	Herpes keratitis
Cherry-red spot on the macula without hepatosplenomegaly	Tay-Sachs disease
Cherry-red spot on the macula with hepatosplenomegaly	Niemann-Pick disease
Bronze skin plus diabetes	Hemochromatosis
Malar rash on the face	Systemic lupus erythematosus
Heliotrope rash (purplish rash on the eyelids)	Dermatomyositis
Clue cells	*Gardnerella vaginalis* infection
Meconium ileus	Cystic fibrosis
Rectal prolapse	Cystic fibrosis

(continued)

Buzz Phrase or Scenario	Condition
Salty-tasting infant	Cystic fibrosis
Café-au-lait spots with normal IQ	Neurofibromatosis
Café-au-lait spots with mental retardation	McCune-Albright syndrome or tuberous sclerosis
Worst headache of the patient's life	Subarachnoid hemorrhage
Abdominal striae	Cushing syndrome or pregnancy
Honey ingestion	Infant botulism
Left lower quadrant tenderness/rebound	Diverticulitis
Children who torture animals	Conduct disorder
Currant jelly stools in children	Intussusception
Ambiguous genitalia and hypotension	21-Hydroxylase deficiency in girls
Cat-like cry in an infant	Cri-du-chat syndrome
Infant weighing more than 10 pounds	Maternal diabetes
Anaphylaxis from immunoglobulin therapy	IgA deficiency
Postpartum fever unresponsive to broad-spectrum antibiotics	Septic pelvic thrombophlebitis
Increased hemoglobin A2 and anemia	Thalassemia
Heavy young woman with papilledema and negative CT/MR scan of head	Pseudotumor cerebri
Low-grade fever in the first 24 hours after surgery	Atelectasis
Vietnam veteran	Posttraumatic stress disorder
Bilateral hilar adenopathy in a black patient	Sarcoidosis
Sudden death in a young athlete	Hypertrophic obstructive cardiomyopathy
Fractures or bruises in different stages of healing in a child	Child abuse
Absent breath sounds in a trauma patient	Pneumothorax
Shopping sprees	Mania
Constant clearing of throat in a child or teenager	Tourette syndrome
Intermittent bursts of swearing	Tourette syndrome
Koilocytosis	Human papillomavirus or cytomegalovirus
Rash develops after administration of ampicillin or amoxicillin for sore throat	Epstein-Barr virus infection
Daytime sleepiness and occasional falling down (cataplexy)	Narcolepsy
Facial port wine stain and seizures	Sturge-Weber syndrome

100. Signs and syndromes

Sign/Syndrome	Explanation
Babinski sign	Stroking the bottom of the foot yields extension of the big toe and fanning of other toes (upper motor neuron lesion)
Beck triad	Jugular venous distention, muffled heart sounds, and hypotension (cardiac tamponade)
Brudzinski sign	Pain on neck flexion with meningeal irritation (meningitis)
Charcot triad	Fever/chills, jaundice, and right upper quadrant pain (cholangitis)
Courvoisier sign	Painless, palpable gallbladder plus jaundice (pancreatic cancer)
Chvostek sign	Tapping on the facial nerve elicits tetany (hypocalcemia)
Cullen sign	Bluish discoloration of periumbilical area (pancreatitis with retroperitoneal hemorrhage)
Cushing reflex	Hypertension, bradycardia, and irregular respirations (high intracranial pressure)
Grey Turner sign	Bluish discoloration of flank (pancreatitis with retroperitoneal hemorrhage)
Homan sign	Calf pain on forced dorsiflexion of the foot (deep venous thrombosis)
Kehr sign	Pain in the left shoulder (ruptured spleen)
Leriche syndrome	Claudication and atrophy of the buttocks with impotence (aortoiliac occlusive disease)
McBurney sign	Tenderness at McBurney point (appendicitis)
Murphy sign	Arrest of inspiration during palpation under the rib cage on the right (cholecystitis)
Ortolani sign/test	Abducting an infant's flexed hips causes a palpable/audible click (congenital hip dysplasia)
Prehn sign	Elevation of a painful testicle relieves pain (epididymitis vs. testicular torsion)
Rovsing sign	Pushing on left lower quadrant then releasing your hand produces pain at McBurney point (appendicitis)
Tinel sign	Tapping on the volar surface of the wrist elicits paresthesias (carpal tunnel syndrome)
Trousseau sign	Pumping up a blood pressure cuff causes carpopedal spasm (tetany from hypocalcemia)
Virchow triad	Stasis, endothelial damage, and hypercoagulability (risk factors for deep venous thrombosis)

CHAPTER 1

ACID-BASE AND ELECTROLYTES

1. **How do you analyze arterial blood gas values?**
   Remember three basic points:
   1. pH tells you whether you are dealing with acidosis or alkalosis as the primary event. The body will compensate as much as it can (secondary event).
   2. Look at the carbon dioxide (CO_2) value. If it is high, the patient either has respiratory acidosis (pH: less than 7.4) or is compensating for metabolic alkalosis (pH: greater than 7.4). If CO_2 is low, the patient either has respiratory alkalosis (pH: greater than 7.4) or is compensating for metabolic acidosis (pH: less than 7.4).
   3. Look at the bicarbonate value. If it is high, the patient either has metabolic alkalosis (pH: greater than 7.4) or is compensating for respiratory acidosis (pH: less than 7.4). If bicarbonate is low, the patient either has metabolic acidosis (pH: less than 7.4) or is compensating for respiratory alkalosis (pH: greater than 7.4).

2. **True or false: The body does not compensate beyond a normal pH.**
   True. For example, a patient with metabolic acidosis will eliminate CO_2 to help restore a normal pH. However, if respiratory alkalosis is a compensatory mechanism (and not a rare, separate primary disturbance), then the pH will not correct to greater than 7.4. Overcorrection does not occur.

3. **List the common causes of acidosis.**
   Respiratory acidosis: chronic obstructive pulmonary disease, asthma, drugs (e.g., opioids, benzodiazepines, barbiturates, alcohol, other respiratory depressants), chest wall problems (paralysis, pain), and sleep apnea.
   Metabolic acidosis: ethanol, diabetic ketoacidosis, uremia, lactic acidosis (e.g., sepsis, shock, bowel ischemia), methanol/ethylene glycol, aspirin/salicylate overdose, diarrhea, and carbonic anhydrase inhibitors.

4. **List the common causes of alkalosis.**
   Respiratory alkalosis: anxiety/hyperventilation and aspirin/salicylate overdose.
   Metabolic alkalosis: diuretics (except carbonic anhydrase inhibitors), vomiting, volume contraction, antacid abuse/milk-alkali syndrome, and hyperaldosteronism.

5. **What type of acid-base disturbance does aspirin overdose cause?**
   Respiratory alkalosis and metabolic acidosis (two different primary disturbances). Look for coexisting tinnitus, hypoglycemia, vomiting, and a history of "swallowing several pills." Alkalinization of the urine (with bicarbonate) speeds excretion.

6. **What happens to the blood gas of patients with chronic lung conditions?**
   In certain people with chronic lung conditions (especially those with sleep apnea), pH may be alkaline during the day because they breathe better when awake. In addition, just after an episode of bronchitis or other respiratory disorder, the metabolic alkalosis that usually compensates for respiratory acidosis is no longer a compensatory mechanism and becomes the primary disturbance (elevated pH and bicarbonate). As a side note, remember that sleep apnea, like other chronic lung diseases, can cause right-sided heart failure (cor pulmonale).

7. **Should you give bicarbonate to a patient with acidosis?**
   For purposes of the Step 2 boards, almost never. First try intravenous fluids and correction of the underlying disorder. If all other measures fail and the pH remains less than 7.0, bicarbonate may be given.

8. **The blood gas of a patient with asthma has changed from alkalotic to normal, and the patient seems to be sleeping. Is the patient ready to go home?**
   For Step 2 purposes, this scenario means that the patient is probably crashing. Remember that pH is initially high in patients with asthma because they are eliminating CO_2. If the patient becomes tired and does not breathe appropriately, CO_2 will begin to rise and pH will begin to normalize. Eventually the patient becomes acidotic and requires emergency intubation if appropriate measures are not taken. If this scenario is mentioned on boards, the appropriate response is to prepare for possible elective intubation and to continue aggressive medical treatment with beta$_2$ agonists, steroids, and oxygen. Fatigue secondary to work of breathing is an indication for intubation. Asthmatic patients are supposed to be slightly alkalotic during an asthma attack. If they are not, you should wonder why.

9. **List the signs and symptoms of hyponatremia.**
   - Lethargy
   - Seizures
   - Mental status changes or confusion
   - Cramps
   - Anorexia
   - Coma

10. **How do you determine the cause of hyponatremia?**
    The first step in determining the cause is to look at the volume status:

	Hypovolemic	Euvolemic	Hypervolemic
Think of	Dehydration, diuretics, diabetes, Addison disease/ hypoaldosteronism (high potassium)	SIADH, psychogenic polydipsia, oxytocin use	Heart failure, nephrotic syndrome, cirrhosis, toxemia, renal failure

    SIADH = syndrome of inappropriate antidiuretic hormone secretion.

11. **How is hyponatremia treated?**
    For hypovolemic hyponatremia, the treatment is normal saline. Euvolemic and hypervolemic hyponatremia are treated with water/fluid restriction; diuretics may be needed for hypervolemic hyponatremia.

12. **What medication is used to treat SIADH if water restriction fails?**
    Demeclocycline, which induces nephrogenic diabetes insipidus.

13. **What happens if hyponatremia is corrected too quickly?**
    You may cause brainstem damage (**central pontine myelinolysis**). Hypertonic saline is used only when a patient has seizures from severe hyponatremia—and even then, only briefly and cautiously. Normal saline is a better choice 99% of the time for board purposes. In chronic severe symptomatic hyponatremia, the rate of correction should not exceed 0.5 to 1 mEq/L/hour.

14. **What causes spurious (false) hyponatremia?**
    - Hyperglycemia (once glucose is greater than 200 mg/dL, sodium decreases by 1.6 mEq/L for each rise of 100 mg/dL in glucose)
    - Hyperproteinemia
    - Hyperlipidemia
    In these instances, the lab value is low, but the total body sodium is normal. Do not give the patient extra salt or saline.

15. **What causes hyponatremia in postoperative patients?**
    The most common cause is the combination of pain and narcotics (causing SIADH) with overaggressive administration of intravenous fluids. A rare cause that you may see on the USMLE is adrenal insufficiency; in this instance, potassium is high and the blood pressure is low.

16. **What is the classic cause of hyponatremia in pregnant patients about to deliver?**
    Oxytocin, which has an antidiuretic hormone-like effect.

17. **What are the signs and symptoms of hypernatremia?**
    Basically the same as the signs and symptoms of hyponatremia:
    - Mental status changes or confusion
    - Seizures
    - Hyperreflexia
    - Coma

18. **What causes hypernatremia?**
    The most common cause is dehydration (free water loss) due to inadequate fluid intake relative to bodily needs. Watch for diuretics, diabetes insipidus, diarrhea, and renal disease as well as iatrogenic causes (administration of too much hypertonic intravenous fluid). Sickle cell disease, which may lead to renal damage and isosthenuria (inability to concentrate urine), is a rare cause of hypernatremia, as are hypokalemia and hypercalcemia, which also impair the kidney's concentrating ability.

19. **How is hypernatremia treated?**
    Treatment involves water replacement, but the patient often is severely dehydrated; therefore, normal saline is used most frequently. Once the patient is hemodynamically stable, he or she often is switched to ½ normal saline. Five percent dextrose in water (D5W) should not be used for hypernatremia.

20. **What are the signs and symptoms of hypokalemia?**
    Hypokalemia causes muscular weakness, which can lead to paralysis and ventilatory failure. When smooth muscles also are affected, patients may develop ileus and/or hypotension. Best known and most tested, however, is the effect of hypokalemia on the heart. EKG findings include loss of the T wave or T-wave flattening, the presence of U waves, premature ventricular and atrial complexes, and ventricular and atrial tachyarrhythmias.

21. **What is the effect of pH on serum potassium?**
    Changes in pH cause changes in serum potassium as a result of cellular shift. Alkalosis causes hypokalemia, whereas acidosis causes hyperkalemia. For this reason, bicarbonate is given to severely hyperkalemic patients. If the pH is deranged, normalization most likely will correct the potassium derangement automatically without the need to give or restrict potassium.

22. **Describe the interaction between digitalis and potassium.**
    The heart is particularly sensitive to hypokalemia in patients taking digitalis. Potassium levels should be monitored carefully in all patients taking digitalis, especially if they are also taking diuretics (a common occurrence).

23. How should potassium be replaced?
Like all electrolyte abnormalities, hypokalemia should be corrected slowly. Oral replacement is preferred, but if the potassium must be given intravenously for severe derangement, do not give more than 20 mEq/hr. Put the patient on an EKG monitor when giving IV potassium because potentially fatal arrhythmias may develop.

24. When hypokalemia persists even after administration of significant amounts of potassium, what should you do?
Check the magnesium level. When magnesium is low, the body cannot retain potassium effectively. Correction of a low magnesium level allows the potassium level to return to normal.

25. What are the signs and symptoms of hyperkalemia?
Weakness and paralysis may occur, but the cardiac effects are the most tested. EKG changes (in order of increasing potassium value) include **tall, peaked T waves,** widening of QRS, prolongation of the PR interval, loss of P waves, and a sine-wave pattern EKG (Fig. 1-1). Arrhythmias include asystole and ventricular fibrillation.

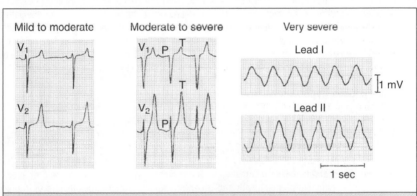

Figure 1-1. The earliest EKG change with hyperkalemia is peaking of the T waves. As the serum potassium concentration increases, the QRS complexes widen, the P waves decrease in amplitude and may disappear, and finally a sine-wave pattern leads to asystole unless emergency therapy is given. (From Goldberger A: Clinical Electrocardiography: A Simplified Approach, 7th ed., Philadelphia, Mosby, 2006, Fig. 10-6.)

26. What causes hyperkalemia?
- Renal failure (acute or chronic)
- Severe tissue destruction (because potassium has a high intracellular concentration)
- Hypoaldosteronism (watch for hyporeninemic hypoaldosteronism in diabetes)
- Medications (stop potassium-sparing diuretics, beta blockers, nonsteroidal antiinflammatory drugs, angiotensin-converting enzyme inhibitors, and angiotensin receptor blockers)
- Adrenal insufficiency (also associated with low sodium and low blood pressure)

27. What should you suspect if an asymptomatic patient has hyperkalemia?
With hyperkalemia, the first consideration (especially if the patient is asymptomatic and the EKG is normal) is whether the lab specimen is hemolyzed. Hemolysis causes a false hyperkalemia due to high intracellular potassium concentrations. Repeat the test.

28. The specimen was not hemolyzed. What is the first treatment?
Get an EKG first to look for cardiotoxicity. In general, the best therapy for hyperkalemia is decreased potassium intake and administration of oral sodium polystyrene resin (Kayexalate).

But if the potassium level is greater than 6.5 or cardiac toxicity is apparent (more than peaked T waves), immediate intravenous therapy is needed. First give **calcium gluconate** (which is cardioprotective, although it does not change potassium levels); then give **sodium bicarbonate** (alkalosis causes potassium to shift inside cells) and **glucose with insulin** (insulin also forces potassium inside cells, and glucose prevents hypoglycemia). Beta$_2$ agonists also drive potassium into cells and can be given if the other choices are not listed on the test. If the patient has renal failure (high creatinine) or initial treatment is ineffective, prepare to institute dialysis emergently.

29. **What are the signs and symptoms of hypocalcemia?**
    Hypocalcemia produces neurologic findings, the most tested of which is tetany. Tapping on the facial nerve at the angle of the jaw elicits contraction of the facial muscles (**Chvostek sign**), and inflation of a tourniquet or blood pressure cuff elicits hand muscle (carpopedal) spasms (**Trousseau sign**). Other signs and symptoms are depression, encephalopathy, dementia, laryngospasm, and convulsions/seizures. The classic EKG finding is QT-interval prolongation.

30. **What should you do if the calcium level is low?**
    First, remember that hypoproteinemia (i.e., low albumin) of any etiology can cause hypocalcemia because the protein-bound fraction of calcium is decreased. In this instance, however, the patient is asymptomatic, because the ionized (unbound, physiologically active) fraction of calcium is unchanged. Thus, you should first check the albumin level and/or the ionized or free calcium level to make sure "true" hypocalcemia is present. For every 1 g/dL decrease in albumin below 4 g/dL, correct the calcium by adding 0.8 mg/dL to the given calcium value.

31. **What causes hypocalcemia?**
    - DiGeorge syndrome (tetany 24 to 48 hours after birth, absent thymic shadow on x-ray)
    - Renal failure (remember the kidney's role in vitamin D metabolism)
    - Hypoparathyroidism (watch for a postthyroidectomy patient; all four parathyroids may have been accidentally removed)
    - Vitamin D deficiency
    - Pseudohypoparathyroidism (short fingers, short stature, mental retardation, and normal levels of parathyroid hormone with end-organ unresponsiveness to parathyroid hormone)
    - Acute pancreatitis
    - Renal tubular acidosis

32. **Describe the relationship between low calcium and low magnesium.**
    It is difficult to correct hypocalcemia until hypomagnesemia (of any cause) also is corrected.

33. **How does pH affect calcium levels?**
    Alkalosis can cause symptoms similar to hypocalcemia through effects on the ionized fraction of calcium (alkalosis causes calcium to shift intracellularly). Clinically, this scenario is most common with hyperventilation/anxiety syndromes, in which the patient eliminates too much CO_2, becomes alkalotic, and develops perioral and extremity tingling. Treat by correcting the pH. Reduce anxiety if hyperventilation is the cause.

34. **Describe the relationship between calcium and phosphorus.**
    Phosphorus and calcium levels usually go in opposite directions (when one goes up, the other goes down), and derangements in one can cause problems with the other. This relationship becomes clinically important in patients with chronic renal failure, in whom you must not only try to raise calcium levels (with vitamin D and calcium supplements) but also restrict/reduce phosphorus.

35. **What are the signs and symptoms of hypercalcemia?**
    Hypercalcemia is often asymptomatic and discovered by routine lab tests. When symptoms are present, recall the following rhyme:

Bones (bone changes such as osteopenia and pathologic fractures)
Stones (kidney stones and polyuria)
Groans (abdominal pain, anorexia, constipation, ileus, nausea, vomiting)
Psychiatric overtones (depression, psychosis, delirium/confusion)
Abdominal pain also may be due to peptic ulcer disease and/or pancreatitis, both of which have an increased incidence with hypercalcemia. The EKG classically shows QT-interval shortening.

36. **What causes hypercalcemia?**
Hypercalcemia in outpatients most commonly is due to hyperparathyroidism. In inpatients, the most common cause is malignancy. Check the parathyroid hormone (PTH) level to differentiate hyperparathyroidism from other causes.
Other causes include vitamin A or D intoxication, sarcoidosis, thiazide diuretics, familial hypocalciuric hypercalcemia (look for low urinary calcium, which is rare with hypercalcemia), and immobilization. Hyperproteinemia (e.g., high albumin) of any etiology can cause hypercalcemia because of an increase in the protein-bound fraction of calcium, but the patient is asymptomatic because ionized (unbound) fraction is unchanged.

37. **Why is asymptomatic hypercalcemia usually treated?**
Prolonged hypercalcemia can cause nephrocalcinosis and renal failure due to calcium salt deposits in the kidney and may result in bone disease secondary to loss of calcium.

38. **How is hypercalcemia treated?**
First, give intravenous fluids. Then, once the patient is well hydrated, give furosemide (i.e., a loop diuretic) to cause calcium diuresis. Thiazides are contraindicated because they increase serum calcium levels. Other treatments include phosphorus administration (use oral phosphorus; intravenous administration can be dangerous), calcitonin, bisphosphonates (e.g., etidronate, which often is used in Paget disease), plicamycin, or prednisone (especially for malignancy-induced hypercalcemia). Correction of the underlying cause of hypercalcemia is the ultimate goal. The previous measures are all temporary until definitive treatment can be given. For hyperparathyroidism, surgery is the treatment of choice.

39. **In what clinical scenario is hypomagnesemia usually seen?**
Alcoholism. Magnesium is wasted through the kidneys.

40. **What are the signs and symptoms of hypomagnesemia?**
Signs and symptoms are similar to those of hypocalcemia (prolonged QT interval on EKG and possibly tetany).

41. **In what clinical scenario is hypermagnesemia seen?**
Hypermagnesemia is classically iatrogenic in pregnant patients who are treated for preeclampsia with magnesium sulfate. It also commonly occurs in patients with renal failure. Patients who receive magnesium sulfate should be monitored carefully, because the physical findings of hypermagnesemia are progressive. The initial sign is a decrease in deep tendon reflexes; then hypotension and respiratory failure occur sequentially.

42. **How is hypermagnesemia treated?**
First, stop any magnesium infusion! Remember the ABCs (airway, breathing, circulation), and intubate the patient if necessary. If the patient is stable, start intravenous fluids. Furosemide can be given next, if needed to cause a magnesium diuresis. The last resort is dialysis.

43. **In what clinical scenarios is hypophosphatemia seen? What are the signs and symptoms?**
Primarily in patients with uncontrolled diabetes (especially diabetic ketoacidosis) and alcoholics. Signs and symptoms of hypophosphatemia include neuromuscular disturbances (encephalopathy, weakness), rhabdomyolysis (especially in alcoholics), anemia, and white blood cell and platelet dysfunction.

44. **What is the intravenous fluid of choice in hypovolemic patients?**
Normal saline or lactated Ringer solution (regardless of other electrolyte problems). First fill the tank; then correct the imbalances that the kidney cannot sort out on its own.

45. **What is the maintenance fluid of choice for patients who are not eating?**
One-half normal saline with 5% dextrose In adults. Typically one-fourth normal saline with 5% dextrose in children under 10 kg; one-third or one-half normal saline with 5% dextrose in children over 10 kg.

46. **Should anything be added to the intravenous fluid for patients who are not eating?**
Usually potassium chloride, 10 or 20 mEq, is added to a liter of intravenous fluid each day to prevent hypokalemia (assuming that the baseline potassium level is normal).

1. **With which cancers is alcohol intake associated?**
Cancers of the oral cavity, larynx, pharynx, esophagus, liver, and lung. It also may be associated with gastric, colon, pancreatic, and breast cancer.

2. **What is the most common cause of cirrhosis and esophageal varices?**
Alcohol.

3. **Describe the relationship between alcohol and accidental or intentional (i.e., suicide and murder) death?**
Alcohol is involved in roughly 50% of fatal car accidents, 67% of drownings, 67% of homicides, 35% of suicides, and 70% to 80% of deaths caused by fire.

4. **What may happen if you give glucose to an alcoholic without giving thiamine first?**
You may precipitate Wernicke encephalopathy. Always give thiamine before glucose to avoid this complication.

5. **What is the difference between Wernicke and Korsakoff syndromes? What causes each?** *(altered mental states)*
Wernicke syndrome is an acute encephalopathy characterized by ophthalmoplegia, nystagmus, ataxia, and/or confusion. It can be fatal but often is reversible with thiamine.
   Korsakoff syndrome is a chronic psychosis characterized by anterograde amnesia (inability to form new memories) and confabulation (lying) to cover up the amnesia. Korsakoff syndrome is generally irreversible and is thought to be due to damage to the mamillary bodies and thalamic nuclei. Both conditions result from thiamine deficiency.

6. **True or false: Alcohol withdrawal can be fatal.**
True. Alcohol withdrawal needs to be treated on an inpatient basis because it can result in death (mortality rate of 1% to 5% with delirium tremens).

7. **How is alcohol withdrawal treated?**
With benzodiazepines (or, in rare cases, barbiturates). The dose is tapered gradually over several days until symptoms have resolved.

8. **What are the stages of alcohol withdrawal?**
Acute withdrawal syndrome (12 to 48 hours after last drink): tremors, sweating, hyperreflexia, and seizures ("rum fits").
   Alcoholic hallucinosis (24 to 72 hours after last drink): auditory and visual hallucinations and illusions without autonomic signs.
   Delirium tremens (2 to 7 days after last drink, possibly longer): hallucinations and illusions, confusion, poor sleep, and autonomic lability (sweating, increased pulse and temperature). Fatality usually is associated with this stage.
   Of course, these stages may overlap. Delirium tremens may occur several days after the last drink. The classic example is a patient who develops delirium on postoperative day 2 but was fine before the surgery. He or she could be a closet alcoholic, assuming other causes for delirium have been ruled out.

9. **What are the classic physical stigmata of liver disease in alcoholics?**
   - Abdominal wall varices (caput medusae)
   - Testicular atrophy
   - Esophageal varices
   - Encephalopathy
   - Hemorrhoids (internal)
   - Asterixis
   - Jaundice
   - Scleral icterus
   - Ascites
   - Edema
   - Palmar erythema
   - Spider angiomas
   - Gynecomastia
   - Terry nails
   - Fetor hepaticus
   - Dupuytren contractures

10. **What are the classic laboratory findings of liver disease in alcoholics?**
    - Anemia (classically macrocytic)
    - Prolonged prothrombin time
    - Hyperbilirubinemia
    - Hypoalbuminemia
    - Thrombocytopenia

11. **What diseases and conditions may be caused by chronic alcohol intake?**
    - Gastritis
    - Fatty change in the liver (Fig. 2-1)
    - Mallory-Weiss tears

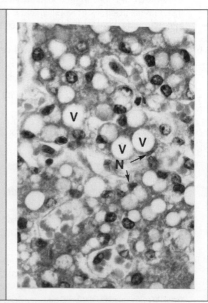

Figure 2-1. Fatty change in the liver. Vacuoles (V) are seen in hepatocytes due to the fact that organic solvents used in standard issue processing dissolves out fat to leave empty, non-staining spaces. These fat vacuoles can be seen to displace nuclei (N) to the periphery of the cell. Commonly seen causes include toxins such as alcohol, diabetes mellitus, obesity and chronic hypoxia. (From Stevens A, et al: Wheater's Basic Histopathology, 4th ed. New York, Churchill Livingstone, 2002, p. 6, with permission.)

- Hepatitis
- Pancreatitis (acute or chronic)
- Cirrhosis
- Peripheral neuropathy (via thiamine deficiency and a direct effect)
- Wernicke or Korsakoff syndrome
- Cerebellar degeneration (ataxia, past-pointing)
- Dilated cardiomyopathy
- Rhabdomyolysis (acute or chronic)

12. **Describe the classic derangement of aspartate aminotransferase (AST) and alanine aminotransferase (ALT) in alcoholic hepatitis.**
The ratio of AST (also known as serum glutamate oxaloacetate transaminase [SGOT]) to ALT (also known as serum glutamate pyruvate transaminase [SGPT]) is at least 2:1, although both may be elevated. Other causes of hepatitis usually are associated with the opposite ratio or equal elevation of both AST and ALT.

13. **What is the best treatment for alcoholism?**
Alcoholics Anonymous or other peer-based support groups have had the best success rates. Disulfiram (an aldehyde dehydrogenase enzyme inhibitor that makes people sick when they drink) can be used in some patients. Be sure to warn patients that metronidazole and certain cephalosporins have a similar effect on those who drink alcohol.

14. **Describe the effects of alcohol on pregnancy.**
Alcohol is a definite teratogen and the most common cause of preventable mental retardation in the United States. You should be able to recognize the classic presentation of a child affected by fetal alcohol syndrome: mental retardation, microcephaly, microphthalmia, short palpebral fissures, midfacial hypoplasia, and cardiac defects. No amount of alcohol consumption can be considered safe during pregnancy. Fetal alcohol syndrome rates vary, but may affect as many as 1 in 1000 births in the United States.

15. **Discuss the epidemiology of alcohol abuse.**
Roughly 10% to 15% of the population abuses alcohol. Alcohol abuse is more common in men. The genetic component is passed most easily from father to son.

16. **What kind of pneumonia should you suspect in a "skid-row" alcoholic?**
Aspiration pneumonia. Look for enteric organisms (anaerobes, *Escherichia coli*, streptococci, staphylococci) as the cause. Think of Klebsiella spp. if sputum resembles currant jelly or thick, mucoid capsules are mentioned in culture reports.

17. **True or false: Alcohol can precipitate hypoglycemia.**
True. But give thiamine first, then glucose in an alcoholic.

18. **What are the classic electrolyte and vitamin/mineral abnormalities in alcoholics?**
Electrolytes: low magnesium, low potassium, low sodium, elevated uric acid (resulting in gout)
   Vitamins: deficiencies of folate and thiamine
   Remember that alcoholics tend to have poor nutrition and may develop just about any deficiency.

19. **How are bleeding esophageal varices treated?**
First, think of the ABCs (airways, breathing, and circulation). Stabilize the patient with intravenous fluids and blood if needed. If indicated, correct clotting factor deficiencies with fresh frozen plasma, fresh blood, and vitamin K. Next, endoscopy is performed to determine

the cause of the upper gastrointestinal bleed (there are many possibilities in an alcoholic). Once varices are identified on endoscopy, sclerotherapy of the veins is attempted with cauterization, banding, or vasopressin. The mortality rate is high, and rebleeding is common. If you must choose, try a transjugular intrahepatic portasystemic shunt (TIPS) over an open surgical portacaval shunt for more definitive management, if needed. The most physiologic shunt type among surgical options is the splenorenal shunt.

20. **How are varices with no history of bleeding treated?**

With nonselective beta-blockers (propranolol, nadolol, timolol), provided that there is no contraindication to the use of beta-blockers.

CHAPTER 3

BIOSTATISTICS

1. **How is the sensitivity of a test defined? What are highly sensitive tests used for clinically?**
   Sensitivity is defined as the ability of a test to detect disease—mathematically, the number of true positives divided by the number of people with the disease. Tests with high sensitivity are used for disease screening. False positives occur, but the test does not miss many people with the disease (low false-negative rate).

2. **How is the specificity of a test defined? What are highly specific tests used for clinically?**
   Specificity is defined as the ability of a test to detect health (or nondisease)—mathematically, the number of true negatives divided by the number of people without the disease. Tests with high specificity are used for disease confirmation. False negatives occur, but the test does not call anyone sick who is actually healthy (low false-positive rate). The ideal confirmatory test must have high sensitivity and high specificity; otherwise, people with the disease may be called healthy.

3. **Explain the concept of a trade-off between sensitivity and specificity.**
   The trade-off between sensitivity and specificity is a classic statistics question. For example, you should understand how changing the cut-off glucose value in screening for diabetes (or changing the value of any of several screening tests) will change the number of true- and false-negative as well as true- and false-positive results. If the cut-off glucose value is raised, fewer people will be called diabetic (more false negatives, fewer false positives), whereas if the cut-off glucose value is lowered, more people will be called diabetic (fewer false negatives, more false positives) (Fig. 3-1).

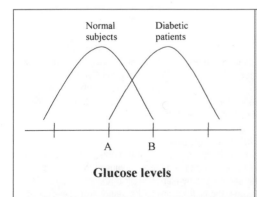

Glucose levels

Figure 3-1. If the cut-off serum glucose value for a diagnosis of diabetes mellitus is set at point A, no cases of diabetes will be missed, but many people without diabetes will be mislabeled as diabetics (i.e., higher sensitivity, lower specificity, lower positive predictive value, higher negative predictive value). If the cut-off is set at B, the diagnosis of diabetes will not be made in healthy people, but many cases of true diabetes will go undiagnosed (i.e., lower sensitivity, higher specificity, higher positive predictive value, lower negative predictive value). The optimal diagnostic value lies somewhere between points A and B.

4. **Define positive predictive value (PPV). On what does it depend?**

   When a test is positive for disease, the PPV measures how likely it is that the patient has the disease (probability of having a condition, given a positive test). PPV is calculated mathematically by dividing the number of true positives by the total number of people with a positive test. PPV depends on the prevalence of a disease (the higher the prevalence, the higher the PPV) and the sensitivity and specificity of the test (e.g., an overly sensitive test that gives more false positives has a lower PPV).

5. **Define negative predictive value (NPV). On what does it depend?**

   When a test comes back negative for disease, the NPV measures how likely it is that the patient is healthy and does not have the disease (probability of not having a condition, given a negative test). It is calculated mathematically by dividing the number of true negatives by the total number of people with a negative test. NPV also depends on the prevalence of the disease and the sensitivity and specificity of the test (the higher the prevalence, the lower the NPV). In addition, an overly sensitive test with lots of false positives makes the NPV higher.

6. **Define attributable risk. How is it measured?**

   Attributable risk is the number of cases of a disease attributable to one risk factor (in other words, the amount by which the incidence of a condition is expected to decrease if the risk factor in question is removed). For example, if the incidence rate of lung cancer is 1/100 in the general population and 10/100 in smokers, the attributable risk of smoking in causing lung cancer is 9/100 (assuming a properly matched control).

7. **You need to develop the habit of drawing a 2 × 2 table for Step 2 statistics questions. Given the 2 × 2 table below, define the formulas for calculating the following test values:**

		Disease		Test Name	Formula
		(+)	(−)	Sensitivity	$A/(A + C)$
				Specificity	$D/(B + D)$
Test	(+)	A	B	PPV	$A/(A + B)$
or				NPV	$D/(C + D)$
Exposure	(−)	C	D	Odds ratio	$(A \times D)/(B \times C)$
				Relative risk	$[A/(A + B)]/[C/(C + D)]$
				Attributable risk	$[A/(A + B)]-[C/(C + D)]$

8. **Define relative risk. From what type of studies can it be calculated?**

   Relative risk compares the disease risk in people exposed to a certain factor with the disease risk in people who have not been exposed to the factor in question. Relative risk can be calculated only after prospective or experimental studies; it cannot be calculated from retrospective data. If a Step 2 question asks you to calculate the relative risk from retrospective data, the answer is "cannot be calculated" or "none of the above."

9. **What is a clinically significant value for relative risk?**

   Any value for relative risk other than 1 is clinically significant. For example, if the relative risk is 1.5, a person is 1.5 times more likely to develop the condition if exposed to the factor in question. If the relative risk is 0.5, the person is only half as likely to develop the condition when exposed to the factor; in other words, the factor protects the person from developing the disease.

10. **Define odds ratio. From what type of studies is it calculated?**
Odds ratio attempts to estimate relative risk with retrospective studies (e.g., case control). An odds ratio compares (the incidence of disease in persons exposed to the factor and the incidence of nondisease in persons not exposed to the factor) with (the incidence of disease in persons unexposed to the factor and the incidence of nondisease in persons exposed to the factor) to see whether there is a difference between the two. As with relative risk, values other than 1 are significant. The odds ratio is a less than perfect way to estimate relative risk (which can be calculated only from prospective or experimental studies).

11. **What do you need to know about standard deviation (SD) for the USMLE?**
You need to know that with a normal or bell-shaped distribution, 1 SD holds 68% of the values, 2 SD hold 95% of the values and 3 SD hold 99.7% of the values. A classic question gives you the mean and standard deviation and asks you what percentage of values will be above a given value. For example, if the mean score on a test is 80 and the standard deviation is 5, 68% of the scores will be within 5 points of 80 (scores of 75 to 85) and 95% of the scores will be within 10 points of 80 (scores of 70 to 90). The question may ask what percentage of scores are over 90. The answer is 2.5% because 2.5% of the scores fall below 70 and 2.5% of the scores are over 90. Variations of this question are common.

12. **Define mean, median, and mode.**
The mean is the average value, the median is the middle value, and the mode is the most common value. A question may give you several numbers and ask you for their mean, median, and mode. For example, if the question gives you the numbers 2, 2, 4, and 8:
The mean is the average of the 4 numbers: $2 + 2 + 4 + 8/4 = 16/4 = 4$.
The median is the middle value. Because there are 4 numbers, there is no true middle value. Therefore, take the average between the two middle numbers (2 and 4). The median $= 3$.
The mode is 2, because the number 2 appears twice (more times than any other value). Remember that in a normal distribution, mean $=$ median $=$ mode.

13. **What is a skewed distribution? How does it affect mean median and mode?**
A skewed distribution implies that the distribution is not normal; in other words, the data do not conform to a perfect bell-shaped curve. **Positive skew** is an asymmetric distribution with an excess of high values; in other words, the tail of the curve is on the right (mean > median > mode) (Fig. 3-2). **Negative skew** is an asymmetric distribution with an excess of low values; in other words, the tail of the curve is on the left (mean < median < mode). Because they are not normal distributions, standard deviation and mean are less meaningful values.

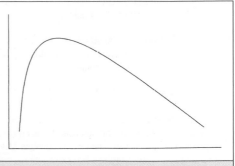

Figure 3-2. Positive skew. An excess of higher values makes this a non-normal distribution.

14. **Define test reliability. How is it related to precision? What reduces reliability?**
Practically speaking, the reliability of a test is synonymous with its precision. Reliability measures the reproducibility and consistency of a test. For example, if the test has good inter-rater reliability, the person taking the test will get the same score if two different people

administer the same test. Random error reduces reliability and precision (e.g., limitation in significant figures).

15. **Define test validity. How is it related to accuracy? What reduces validity?**
Practically speaking, the validity of a test is synonymous with its accuracy. Validity measures the trueness of measurement; in other words, whether the test measures what it claims to measure. For example, if you give a valid IQ test to a genius, the test should not indicate that he or she is retarded. Systematic error reduces validity and accuracy (e.g., when the equipment is miscalibrated).

16. **Define correlation coefficient. What is the range of its values?**
A correlation coefficient measures to what degree two variables are related. The value of the correlation coefficient ranges from −1 to +1.

17. **True or false: A correlation coefficient of −0.6 is a stronger correlation coefficient than +0.4.**
True. The important factor in determining the strength of the relationship between the two variables is the distance of the value from zero. A zero correlation equals no association whatsoever; the two variables are totally unrelated. Positive 1 equals a perfect positive correlation (when one variable increases, so does the other), whereas negative 1 equals a perfect negative correlation (when one variable increases, the other decreases). Therefore use the absolute value to give you the strength of the correlation (e.g., −0.3 is equal to +0.3).

18. **Define confidence interval. Why is it used?**
When you take a set of data from a subset of the population and calculate its mean, you want to say that it is equivalent to the mean of the whole population. In fact, however, the two means usually are not exactly equal. A confidence interval of 95% (the value used in most medical literature before data are accepted by the medical community) says that you are 95% confident that the mean of the entire population is within a certain range (usually two SD of your experimental or derived mean, calculated from the subset of the population that you examined). For example, if you sample the heart rate of 100 people and calculate a mean of 80 beats per minute and a standard deviation of 2, your confidence interval (also known as confidence limits) is written as $76 < X < 84 = 0.95$. In other words, you are 95% certain that the mean heart rate of the whole population (X) is between 76 and 84.

19. **What five types of studies should you know for the Step 2 exam?**
From highest to lowest quality and desirability: (1) experimental studies, (2) prospective studies, (3) retrospective studies, (4) case series, and (5) prevalence surveys.

20. **What is an experimental study?**
Experimental studies are the gold standard. They compare two equal groups in which one variable is manipulated and its effect is measured. Experimental studies use double-blinding (or at least single-blinding) and well-matched controls to ensure accurate data. It is not always possible to do experimental studies because of ethical concerns.

21. **What are prospective studies? Why are they important?**
Prospective studies (also known as observational, longitudinal, cohort, incidence, or follow-up studies) involve choosing a sample and dividing it into two groups based on the presence or absence of a risk factor and following the groups over time to see what diseases they develop. For example, you can follow people with and without asymptomatic hypercholesterolemia to see if people with hypercholesterolemia have a higher incidence of myocardial infarction later in life. You can calculate relative risk and incidence from this type of study. Prospective studies are time-consuming and expensive but practical for common diseases.

22. **What are retrospective studies? Discuss their advantages and disadvantages.**
Retrospective (case-control) studies choose population samples after the fact, based on the presence (cases) or absence (controls) of disease. Information can be collected about risk factors. For example, you can compare people with lung cancer and people without lung cancer to see if people with lung cancer smoked more before they developed lung cancer. With a retrospective study you can calculate an odds ratio, but you cannot calculate a true relative risk or measure incidence. Compared with prospective studies, retrospective studies are less expensive, less time-consuming, and more practical for rare diseases.

23. **What is a case series study? How is it used?**
A case series study simply describes the clinical presentation of people with a certain disease. This type of study is good for extremely rare diseases (as are retrospective studies) and may suggest a need for a retrospective or prospective study.

24. **What is a prevalence survey? How is it used?**
Prevalence (cross-sectional) surveys look at the prevalence of a disease and the prevalence of risk-factors. When used to compare two different cultures or populations, a prevalence survey may suggest a possible cause of a disease. The hypothesis then can be tested with a prospective study. For example, researchers have found a higher prevalence of colon cancer and a diet higher in fat in the United States versus a lower prevalence of colon cancer and a diet lower in fat in Japan.

25. **What is the difference between incidence and prevalence?**
Incidence is the number of new cases of a disease in a unit of time (generally 1 year, but any time frame can be used). The incidence of a disease is equal to the absolute (or total) risk of developing a condition (as distinguished from relative or attributable risk).
Prevalence is the total number of cases of a disease (new or old) at a certain point in time.

26. **If a disease can be treated only to the point that people can be kept alive longer without being cured, what happens to the incidence and prevalence of the disease?**
This is the classic question about incidence and prevalence on the Step 2 exam. Nothing happens to the incidence (the same number of people contract the disease every year), but the prevalence will increase, because people with the disease live longer. In short-term diseases (e.g., influenza), the incidence may be higher than the prevalence, whereas in chronic diseases (e.g., diabetes or hypertension), the prevalence is greater than the incidence.

27. **Define epidemic.**
In an epidemic the observed incidence greatly exceeds the expected incidence.

28. **When do you use a chi-squared test, T-test, and analysis of variance test?**
All of these tests are used to compare different sets of data.
Chi-squared test: used to compare percentages or proportions (nonnumeric or nominal data).
T-test: used to compare two means.
Analysis of variance (ANOVA): used to compare three or more means.

29. **What is the difference between nominal, ordinal, and continuous types of data?**
Nominal data have no numeric value; for example, the day of the week. Ordinal data give a ranking but no quantification; for example, class rank, which does not specify how far number 1 is ahead of number 2. Most numerical measurements are continuous data; for example, weight, blood pressure, and age. This distinction is important because of question 28: chi-squared tests must be used to compare nominal or ordinal data, whereas a T-test or ANOVA test is used to compare continuous data.

30. Define p-value.

The significance of the p-value is high-yield on the Step II exam. If $p < 0.05$ for a set of data, there is less than a 5% chance ($0.05 = 5\%$) that the data were obtained by random error or chance. If $p < 0.01$, the chance is less than 1%. For example, if the blood pressure in my control group is 180/100 mmHg but falls to 120/70 mmHg after drug X is given, a p-value < 0.10 means that the chance that this difference was due to random error or chance is less than 10%. It also means, however, that the chance that the result is random and unrelated to the drug may be as high as 9.99%. A $p < 0.05$ is generally used as the cutoff for statistical significance in the medical literature.

31. What three points about p-value should be remembered for the Step 2 exam?

1. A study with a p-value < 0.05 may still have serious flaws.
2. A low p-value does not imply causation.
3. A study that has statistical significance does not necessarily have clinical significance. For example, if I tell you that drug X can lower blood pressure from 130/80 to 129/80 mmHg with $p < 0.0001$, you still would not use drug X because the result is not clinically important given the minimal blood pressure reduction, the costs, and probable side effects.

32. Explain the relationship of the p-value to the null hypothesis.

The p-value also is related to the null hypothesis (the hypothesis of no difference). For example, in a study of hypertension, the null hypothesis says that the drug under investigation does not work; therefore, any difference in blood pressure is due to random error or chance. When the drug works beautifully and lowers blood pressure by 60 points, the null hypothesis must be rejected because clearly the drug works. When $p < 0.05$, I can confidently reject the null hypothesis, because the p-value tells me that there is less than a 5% chance that the null hypothesis is correct. If the null hypothesis is wrong, the difference in blood pressure is not due to chance; therefore, it must be due to the drug.

In other words, the p-value represents the chance of making a type I error—that is, claiming an effect or difference when none exists or rejecting the null hypothesis when it is true. If $p < 0.07$, there is less than a 7% chance that you are making a type I error if you claim a true difference (not due to random error) in blood pressure between the control and experimental groups.

33. What is a type II error?

In a type II error the null hypothesis is accepted when in fact it is false. In the above example, it would mean that the antihypertensive drug works but the experimenter says that it does not.

34. What is the power of a study? How do you increase the power of a study?

Power measures the probability of rejecting the null hypothesis when it is false (a good thing). The best way to increase power is to **increase the sample size.**

35. What are confounding variables?

Confounding variables are unmeasured variables that affect both the independent (manipulated, experimental) variable and dependent (outcome) variables. For example, an experimenter measures the number of ashtrays owned and the incidence of lung cancer and finds that people with lung cancer have more ashtrays. He concludes that ashtrays cause lung cancer. Smoking tobacco is the confounding variable, because it causes the increase in ashtrays and lung cancer.

36. Discuss nonrandom or nonstratified sampling.

City A and City B can be compared, but they may not be equivalent. For example, if city A is a retirement community and city B is a college town, of course city A will have higher rates of mortality and heart disease if the groups are not stratified into appropriate age-specific comparisons.

37. **What is nonresponse bias?**
Nonresponse bias occurs when people do not return printed surveys or answer the phone in a phone survey. If nonresponse accounts for a significant percentage of the results, the experiment will suffer. The first strategy in this situation is to visit or call the nonresponders repeatedly. If this strategy is unsuccessful, list the nonresponders as unknown in the data analysis and see if any results can be salvaged. *Never* make up or assume responses.

38. **Explain lead-time bias.**
Lead-time bias is due to time differentials. The classic example is a cancer screening test that claims to prolong survival compared with older survival data, when in fact the difference is due only to earlier detection—*not* to improved treatment or prolonged survival.

39. **Explain admission rate bias.**
The classic admission rate bias occurs when an experimenter compares the mortality rates for myocardial infarction (or some other disease) in hospitals A and B and concludes that hospital A has a higher mortality rate. But the higher rate may be due to tougher admission criteria at hospital A, which admits only the sickest patients with myocardial infarction. Hence, they have higher mortality rates, although their care may be superior. The same bias can apply to a surgeon's mortality and morbidity rates if he or she takes only tough cases.

40. **Explain recall bias.**
Recall bias is a risk in all retrospective studies. When people cannot remember exactly, they may inadvertently over- or underestimate risk factors. For example, John died of lung cancer and his angry widow remembers him as smoking "like a chimney," whereas Mike died of non–smoking-related causes and his loving wife denies that he smoked "much." In fact, both men smoked one pack per day.

41. **Explain interviewer bias.**
Interviewer bias occurs in the absence of blinding. The scientist receives big money to do a study and wants to find a difference between cases and controls. Thus, he or she inadvertently calls the same patient comment or outcome "not significant" in the control group and "significant" in the treatment group.

42. **What is unacceptability bias?**
Unacceptability bias occurs when people do not admit to embarrassing behavior or claim to exercise more than they do to please the interviewer—or they may claim to take experimental medications when they spit them out.

CHAPTER 4

CARDIOLOGY

1. **What is your job when the Step 2 exam describes a patient with chest pain?**
   To make sure that the chest pain is not due to any life-threatening condition. Usually you must try to make sure that the patient has not had a heart attack.

2. **What elements of the history and physical exam steer you away from a diagnosis of myocardial infarction (MI)?**
   Wrong age: in the absence of known heart disease, strong family history, or multiple risk factors for coronary artery disease, a patient under the age of 40 is extremely unlikely to have an MI.

   Lack of risk factors: a 60-year-old marathon runner who eats well and has a high level of high-density lipoprotein (HDL) and no cardiac risk factors (other than age) is unlikely to have a heart attack.

   Physical characteristics of pain: if the pain is reproducible by palpation, it is from the chest wall, not the heart. The pain associated with an MI is usually not sharp or well localized. The pain should not be related to certain foods or eating.

   Having said all of this, many physicians still want to make sure that a heart attack has not occurred with at least an EKG and possibly one or more sets of cardiac enzyme levels. For the Step 2 exam, however, these clues should steer you toward an alternative diagnosis.

3. **What findings on EKG should make you suspect an MI?**
   After a heart attack you should see flipped or flattened T waves, ST-segment elevation (depression means ischemia; elevation means injury), and/or Q waves in a segmental distribution (e.g., leads II, III, and AVF for an inferior infarct) (Fig. 4-1).

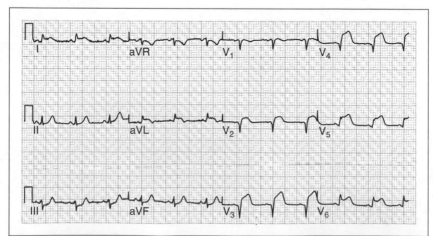

Figure 4-1. This figure shows an anterolateral acute myocardial infarction caused by a lesion in the proximal left anterior descending artery. ST segment elevation is seen in leads I, aVL, V_5, and V_6. (From Marx J, Hockberger R, Walls R: Rosen's Emergency Medicine: Concepts and Clinical Practice, 6th ed. Philadelphia, Mosby, 2006, Fig. 77-6.)

4. **Describe the classic pattern of chest pain in an MI.**
   The pain is classically described as a crushing or pressure sensation; it is a poorly localized substernal pain that may radiate to the shoulder, arm, or jaw. The pain usually is not reproducible on palpation and in patients with a heart attack often does not resolve with nitroglycerin (as it often does in angina). The pain usually lasts at least half an hour.

5. **What tests are used to diagnose an MI?**
   Other than an EKG, the patient with a possible MI should have serial determinations of the MB fraction of creatine kinase (CK-MB), troponin I or T, or myoglobin (usually drawn every 8 hours 3 times before a heart attack is ruled out). Elevation of lactate dehydrogenase (LDH) and a reversed ratio (LDH1 > LDH2) are now uncommonly used for a late MI presentation because the troponin levels stay elevated for more than 24 hours. Aspartate aminotransferase (AST) usually is elevated, but this parameter is not used clinically for detection of cardiac injury. Radiographs may show cardiomegaly and/or pulmonary congestion; echocardiography may show ventricular wall motion abnormalities.

6. **Describe the classic physical exam findings in patients with MI.**
   Patients are often diaphoretic, anxious, tachycardic, tachypneic, and pale; they may have nausea and vomiting. With large heart attacks that cause heart failure, look for bilateral pulmonary rales in the absence of other pneumonia-like symptoms, distended neck veins, S3 or S4 heart sound, new murmurs, hypotension, and/or shock.

7. **What historical points should steer you toward a diagnosis of MI?**
   Patients often have a history of angina or previous chest pain, murmurs, arrhythmias, risk factors for coronary artery disease, hypertension, or diabetes. They also may be taking digoxin, furosemide, cholesterol medications, anti-hypertensives, or other medications.

8. **Describe the treatment for an MI.**
   Treatment involves admission to the intensive or cardiac care unit. Several basic principles should be kept in mind:
   1. Early reperfusion is indicated if the time from onset of symptoms is less than 12 hours, and choice of reperfusion therapy is determined by patient and medical center criteria. Early reperfusion (fewer than 4 to 6 hours) is preferred to try to salvage myocardium. Reperfusion may be accomplished by fibrinolysis or percutaneous coronary intervention (i.e., balloon angioplasty/stent). Coronary artery bypass grafting may be required.
   2. EKG monitoring is essential. If ventricular tachycardia occurs, use amiodarone.
   3. Give oxygen by nasal cannula, and maintain an oxygen saturation > 90%.
   4. Control pain with **morphine**, which may improve pulmonary edema, if present.
   5. Administer **aspirin**.
   6. Administer **nitroglycerin**.
   7. **Beta blockers**, which patients without contraindications should take for life, reduce the mortality rate of MI as well as the incidence of a second heart attack.
   8. Administer **clopidogrel.** (plavix)
   9. Administer **unfractionated or low molecular weight heparin**.
   10. An **angiotensin-converting enzyme (ACE) inhibitor** or **angiotensin receptor blocker (ARB)** should be started within 24 hours.
   11. Administer an **HMG-CoA reductase inhibitor** (statin).

9. **True or false: With good management, patients with an MI will not die in the hospital.**
False. Even with the best of medical management, patients may die from an MI. They also may have a second heart attack during hospitalization. Watch for sudden deterioration!

10. **When is heparin indicated in the setting of chest pain and MI?**
Heparin should be started if unstable angina is diagnosed, if the patient has a cardiac thrombus, or if severe congestive heart failure is seen on echocardiogram. The Step 2 exam will not ask about other indications, which are not as clear-cut. Do not give heparin to patients with contraindications to its use (e.g., active bleeding).

11. **What clues suggest the common noncardiac causes of chest pain?**
Gastroesophageal reflux/peptic ulcer disease: look for a relation to certain foods (spicy, chocolate), smoking, caffeine, or lying down. Pain is relieved by antacids or acid-reducing medications. Patients with peptic ulcer disease test positive for Helicobacter pylori.

    Chest wall pain (costochondritis, bruised or broken ribs): pain is well localized and reproducible on chest wall palpation.

    Esophageal problems (achalasia, nutcracker esophagus, or esophageal spasm): often a difficult differential. The question probably will give a negative work-up for MI or mention the lack of atherosclerosis risk factors. Look for abnormalities with barium swallow (achalasia) or esophageal manometry. Treat achalasia with pneumatic dilatation or botulism toxin administration, and treat nutcracker esophagus or esophageal spasm with calcium channel blockers. If medical treatments are ineffective, surgical myotomy may be needed.

    Pericarditis: look for viral upper respiratory infection prodrome. The EKG shows diffuse ST-segment elevation, the erythrocyte sedimentation rate is elevated, and a low-grade fever is present. Classically the pain is relieved by sitting forward. The most common cause is infection with coxsackievirus. Other causes include tuberculosis, uremia, malignancy, and lupus erythematosus or other autoimmune diseases (Fig. 4-2).

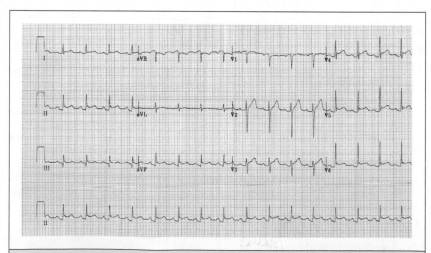

Figure 4-2. Acute pericarditis in a 30-year-old man presenting with pleuritic chest pain. The EKG demonstrates ST segment elevation most clearly seen in leads I, II, aVF, V3–V6, diffuse PR segment depression, and PR segment elevation in lead aVR. (From Demangone D: ECG Manifestations: Noncoronary Heart Disease, Emergency Medicine Clinics of North America. 24(1):113-131, Fig. 1, 2006.)

Pneumonia: chest pain is due to pleuritis. Patients also have cough, fever, and/or sputum production. Ask about possible sick contacts.

Aortic dissection: associated with severe tearing or ripping pain that may radiate to the back. Look for hypertension or evidence of Marfan's syndrome (tall, thin patient with hyperextensible joints). Blunt chest trauma can cause aortic laceration and pseudoaneurysm, which are different condition that are often managed similarly (Fig. 4-3).

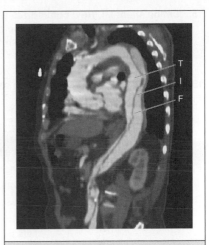

Figure 4-3. Aortic dissection is seen in this contrast-enhanced spiral CT scan of the chest at the level of the pulmonary artery showing an intimal flap (I) in the descending thoracic aorta separating the two lumina in a type B aortic dissection. F = false lumen; T = true lumen. (From Libby P, et al.: Braunwald's Heart Disease: A Textbook of Cardiovascular Medicine, 8th ed. Philadelphia, Saunders, 2008, Fig. 56-19.)

12. **How can you recognize stable angina?**

The chest pain of stable angina begins with exertion or stress and remits with rest or calming down. The pain is described as a pressure or squeezing pain in the substernal area and may radiate to the shoulders, neck, and/or jaw. It often is accompanied by shortness of breath, diaphoresis, and/or nausea. The pain usually is relieved by nitroglycerin. An EKG done during an acute attack often shows ST-segment depression, but in the absence of pain the EKG is often normal. The pain should last less than 20 minutes or be relieved after a sublingual nitroglycerin; otherwise, there may be progression to unstable angina or MI.

13. **Define unstable angina. How is it diagnosed and treated?**

In strict terms, unstable angina is defined as a change from previously stable angina. If a patient used to experience angina once a week and now experiences it once a day, the patient technically has unstable angina. Unstable angina usually presents with normal or only minimally elevated cardiac enzymes, EKG changes (ST depression), and prolonged chest pain that does not respond to nitroglycerin initially (like a heart attack). The pain often begins at rest. Treatment is similar to that for MI. The patient is admitted to the coronary or intensive care unit. Initial treatment begins with oxygen, aspirin, and nitroglycerin. The patient should be given a beta-blocker, clopidogrel, heparin (unfractionated or low molecular weight) and a glycoprotein IIb/IIIa receptor inhibitor. An angiotensin-converting enzyme (ACE) inhibitor or angiotensin receptor blocker (ARB) should be given as well. Consider emergent PTCA if the pain does not resolve. Almost all patients have a history of stable angina and coronary artery disease risk factors.

14. **Describe variant (Prinzmetal) angina.**

This rare type of angina is characterized by pain at rest (unrelated to exertion) and ST elevation; cardiac enzymes are normal. The cause is coronary artery spasm. Prinzmetal angina usually responds to nitroglycerin and is treated over the long term with calcium channel blockers, which reduce arterial spasm.

15. Define silent MI. How common is it?

Patients with a silent MI do not develop chest pain. They present with congestive heart failure, shock, or confusion and delirium (especially elderly patients). MIs are silent in up to 25% of cases (especially in diabetics with neuropathy).

16. What physical exam findings are associated with various heart valve abnormalities?

Valve Problem	Physical Characteristics	Other Findings
Mitral stenosis	Late diastolic blowing murmur (best heard at apex)	Opening snap, loud S1, AF, LAE, PH
Mitral regurgitation	Holosystolic murmur (radiates to axilla)	Soft S1, LAE, PH, LVH
Aortic stenosis	Harsh systolic ejection murmurs (best heard in aortic area; radiates to carotids)	Slow pulse upstroke, S3/S4, ejection click, LVH, cardiomegaly; syncope, angina, heart failure
Aortic regurgitation	Early diastolic decrescendo murmur (best heard at apex)	Widened pulse pressure, LVH, LV dilatation, S3
Mitral prolapse	Midsystolic click, late systolic murmur	Panic disorder

AF = atrial fibrillation; LAE = left atrial enlargement; PH = pulmonary hypertension; LVH = left ventricular hypertrophy; LV = left ventricle.

17. True or false: An understanding of the pathophysiology behind the various changes associated with long-standing valvular heart disease is high-yield for the Step 2 exam.

True. For example, it is advisable to understand why right-heart failure may occur with long-standing mitral stenosis. This is not memorization but rather the ability to determine rationally which changes are associated with each type of valvular dysfunction.

18. Who should receive endocarditis prophylaxis?

The 2008 American Heart Association recommendations conclude that only an extremely small number of cases of infective endocarditis might be prevented by antibiotic prophylaxis for dental procedures. Cardiac conditions for which prophylaxis with dental procedures is recommended includes prosthetic cardiac valve, previous infectious endocarditis, congenital heart disease, and cardiac transplant recipients who develop valvulopathy. Antibiotic prophylaxis is no longer recommended for genitourinary or gastrointestinal procedures.

19. Describe the protocols for endocarditis prophylaxis.

An antibiotic for prophylaxis should be administered in a single dose before the procedure. Amoxicillin is the preferred choice for oral therapy. Cephalexin, clindamycin, azithromycin, or clarithromycin may be used in patients with penicillin allergy. Ampicillin, cefazolin, ceftriaxone, or clindamycin may be used for patients unable to take oral medication.

20. What is Virchow's triad?

Virchow's triad consists of three findings associated with deep venous thrombosis (DVT): endothelial damage, venous stasis, and hypercoagulable state. These three broad categories should help you remember when to think about the possibility of DVT.

21. List the common clinical scenarios for development of DVT.

- Surgery (especially orthopedic, pelvic, abdominal, or neurosurgery)
- Malignancy
- Trauma
- Immobilization
- Pregnancy
- Use of birth control pills
- Disseminated intravascular coagulation
- Hypercoagulable states such as factor V (Leiden), antithrombin III deficiency, protein C deficiency, protein S deficiency, prothrombin G20210A gene mutation, hyperhomocysteinemia, or antiphospholipid antibodies

22. Describe the physical signs and symptoms of DVT. How is it diagnosed?

Signs and symptoms include unilateral leg swelling, pain or tenderness, and/or **Homan sign** (present in 30% of cases). Superficial palpable cords imply superficial thrombophlebitis rather than DVT (see below). DVT is best diagnosed by compression ultrasonography or impedance plethysmography of the veins of the extremity. The gold standard is venography, but this invasive test is reserved for situations in which the diagnosis is not clear.

23. True or false: Superficial thrombophlebitis is a risk factor for pulmonary embolus.

False. Superficial thrombophlebitis (erythema, tenderness, edema, and palpable clot in a superficial vein) affects superficial veins and does not cause pulmonary emboli. It is considered a benign condition, although recurrent superficial thrombophlebitis can be a marker for underlying malignancy (e.g., Trousseau syndrome, or migratory thrombophlebitis, is a classic marker for pancreatic cancer). Treat affected patients with nonsteroidal anti-inflammatory drugs (e.g., aspirin) and warm compresses.

24. How is DVT treated? For how long?

Systemic anticoagulation is necessary. Use intravenous heparin or subcutaneous low-molecular-weight heparin initially, followed by crossover to oral warfarin. Patients should be maintained on warfarin for at least 3 to 6 months—and possibly for life if more than one episode of clotting occurs.

25. What is the best way to prevent DVT in patients undergoing surgery?

Prophylactic measures for patients undergoing surgery depend on the risk for developing deep venous thrombosis or pulmonary embolism. Early ambulation is recommended for low risk patients. Low molecular weight heparin, low dose unfractionated heparin, or fondaparinux is recommended for patients at moderate risk. High risk patients should be given low molecular weight heparin, fondaparinux, or an oral vitamin K antagonist. Pneumatic compression stockings should be used instead if the patient is moderate risk or higher and is at high risk of bleeding.

26. In what clinical settings does pulmonary embolus (PE) occur? Describe the symptoms and signs.

PE commonly follows DVT, delivery (amniotic fluid embolus), or fractures (fat emboli). The classic patient recently went on a long car ride or took a long airplane flight. Symptoms include tachypnea, dyspnea, chest pain, hemoptysis (if a lung infarct has occurred), and hypotension, syncope, or death in severe cases. In rare instances, the chest radiograph shows a wedge-shaped defect due to pulmonary infarct (Fig. 4-4).

27. **True or false: DVT can lead to a stroke.**
False—with one rare exception. Embolization of left-sided heart clots (due to atrial fibrillation, ventricular wall aneurysm, severe congestive heart failure, or endocarditis) causes arterial infarcts (stroke and renal, gastrointestinal, or extremity infarcts)—**not** pulmonary emboli. Deep venous thrombi (or right-sided heart clots) that embolize cause pulmonary emboli—**not** arterial emboli.

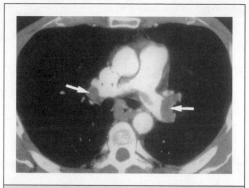

Figure 4-4. Spiral computed tomographic image of acute pulmonary emboli in both main pulmonary arteries in a postoperative patient who suddenly developed dyspnea, hypoxemia, and hypotension. (From Goldman L, Ausiello D: Cecil Medicine, 23rd ed. Philadelphia, Saunders, 2008, Fig. 99-1.)

The exception is patients with a right-to-left shunt, such as a patent foramen ovale, atrial or ventricular septal defect, or pulmonary arteriovenous fistula. In such patients, a venous clot may embolize and cross over to the left side of the circulation, causing an arterial infarct. This event is quite rare.

28. **How is PE diagnosed?**
Use a ventilation/perfusion (V/Q) scan or CT pulmonary angiogram to screen for PE. If the test is positive, PE is diagnosed and treatment is started. If the test is indeterminate, a conventional pulmonary angiogram is used to clinch the diagnosis. Conventional pulmonary angiography is the gold standard, but it is invasive and carries substantial risks. If a V/Q scan or CT angiogram is negative, it is highly unlikely that the patient has a significant PE; thus, no treatment is needed. In the setting of a low-probability V/Q scan and high clinical suspicion, a CT angiogram or conventional pulmonary angiogram is needed.

29. **How is PE treated?**
PE is treated initially with low molecular weight heparin or intravenous unfractionated heparin to prevent further clots and emboli. Then the patient switches gradually to oral warfarin, which must be taken for at least 3 to 6 months. In patients with recurrent clots on anticoagulation or contraindications to anticoagulation, an inferior vena cava filter (e.g., Greenfield filter) should be used. In rare patients with massive PE, surgical embolectomy or pharmacologic thrombolysis (e.g., giving t-PA) may be attempted.

30. **What is the most important side effect of heparin?**
Heparin can cause thrombocytopenia that in some unlucky patients is associated with arterial thrombosis. Measure complete blood counts to monitor for this side effect, which usually occurs on day 3 to day 7 of heparin administration. Discontinue heparin immediately if platelet counts begin to fall.

31. **How are the effects of aspirin, heparin, and warfarin monitored?**
Heparin is monitored with the **partial thromboplastin time (PTT),** a measure of the internal coagulation pathway. Warfarin is monitored with the **prothrombin time (PT),** a measure of the external coagulation pathway. Aspirin prolongs the **bleeding time,** a measure of platelet

function. Clinically, the effect of aspirin is not monitored with lab testing, but be aware that it prolongs the bleeding time test.

32. **How are the effects of low-molecular-weight heparin monitored?**
Low-molecular-weight heparin does not affect any of the coagulation parameters mentioned in the previous question, and its effect is not clinically monitored. Rarely, a special type of factor X assay (anti-Xa) is used to measure the effect.

33. **In an emergency, how can you reverse the effects of heparin, warfarin, and aspirin?**
Heparin and low-molecular-weight heparin can be reversed with **protamine;** warfarin with fresh frozen plasma (contains clotting factors; immediate effect) and/or vitamin K (takes a few days to work); and aspirin with platelet transfusions.

34. **How do the conditions below affect coagulation tests?**

Condition	Prolongs	Aids to Diagnosis
Hemophilia A	PTT	Low levels of factor 8; normal PT and bleeding time; X-linked
Hemophilia B	PTT	Low levels of factor 9; normal PT and bleeding time; X-linked
vWF deficiency	Bleeding time and PTT	Normal or low levels of factor 8; normal PT; autosomal dominant
Disseminated intravascular coagulation	PT, PTT, bleeding time	Positive p-dimer or FDPs; postpartum, infection, malignancy; schistocytes and fragmented cells on peripheral smear
Liver disease	PT	PTT normal or prolonged; all factors but 8 are low; stigmata of liver disease; no correction with vitamin K
Vitamin K deficiency	PT, PTT (slight)	Normal bleeding time; low levels of factors 2, 7, 9, and 10, as well as proteins C and S; look for neonate who did not receive prophylactic vitamin K; malabsorption, alcoholism, or prolonged antibiotic use (which kills vitamin K-producing bowel flora)

PT = prothrombin time; PTT = partial thromboplastin time; FDPs = fibrin degradation products; vWF = von Willebrand factor.

Remember also that uremia causes a qualitative platelet defect and that vitamin C deficiency and chronic corticosteroid therapy can cause bleeding tendency with normal coagulation tests.

35. **What are the general symptoms and signs of congestive heart failure (CHF)?**
- Fatigue
- Ventricular hypertrophy on EKG
- Dyspnea
- S3 or S4 on cardiac exam
- Cardiomegaly on chest radiograph
- Specific left and right-sided findings (see next question)

36. **What symptoms and signs help to determine whether CHF is due to left or right ventricular failure?**

Left ventricular failure: orthopnea (shortness of breath when lying down; the patient sleeps on more than one pillow or even sitting up); paroxysmal nocturnal dyspnea; pulmonary congestion (rales); Kerley B lines on chest radiograph; pulmonary vascular congestion and edema; bilateral pleural effusions.

Right ventricular failure: peripheral edema, jugular venous distention, hepatomegaly, ascites, underlying lung disease (cor pulmonale; see below)

Note: Both ventricles are commonly affected, so a mixed pattern is commonly seen.

37. **How is chronic CHF treated?**

Chronic CHF is treated on an outpatient basis with sodium restriction, ACE inhibitors (first- line agents that reduce mortality rate), beta blockers (somewhat counterintuitive but proven to work), diuretics, spironolactone, digoxin (not used in diastolic dysfunction; usually reserved for moderate-to-severe CHF with low ejection fraction or systolic dysfunction), and vasodilators (arterial and venous).

38. **How is acute congestive heart failure treated?**

Acute CHF is treated on an inpatient basis with oxygen, diuretics, and positive inotropes. Digoxin may be used if the patient is stable. Intravenous sympathomimetics (dobutamine, dopamine, amrinone) are used for severe CHF.

39. **What factors precipitate exacerbations in previously stable patients with CHF?**

The most common is noncompliance with diet or medications, but watch for **myocardial infarction,** severe hypertension, arrhythmias, infections and fever, pulmonary embolus, anemia, thyrotoxicosis, and myocarditis.

40. **Define cor pulmonale. With what clinical scenarios is it associated?**

Cor pulmonale is right ventricular enlargement, hypertrophy, and failure due to primary lung disease. Common causes are chronic obstructive pulmonary disease and pulmonary embolus. In a young woman (20 to 40 years old) with no other medical history or risk factors, think of idiopathic pulmonary arterial hypertension. Treat with prostacyclins (parenteral epoprostenol), antiendothelins (bosentant), phosphodiesterase 5 inhibitors, and calcium channel blockers while awaiting heart-lung transplantation. Sleep apnea also can cause cor pulmonale; look for an obese snorer who is sleepy during the day. Patients with cor pulmonale may have tachypnea, cyanosis, clubbing, parasternal heave, loud P2, and right-sided S4 in addition to the signs and symptoms of pulmonary disease.

41. **What causes restrictive cardiomyopathy? How is it different from constrictive pericarditis?**

Restrictive cardiomyopathy involves a problem with the ventricles and usually is due to amyloidosis, sarcoidosis, hemochromatosis, or myocardial fibroelastosis. A ventricular biopsy is abnormal in all of these conditions. **Constrictive pericarditis** can be fixed simply by removing an abnormal pericardium; look for a pericardial knock on exam, calcification of the pericardium, and a normal ventricular biopsy. Watch for an S4 (which indicates stiff ventricles) and signs of right-sided heart failure (jugular venous distention and peripheral edema) in both conditions. These two disorders are mentioned together because both can cause a "restrictive"-type cardiac physiology, but the treatments are quite different.

42. **What is the most common kind of cardiomyopathy? What causes it?**
Dilated cardiomyopathy, which most commonly is caused by chronic coronary artery disease or ischemia, though by strict definition this is not a true cardiomyopathy. For the USMLE, watch for alcohol, myocarditis, or doxorubicin as the cause of dilated cardiomyopathy.

43. **Which cardiomyopathy is likely in a young person who passes out or dies while exercising or playing sports and has a family history of sudden death?**
Hypertrophic cardiomyopathy, which may be autosomal dominant. This idiopathic condition causes an asymmetric ventricular hypertrophy that reduces cardiac output (an example of diastolic dysfunction). Treat with beta blockers, or disopyramide (to allow the ventricle more time to fill). Competitive sports should be avoided. Positive inotropes (e.g., digoxin), diuretics, and vasodilators are contraindicated because they worsen the condition.

44. **What EKG abnormalities do I need to know about for the Step 2 exam? How are they treated?**
See an EKG book for tracings not shown in Figs 4-5 through 4-9. Always check for electrolyte disturbances as a cause for any arrhythmia.

Arrhythmia	Treatment and Warnings
Atrial fibrillation	In symptomatic patients, first slow ventricular rate with beta blocker, calcium channel blocker, or digoxin: ■ If acute (onset < 24 hr), cardiovert with amiodarone, procainamide, or DC cardioversion. ■ If chronic, first anticoagulate, then cardiovert; if this approach fails or atrial fibrillation recurs, leave the patient on rate control medications (beta-blocker, calcium channel blocker, or digoxin) and warfarin.
Atrial flutter	Treat like atrial fibrillation. You may try to stop arrhythmia with vagal maneuvers (e.g., carotid massage).
Heart block: First-degree	No treatment, but avoid beta blockers and calcium channel blockers, both of which slow conduction.
Second-degree	For Mobitz type I, use pacemaker or atropine only in symptomatic patients; use pacemaker in all patients with Mobitz type II.
Third-degree	Use pacemaker.
WPW syndrome	Use procainamide or quinidine; avoid digoxin and verapamil.
Ventricular tachycardia	If pulseless, treat with immediate defibrillation followed by epinephrine, vasopressin, amiodarone, or lidocaine. If a pulse is present, treat with amiodarone and synchronized cardioversion.
Ventricular fibrillation	Immediate defibrillation.

(continued)

Arrhythmia	Treatment and Warnings
PVCs	Usually not treated; if severe and symptomatic, consider beta blockers or amiodarone.
Sinus bradycardia	Usually not treated; use atropine if severe and symptomatic (e.g., after-heart attack). Avoid beta blockers, calcium channel blockers, and other conduction-slowing medications.
Sinus tachycardia	Usually none; correct underlying cause. Use beta blocker or calcium channel blocker if symptomatic.

DC = direct current; WPW = Wolff-Parkinson-White; PVCs = premature ventricular complexes.

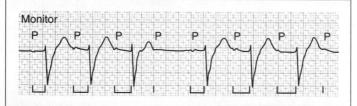

Figure 4-5. First-degree atrioventricular block with a PR interval of 0.32 seconds (normal is 0.12 to 0.20 seconds). (From Goldberger E: Treatment of Cardiac Emergencies, 5th ed. St. Louis, Mosby, 1990.)

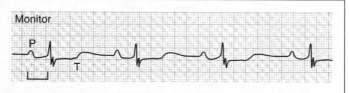

Figure 4-6. Mobitz type I second-degree atrioventricular block (Wenckebach). Notice the progression of the PR interval before the impulse is completely blocked. (From Goldberger E: Treatment of Cardiac Emergencies, 5th ed. St. Louis, Mosby, 1990.)

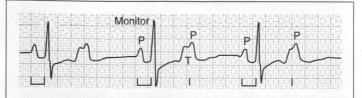

Figure 4-7. Mobitz type II second-degree atrioventricular block. Notice that every alternate P wave is blocked. (From Goldberger E: Treatment of Cardiac Emergencies, 5th ed. St. Louis, Mosby, 1990.)

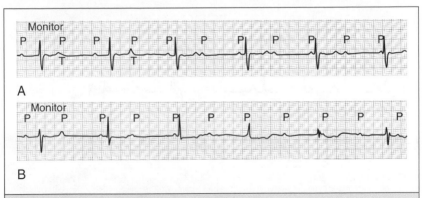

Figure 4-8. Third-degree atrioventricular block. Strips **A** and **B** were taken several hours apart. Strip **A** demonstrates an atrial rate of 75 bpm but the ventricles are beating independently at a slow rate of approximately 40 bpm. Strip **B**, taken a few hours later in the same patient demonstrates variations in the shape of QRS complex from beat to beat. (From Goldberger E: Treatment of Cardiac Emergencies, 5th ed. St. Louis, Mosby, 1990.)

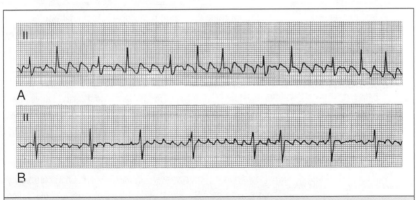

Figure 4-9. Atrial flutter with variable block (**A**) and coarse atrial fibrillation (**B**) may be easily confused. Notice that with atrial fibrillation the ventricular rate is erratic and the atrial waves are not identical from segment to segment, while these atrial waves are identical with atrial flutter. (From Goldberger A: Clinical Electrocardiography: A Simplified Approach, 7th ed., Philadelphia, Mosby, 2006, Fig. 23-3.)

45. **What endocrine disease is suggested when a patient presents with sinus tachycardia or atrial fibrillation?**
    Hyperthyroidism. Check the level of thyroid-stimulating hormone (TSH) as a screening test.

46. **How does Wolff-Parkinson-White syndrome classically present?**
    A child becomes dizzy or dyspneic or passes out after playing, then recovers and has no other symptoms. The cause is a transient arrhythmia via the accessory pathway. EKG shows the infamous delta wave (Fig. 4-10).

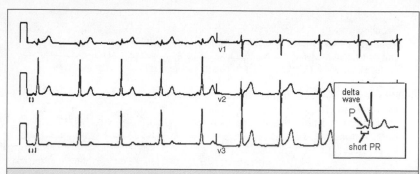

Figure 4-10. Electrocardiogram of Wolff-Parkinson-White syndrome demonstrating the classic shortened PR interval and delta wave (slurred upstroke of the QRS complex). (From DeLee J, Drez D, Miller M: DeLee and Drez's Orthopaedic Sports Medicine, 2nd ed. Philadelphia, Saunders, 2003, Fig. 7C-3.)

47. What do you need to know about the common congenital heart defects?

Defect	Symptoms, Treatment, and Other Information
Patent ductus arteriosus	Constant, machine-like murmur in upper left sternal border; dyspnea and possible CHF. Close with indomethacin or surgery (if indomethacin fails). Keep open with prostaglandin E_1. Associated with congenital rubella and high altitudes.
Ventricular septal defect (VSD)	*Most common congenital heart defect.* Characterized by holosystolic murmur next to sternum. Most cases resolve on their own. Watch for fetal alcohol, TORCH, or Down syndrome.
Atrial septal defect	Often asymptomatic until adulthood. Characterized by fixed, split S2 and palpitations. Most defects do not require correction (unless very large).
Tetralogy of Fallot	*Most common **cyanotic** congenital heart defect.* Characterized by four-anomalies: VSD, RVH, pulmonary stenosis, and overriding aorta. Look for "tet" spells (squatting after exertion).
Coarctation of aorta	Upper extremity hypertension only; radiofemoral delay; systolic murmur heard over mid-upper back; rib notching on radiograph; associated with Turner syndrome.

CHF = congestive heart failure; TORCH = toxoplasma, other, rubella, cytomegalovirus, and herpes infections; RVH = right ventricular hypertrophy.

Note: Endocarditis prophylaxis is required for all of these cardiac defects except asymptomatic secundum-type atrial septal defect.

48. What is important to remember about tachycardia in children?

Heart rates over 100 beats per minute may be normal in a child, as may respiratory rates greater than 20 respirations per minute.

49. In the fetal circulation, where is the highest and lowest oxygen content?

The highest oxygen content in fetal circulation is in the umbilical vein (the blood coming from the mother), and the lowest is in the umbilical arteries. Remember also that oxygen content is higher in blood going to the upper extremities than in blood going to the lower extremities.

50. What changes occur in the circulation as an infant goes from intrauterine to extrauterine life?

The first breaths inflate the lungs and cause decreased pulmonary vascular resistance, which increases blood flow to the pulmonary arteries. This and the clamping of the cord increase left-sided heart pressures, causing functional closure of the foramen ovale. Increased oxygen concentration shuts off prostaglandin production in the ductus arteriosus, causing gradual closure.

CHAPTER 5

CHOLESTEROL

1. **When is cholesterol screening done?**
   Although no protocol is universally accepted, measurement of total cholesterol and high-density lipoprotein (HDL) cholesterol every 5 years once a person turns 20 years old is considered reasonable by most authorities. Start sooner and screen more frequently for obese patients and patients with a family history of hypercholesterolemia.

2. **What physical findings will the Step 2 test use as clues to hypercholesterolemia?**
   Xanthelasma (Fig. 5-1), tendon xanthomas (cholesterol deposits in the skin, classically over tendons in the lower extremities), corneal arcus in younger patients, "milky"-appearing serum, and obesity are possible markers for familial hypercholesterolemia. Family members should be tested if a case of familial hypercholesterolemia is found. Pancreatitis in the absence of obvious risk factors may be a marker for familial hypertriglyceridemia.

3. **What are the current recommendations for management of cholesterol levels?**
   The following information is from the Third Report of the National Cholesterol Education Panel, Adult Treatment Panel III (ATP III). Total cholesterol goal is less than 200 mg/dL with more than 240 considered high, and normal triglycerides levels are less than 150 mg/dL with more than 200 considered high, but LDL is usually the main player for treatment decisions. The numbers in the chart below represent mg/dL:

No CHD Risk Factors	≥2 CHD Risk Factors*	Known CAD/ Equivalent†	Very High Risk‡	Intervention
LDL < 160	LDL < 100	LDL < 100	LDL < 70	None (meets goal)
LDL 160–189	LDL 100–129		LDL 70–99	Diet ± medications§
LDL ≥ 190	LDL ≥ 130	LDL ≥ 100	LDL ≥ 100	Medications (+ diet)

*CHD = coronary heart disease. Risk factors for CHD are listed in question 4.
†CAD = coronary artery disease. CHD equivalents include diabetes mellitus, peripheral arterial atherosclerotic disease, symptomatic carotid artery disease, and abdominal aortic aneurysm.
‡"Very" high-risk patients are those with CAD who have a heart attack, diabetes or other severe and poorly controlled risk factors (e.g., metabolic syndrome, heavy smoking).
§"Diet" includes general lifestyle modifications such as eating less and healthier, decreasing alcohol intake, exercising, etc. The trend is toward more aggressive intervention, so you will not be faulted for initiating medications at these "gray area" LDL levels, particularly in higher risk people.

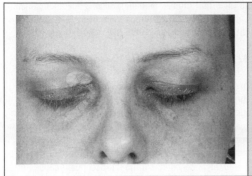

Figure 5-1. Xanthelasma is usually a normal finding with no significance but is classically seen on the USMLE because of its association with hypercholesterolemia. Screen affected patients with a fasting lipid profile. (From du Vivier A: Atlas of Clinical Dermatology, 3rd ed. New York, Churchill Livingstone, 2002, p 523, with permission.)

4. **List the major risk factors for coronary heart disease.**

Although elevated levels of LDL and total cholesterol are risk factors for CHD, do not count them as risk factors when deciding to treat or not to treat high cholesterol. The following factors should be counted:

- **Age** (men aged 45 years and older; women aged 55 years and older or with premature menopause and no estrogen replacement therapy)
- **Family history of premature heart attacks** (defined as definite myocardial infarction or sudden death in father or first-degree male relative less than 55 years old or mother or first-degree female relative less than 65 years old)
- **Cigarette smoking**
- **Hypertension** (greater than or equal to 140/90 mm Hg or prescription for antihypertensive medications)
- **Diabetes mellitus**
- **Low HDL** (less than 40 mg/dL)

Note: An HDL level greater than or equal to 60 mg/dL is considered protective and negates one risk factor.

5. **Discuss other possible risk factors for heart disease.**

C-reactive protein and homocysteine are hot topics right now, but ATP III does not list elevated CRP or homocysteine as major risk factors for coronary artery disease. Obesity and type A personality (the hard-driving attorney) are weaker risk factors, as are stress and physical inactivity. Hypertriglyceridemia alone is not a significant risk factor but in association with high cholesterol causes more coronary heart disease than high cholesterol alone. For Step 2 boards, use only the definite risk factors mentioned in the previous question (especially when deciding how to treat a patient with high cholesterol), but keep these other factors in mind.

6. **How is LDL calculated?**

Lipoprotein analysis involves measuring total cholesterol, HDL, and triglycerides. LDL then can be calculated from the following formula:

$LDL = \text{total cholesterol} - HDL - (\text{triglycerides}/5)$

7. **Describe the treatment for hypercholesterolemia.**

As with hypertension, give patients a few months to try lifestyle modifications (decreased calories, cholesterol, and saturated fat in diet; decreased alcohol and smoking; exercise and weight loss) before initiating drug therapy. If the patient has coronary artery disease or a coronary artery disease equivalent (e.g., diabetes, peripheral vascular disease) and the LDL is greater than or equal to 100, medication therapy is indicated. Once the decision to start medications is made, first-line agents are HMG CoA reductase inhibitors (statins); watch for rare but potentially serious side effects (liver and muscle damage). Second line agents include niacin (poorly tolerated, but effective and raises HDL), ezetimibe (selectively inhibits the intestinal absorption of cholesterol), and bile acid-binding resins (e.g., cholestyramine).

8. **How is HDL affected by alcohol? Estrogens? Exercise? Smoking? Progesterone?**

High HDL is protective against atherosclerosis and is increased by moderate alcohol consumption (1 to 2 drinks/day; but not by high alcohol intake), exercise, and estrogens. HDL is decreased by smoking, androgens, progesterone, and hypertriglyceridemia.

9. **What causes hypercholesterolemia?**

Genetics certainly plays a role (e.g., familial hyperlipidemia), but most cases are thought to be multifactorial. Western diet and inactive lifestyle certainly contribute. Secondary causes of increased cholesterol include uncontrolled diabetes, hypothyroidism, uremia, nephrotic syndrome, obstructive liver disease, excessive alcohol intake (which increases triglycerides), and medications (e.g., birth control pills, glucocorticoids, thiazides, beta blockers).

10. **Why is cholesterol so important?**

Cholesterol is one of the main known modifiable risk factors for atherosclerosis. Atherosclerosis is involved in about one-half of all deaths in the United States and one-third of deaths between the ages of 35 and 65 years. Atherosclerosis is the most important cause of permanent disability and accounts for more hospital days than any other illness. (*Translation: Atherosclerosis and high cholesterol are high-yield USMLE topics.*)

CHAPTER 6

DERMATOLOGY

1. **Cover the two right-hand columns and define the following common terms used in dermatology to describe skin findings:**

Term	Definition	Examples
Macule	Flat spot less than 1 cm (nonpalpable, just visible)	Freckles, tattoos
Patch	Same as macule but greater than 1 cm	Port-wine birthmarks
Papule	Solid, elevated lesion less than 1 cm (palpable)	Wart, acne, lichen planus
Plaque	Same as papule but greater than 1 cm and flat-topped	Psoriasis
Nodule	Palpable, solid lesion greater than 1 cm and not flat-topped	Small lipoma, erythema nodosum
Vesicle	Elevated, circumscribed lesion less than 5 mm containing clear fluid (small blister)	Chickenpox, genital herpes
Bulla	Same as vesicle but greater than 5 mm (large blister)	Contact dermatitis, pemphigus
Wheal	Itchy, transiently edematous area	Allergic reaction

2. **Define vitiligo. With what diseases is it associated?**
   Vitiligo is characterized by skin depigmentation of unknown etiology. It is associated with autoimmune conditions such as pernicious anemia, hypothyroidism, Addison's disease, and type I diabetes. Patients often have antibodies to melanin, parietal cells, thyroid, or other factors.

3. **Name several conditions to think about on the Step 2 exam in patients with pruritus.**
   Think of serious conditions first, such as obstructive biliary disease, uremia, and polycythemia rubra vera (classically seen after a warm shower or bath). Pruritus also may be caused by contact or atopic dermatitis, scabies, and lichen planus.

4. **Define contact dermatitis. How do you recognize it? What are the classic culprits?**
   Contact dermatitis is usually due to a type IV hypersensitivity reaction, although it also may be due to an irritating or toxic substance. Look for new exposure to a classic offending agent, such as poison ivy, nickel earrings, or deodorant. The rash is well circumscribed and occurs only in the area of exposure. The skin is red and itchy and often has vesicles or bullae (Fig. 6-1). Avoidance of the agent is required. Patch testing can be done, if needed, to determine the antigen.

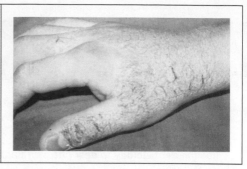

Figure 6-1. Primary irritant dermatitis. The skin is dry, pink, scaly, and fissured. The backs of the hands are particularly affected. This patient was working as a mechanic. (From du Vivier A: Atlas of Clinical Dermatology, 3rd ed. New York, Churchill Livingstone, 2002, p 57, with permission.)

5. Define atopic dermatitis. What history points to this diagnosis?

Atopic dermatitis is a chronic allergic-type condition that begins in the first year of life with red, itchy, weeping skin on the head, upper extremities, and sometimes around the diaper area. The clue to diagnosis is a family and/or personal history of allergies (e.g., hay fever) and asthma. The biggest problem is scratching of affected skin, which leads to skin breaks and possible bacterial infection. Treatment involves avoidance of drying soaps and use of antihistamines and topical steroids.

6. Define seborrheic dermatitis. What part of the body does it involve? How is it treated?

Seborrheic dermatitis causes the common conditions known as cradle cap and dandruff as well as blepharitis (eyelid inflammation). Look for scaling skin with or without erythema on the hairy areas of the head (scalp, eyebrows, eyelashes, mustache, beard) as well as on the forehead, nasolabial folds, external ear canals, and postauricular creases. Treat with dandruff shampoo (e.g., selenium or tar shampoo), topical corticosteroids, and/or ketoconazole cream.

7. Name the various dermatologic fungal infections.

Known as dermatophytosis, tinea, and ringworm, fungal infections include the following:

Tinea corporis (body/trunk): look for red ring-shaped lesions with raised borders that tend to clear centrally while they expand peripherally (Fig. 6-2).

Tinea pedis (athlete's foot): look for macerated, scaling web spaces between the toes that often itch and may be associated with thickened, distorted toenails (onychomycosis). Good foot hygiene is part of treatment.

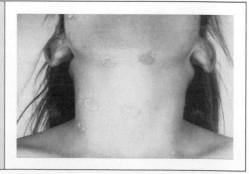

Figure 6-2. Tinea corporis. This child has classic annular ringworm, with well-defined scaly margins that contrast with healing centers. (From du Vivier A: Atlas of Clinical Dermatology, 3rd ed. New York, Churchill Livingstone, 2002, p 324, with permission.)

Tinea unguium (onychomycosis): thickened, distorted nails with debris under the nail edges.

Tinea capitis (scalp): mainly affects children (highly contagious), who have scaly patches of hair loss and may have an inflamed, boggy granuloma of the scalp (known as a kerion) that usually resolves on its own.

Tinea cruris (jock itch): more common in obese males; usually is found in the crural folds of the upper, inner thighs.

8. **What organisms cause fungal infections?**

   Most fungal infections are due to *Trichophyton* species. In tinea capitis, if the hair fluoresces under the Wood's lamp, *Microsporum* species is the cause; if not, probably *Trichophyton*.

9. **How are fungal infections diagnosed and treated?**

   Formal diagnosis of any fungal infection can be made by scraping the lesion and doing a potassium hydroxide (KOH) preparation to visualize the fungus via a microscope or by doing a culture. Because they are so common clinically, empiric treatment without a formal diagnosis is common, but for the USMLE, get a formal diagnosis before treating. Oral antifungals must be used to treat tinea capitis and onychomycosis; the others can be treated with topical antifungals (imidazoles such as miconazole, clotrimazole, or ketoconazole) or griseofulvin, which is better for severe or persistent infections.

10. **True or false: Candidiasis is often a normal finding in some women and children.**

    True. Oral thrush (creamy white patches on the tongue or buccal mucosa that can be scraped off) is seen in normal children and *Candida* vulvovaginitis is seen in normal women, especially during pregnancy or after taking antibiotics. However, at other time periods and in different patients, candidal infections may be a sign of diabetes or immunodeficiency; for example, thrush in a man should make you think about the possibility of AIDS.

11. **How is candidiasis treated?**

    Treat with local/topical nystatin or imidazoles (e.g., miconazole, clotrimazole). Oral therapy (nystatin or ketoconazole) is used for extensive or resistant disease.

12. **What causes scabies? How do you recognize it?**

    Scabies is caused by the mite *Sarcoptes scabei,* which tunnels into the skin and leaves visible burrows on the skin, classically in the finger web spaces and flexor surface of the wrists. You should know what these burrows look like. Facial involvement sometimes is seen in infants. Patients also have severe pruritus, and scratching can lead to secondary bacterial infection.

13. **How do you diagnose and treat scabies?**

    Diagnosis is made by scraping a mite out of a burrow and viewing it under a microscope. Treat scabies with permethrin cream applied to the whole body. Remember to treat all contacts (e.g., the whole family). Do *not* use lindane unless permethrin is not an option. Lindane used to be treatment of choice but can cause neurotoxicity, especially in young children.

14. **How do you recognize and treat tinea versicolor?**

    Tinea versicolor (also known as pityriasis versicolor) is a *Pityrosporum* fungal infection that presents most commonly with multiple patches of various size and color (brown, tan, and white) on the torso of young adults. Often it becomes noticeable in the summer because the affected areas fail to tan and look white. Diagnose from lesion scrapings (KOH preparation). Treat with selenium sulfide shampoo or topical imidazoles.

15. **What causes lice? How are they treated?**

    Lice (pediculosis) can involve the head (caused by *Pediculus capitis;* common in school-aged children), body (caused by *Pediculus corporis;* unusual in people with good hygiene), or pubic area (crabs, caused by *Phthirus pubis* and transmitted sexually). Infected areas tend to itch. Diagnosis is made by seeing the lice on hair shafts. Treat with permethrin cream (preferred over lindane because of lindane's neurotoxicity), and decontaminate sources of reinfection (wash or sterilize combs, hats, bed sheets, clothing).

16. **What causes warts? How are they treated?**

    Warts are caused by the human papillomavirus (HPV). They are infectious and are most commonly seen in older children, classically on the hands. The most common serotypes are 6 and 11. Multiple treatments are available, including salicylic acid, liquid nitrogen, and curettage. Genital warts also are caused by HPV; serotypes 16 and 18 are associated with cervical cancer.

17. **Define molluscum contagiosum. How do you recognize it? How is it treated?**

    Molluscum contagiosum is a poxvirus infection that is common in children but also may be transmitted sexually. Diagnosis is made by the characteristic appearance of the lesions (skin-colored, smooth, waxy papules with a central depression [umbilicated] that are roughly 0.5 cm) or by looking at contents of the lesion, which include cells with characteristic inclusion bodies. The usual treatment is freezing or curettage.

18. **True or false: A child with genital molluscum is probably a victim of sexual abuse.**

    False. A child who has genital molluscum may or may not have contracted the disease from sexual contact. The more common mechanism is autoinoculation, in which the child has a lesion on the hand that spreads to the genital area from scratching. Do *not* automatically assume child abuse, although it must be ruled out.

19. **How is acne described in medical terms? What bacteria may be partially involved in its pathogenesis?**

    The description of acne includes comedones (whiteheads and blackheads), papules, pustules, inflamed nodules, superficial pus-filled cysts, and/or possible inflammatory skin changes, including scar formation. *Propionibacterium acnes* is thought to be partially involved in pathogenesis, as is blockage of pilosebaceous glands.

20. **True or false: Acne is not related to food, exercise, or sex.**

    True. Acne has *not* been proven to be related to food, exercise, or sex (including masturbation). However, if the patient relates acne to a food, you can try discontinuing it. Cosmetics may aggravate acne.

21. **What are the treatment options for acne?**

    Treatment options are multiple. Start with topical benzoyl peroxide; then try topical clindamycin, oral tetracycline, or oral erythromycin (for *Propionibacterium acnes* eradication). The third option is topical tretinoin; oral isotretinoin is the *last resort*. Although highly effective, isotretinoin is teratogenic; pregnancy testing in women before and during therapy as well as contraceptive use is mandatory. In addition, it may cause dry skin and mucosae, muscle and joint pain, and liver function test abnormalities.

22. **Define rosacea. In what age group is it seen? How do you treat it?**

    Rosacea often looks like acne but begins in middle age. Look for **rhinophyma** (bulbous red nose) and coexisting blepharitis. Treat with topical metronidazole or oral tetracycline. The pathogenesis is incompletely understood, but rosacea is not related to diet.

23. What should you think about if hirsutism is described on the Step 2 exam?
Hirsutism is most commonly idiopathic, but other signs of virilization (e.g., deepening voice, clitoromegaly, frontal balding) suggest an androgen-secreting ovarian tumor. In the absence of virilization, consider Cushing syndrome, polycystic ovary syndrome (Stein-Leventhal syndrome), and drugs (minoxidil, corticosteroids, and phenytoin).

24. What are the common pathologic causes of baldness?
Watch out for trichotillomania (a psychiatric disorder in which patients pull out their hair; baldness is patchy and irregular) and alopecia areata (idiopathic but associated with antimicrosomal and other autoantibodies). Baldness also may be seen in patients with lupus erythematosus or syphilis and after cancer chemotherapy.

25. What causes ordinary male pattern baldness?
Although the exact pathophysiology is still not clear, male-pattern baldness is considered a genetic disorder that requires androgens for expression.

26. Describe the classic psoriatic lesion.
Psoriatic lesions classically are described as dry, well-circumscribed, silvery, scaling papules and plaques that are *not* pruritic. Classic lesions are found on the scalp and extensor surfaces of the elbows and knees.

27. What other historical points and physical findings may be seen with psoriasis? How is it diagnosed and treated?
A family history of psoriasis is often present, and the disease occurs mostly in caucasians with onset in early adulthood. Affected patients may have pitting of the nails and an arthritis that resembles rheumatoid arthritis but is rheumatoid factor-negative. Diagnosis of psoriasis can often be made by appearance alone, but a biopsy can be used in doubtful cases. Treatment is complex but involves exposure to ultraviolet light, lubricants, topical corticosteroids, and keratolytics (e.g., coal tar, salicylic acid, anthralin).

28. Give the classic description and natural course of pityriasis rosea.
Pityriasis rosea is typically seen in young adults. Look for a herald patch (slightly erythematous, scaly, ring-shaped or oval patch classically seen on the trunk), followed 1 week later by many similar lesions that tend to itch. Look for lesions on the back with a long axis that parallels the Langerhans skin cleavage lines, typically in a "Christmas tree" pattern. The condition usually remits spontaneously in 1 month. Think about syphilis in the differential diagnosis. Treat with reassurance.

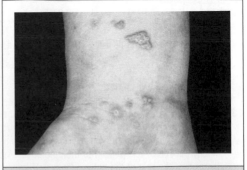

29. What are the "four Ps" that clinch a diagnosis of lichen planus?
Pruritic, purple, polygonal papules classically on the wrists or lower legs, usually of adults (Fig. 6-3). Oral mucosal lesions (whitish, with a lace-like pattern) also may be present.

Figure 6-3. Lichen planus. This disorder has a predilection for the wrists and other portions of the distal extremities. Purple or violaceous, polygonal, flat-topped papules are characteristic, and these are classically pruritic. (From du Vivier A: Atlas of Clinical Dermatology, 3rd ed. New York, Churchill Livingstone, 2002, p 97, with permission.)

30. **List the classic drugs that cause photosensitivity of the skin.**
Tetracyclines, phenothiazines, and birth control pills.

31. **Describe the classic lesion of erythema multiforme. What drugs classically cause it?**
Look for the classic target (iris) lesions. The classic cause is sulfa drugs or penicillins, but herpes infections may also cause erythema multiforme, and some cases are idiopathic. In its severe form, erythema multiforme is known as **Stevens-Johnson syndrome,** which often is fatal because of severe, widespread skin involvement. Treat supportively.

32. **Describe the classic lesion of erythema nodosum. With what diseases is it commonly associated?**
Erythema nodosum (Fig. 6-4) is an inflammation of the subcutaneous tissue and skin, classically over the shins (pretibial). Look for tender, red nodules. Sarcoidosis, coccidioidomycosis, or ulcerative colitis classically accompany this condition on the USMLE, though multiple other infections (e.g., streptococcal, tuberculosis) and drugs (e.g., sulfonamides) can also result in this finding.

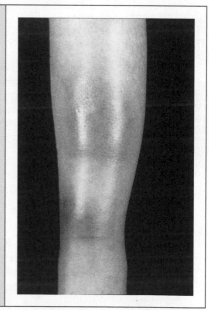

Figure 6-4. Erythema nodosum. Tender red nodules over the shins are classic, and are due to panniculitis (inflammation of [the subcutaneous] fat). (From du Vivier A: Atlas of Clinical Dermatology, 3rd ed. New York, Churchill Livingstone, 2002, p 391, with permission.)

33. **Define and describe pemphigus vulgaris. How is it different from bullous pemphigoid?**
Pemphigus vulgaris is a potentially life-threatening autoimmune disease of middle-aged and elderly patients. It presents with multiple bullae, starting in the oral mucosa and spreading to the skin of the rest of the body. Biopsy can be stained for antibody (an IgG antibody to desmoglein III, which is associated with desmosomes) and shows a "lace-like" or "fishnet" immunofluorescence pattern. Treat with oral corticosteroids. Bullous pemphigoid is a similar, but milder, condition that results in a linear immunofluorescence pattern (different antibody) and is treated similarly (Fig. 6-5).

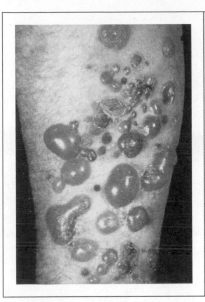

Figure 6-5. Bullous pemphigoid. Many blisters are present at various stages of development. (From du Vivier A: Atlas of Clinical Dermatology, 3rd ed. New York, Churchill Livingstone, 2002, p 419, with permission.)

34. **What skin disease is associated with celiac disease (gluten intolerance or sensitivity)? How is it treated?**
Dermatitis herpetiformis is associated with celiac sprue. Patients have intensely pruritic vesicles, papules, and wheals on the extensor aspects of the elbows and knees and possibly on the face or neck. Look for diarrhea and weight loss (due to gluten sensitivity).
On biopsy, the skin has IgA deposits even in unaffected areas. Treat both conditions with a gluten-free diet.

35. **What are decubitus ulcers? What is the best method of prevention?**
Decubitus ulcers (bedsores or pressure sores) are skin ulcers due to prolonged pressure against the skin. The best treatment is prophylaxis. Periodic turning of paralyzed, bedridden, or debilitated patients (the populations in which they are most common) and use of special air mattresses prevents bedsores. Cleanliness and dryness also help to prevent decubitus ulcers. Periodic skin inspection makes sure that the problem is recognized early. When missed, the lesions can ulcerate down to the bone and become infected, possibly leading to sepsis and death. Treat major skin breaks with aggressive surgical debridement; if signs of infection are present, administer antibiotics.

36. **What conditions should excessive perspiration suggest on the USMLE?**
We all know people who sweat too much for no apparent reason. On the Step 2 exam, however, look for a serious cause, such as a myocardial infarction, tuberculosis or infection, hyperthyroidism, or pheochromocytoma.

37. **True or false: Most melanomas start out as simple moles.**
True. Moles are common and benign, but malignant transformation is possible (Fig. 6-6). Excise any mole (or do a biopsy if the lesion is very large) if it enlarges suddenly, develops irregular borders, darkens or becomes inflamed, changes color (even if only one small area of the mole changes color), begins to bleed, begins to itch, or becomes painful.

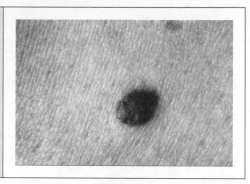

Figure 6-6. Melanoma. This solitary black papule was proved to represent vertical growth phase invasive malignant melanoma. (From du Vivier A: Atlas of Clinical Dermatology, 3rd ed. New York, Churchill Livingstone, 2002, p 4, with permission.)

38. Define dysplastic nevi syndrome. How is it managed?

Dysplastic nevus syndrome is a genetic condition with multiple dysplastic-appearing nevi (usually more than 100 moles). Also look for a family history of melanoma. Treat with careful follow-up, excision or biopsy of any suspicious lesions, avoidance of sun exposure, and sunscreen use.

39. Why is keratoacanthoma of note?

Keratoacanthoma can mimic skin cancer (especially squamous cell cancer). Look for a flesh-colored lesion with a central crater that contains keratinous material, classically on the face (Fig. 6-7). Keratoacanthoma has a very rapid onset, and grows to its full size in 1 to 2 months (which almost never happens with squamous cell cancer). The lesion involutes spontaneously in a few months and requires no treatment. If unsure, the best step is a biopsy, but choose observation as the answer in patients with a classic history of keratoacanthoma.

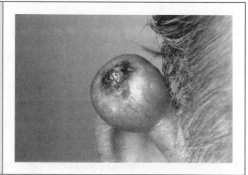

Figure 6-7. Keratoacanthoma. Though this nodule on a sun-exposed site with a warty (keratinous) center could reflect a malignancy, it grew rapidly over three weeks, allowing the correct diagnosis of keratoacanthoma to be made. (From du Vivier A: Atlas of Clinical Dermatology, 3rd ed. New York, Churchill Livingstone, 2002, p 5, with permission.)

40. When and where are keloids seen?

Keloids are overgrowths of scar tissue after an injury; they are seen most frequently seen in blacks. They are usually slightly pink and classically appear on the upper back, chest, and deltoid area. Also look for keloids to develop after ear piercing. Do not excise these lesions, because it may worsen scarring.

41. **Describe the classic lesion of basal cell cancer. What should you do if you suspect it?**

Basal cell cancer classically begins as a shiny papule on a skin-exposed area (the head is classic) and slowly enlarges and develops an umbilicated center (which later may ulcerate) with peripheral telangiectasias. Like all skin cancers, sunlight exposure increases the risk. It is more common in elderly, light-skinned people. Treat with excision. Biopsy any suspicious skin lesions in the elderly.

42. **True or false: Basal cell skin cancer almost never develops metastases.**

True. However, it may be locally invasive and destructive.

43. **From what lesion does squamous cell cancer classically develop? What is Bowen disease?**

Squamous cell cancer often develops in areas with preexisting actinic keratoses (hard, sharp, red, often scaly lesions in sun-exposed areas) or burn scars (Fig. 6-8). The lesions become nodular, warty, or ulcerated; do a biopsy if such transformation occurs. Squamous cell cancer in situ is known as Bowen disease. Although metastases are rare in squamous cell cancer, they occur more frequently than in basal cell cancer.

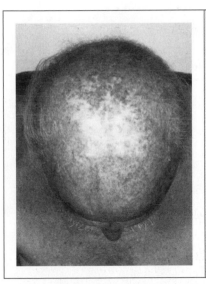

Figure 6-8. Actinic or solar keratosis. The typical appearance of red plaques with rough, adherent scales on a chronically sun-exposed area is shown. Men who become bald at an early age are at increased risk for this premalignant condition, as hair is protective. (From du Vivier A: Atlas of Clinical Dermatology, 3rd ed. New York, Churchill Livingstone, 2002, p 167, with permission.)

44. **To what parameter is the prognosis of a malignant melanoma most closely related?**

The vertical depth of invasion into the skin.

45. **What type of melanoma do black patients tend to develop? How do you recognize it?**

Although uncommon in blacks, melanoma tends to be of the acrolentiginous type. Look for black dots on the palms or soles or under the fingernail that start to change in appearance or cause symptoms.

46. **Describe Paget disease of the nipple. What is its significance?**

    Paget disease of the nipple presents as a unilateral, red, oozing or crusting nipple in an adult woman that fails to respond to typical dermatology treatments. Though rare (roughly 1% to 2% of breast cancers), it signifies an underlying breast cancer (usually invasive ductal carcinoma or ductal carcinoma in situ) with extension to the skin.

47. **Define stomatitis. What does it suggest?**

    Stomatitis is an inflammation of the mucous membranes of the mouth. The classic finding is fissuring of the corners of the mouth (angular stomatitis). Watch for deficiencies of B-complex vitamins (riboflavin, niacin, pyridoxine) or vitamin C.

CHAPTER 7

DIABETES MELLITUS

1. **Outline the current recommendations for diabetes mellitus screening.**
   Universal screening is not generally recommended. Screening is more accepted, but not universal, in patients who are obese, people over 45 years of age, people with a family history of diabetes, and members of certain minority groups (blacks, Hispanics, Pima Indians). Screening in pregnancy is mandatory!

2. **Define diabetes.**
   Diabetes is defined as (1) a glucose level greater than or equal to 126 mg/dL after an overnight (or 8-hour) fast on two separate occasions or (2) a random glucose level greater than 200 mg/dL or (3) an A1C level of greater than 6.5 percent on two separate occasions. If the patient has classic symptoms of diabetes (see hereafter), one test is sufficient to make the diagnosis. In an asymptomatic patient, it is best to repeat the test. An oral glucose tolerance test is common in pregnancy; otherwise, it is rarely used because of poor reproducibility and patient compliance. With a glucose tolerance test, diabetes is diagnosed when glucose levels in the blood reach or exceed 200 mg/dL within 2 hours of receiving a 75 g oral dose of glucose.

3. **What are the classic differences between type 1 and type 2 diabetes?**

	Type 1 (10% of Cases)	Type 2 (90% of Cases)
Age at onset	Most commonly < 30 yrs	Most commonly > 30 yrs
Associated body habitus	Thin	Obese
Development of ketoacidosis	Yes	No
Development of hyperosmolar state	No	Yes
Level of endogenous	Low to none	Normal to high (insulin resistance)
Twin concurrence	< 50%	> 50%
HLA association	Yes	No
Response to oral hypoglycemics	No	Yes
Antibodies to insulin	Yes (at diagnosis)	No
Risk for diabetic complications	Yes	Yes
Islet-cell pathology	Insulitis (loss of most B cells)	Normal number, but with amyloid deposits

Remember, however, that these findings may overlap.

4. **What are the goals of treatment in terms of glucose levels?**
   The goals are to keep postprandial glucose levels less than 180 mg/dL and fasting glucose levels 70–130 mg/dL. Attempts at stricter control may result in hypoglycemia; watch for symptoms of sympathetic nervous system activation and mental status changes.

5. **What is a good measure of long-term diabetes control?**
   Hemoglobin A_{1c} measures the "average" control of blood glucose level over the prior 2 to 3 months. The current recommendation is to keep the hemoglobin A_{1c} level below 7. This is a good way to catch patients with nocturnal hyperglycemia or less-than-honest patients who falsely record low glucose test readings. A rough rule of thumb is that hemoglobin A_{1c} times 20 equals the average blood glucose level.

6. **When a nondiabetic patient presents with hypoglycemia, how can you distinguish between factitious disorder (exogenous insulin) and an insulinoma (endogenous insulin)?**
   Measure the **C-peptide level.** C-peptide is produced whenever the body makes insulin, but it is absent in prescription insulin preparations. Therefore, C-peptide is high with an insulinoma and low with factitious disorder. This is a classic USMLE question.

7. **What should you remember before giving intravenous iodinated contrast material to a diabetic patient or a patient with renal insufficiency?**
   Diabetic patients and patients with renal insufficiency are prone to acute renal failure from the intravenously administered iodinated contrast agents used for intravenous pyelography (IVP), conventional angiography, and computed tomography (CT). You need to weigh carefully the risk-to-benefit ratio of using intravenous contrast agents. If you choose to give contrast, first hydrate the patient well with intravenous fluids to avoid renal shutdown. Acetylcysteine and bicarbonate may decrease the risk of contrast nephropathy in patients at high risk. The concerns about intravenous iodinated contrast do not apply to oral contrast agents (e.g., barium).

8. **What is diabetic ketoacidosis (DKA)? How is it treated?**
   All type I diabetics will die without insulin. DKA is what happens before they die. Clinically, look for Kussmaul breathing (deep, rapid respirations), dehydration, hyperglycemia, acidosis (due to excessive ketone formation), and increased ketones in the serum (often associated with a fruity odor of the breath) and urine.
   Treatment involves intravenous fluids, insulin, and replacement of electrolytes (especially potassium and phosphate). For the boards, do not use bicarbonate to correct acidosis. Remember to search for the cause of DKA, which most commonly is noncompliance with insulin therapy. The second most common cause is an infection. The mortality rate of DKA with current treatment efforts is less than 10%.

9. **What is nonketotic hyperglycemic hyperosmolar state? How is it treated?**
   It is what happens to type II diabetics who go without adequate treatment before they die. Hyperglycemia and increased serum osmolarity are present in the absence of ketones and acidosis. Most patients are severely dehydrated; the first three treatments are thus "fluids, fluids, and fluids" (i.e. intravenous hydration with normal saline). Insulin and electrolyte replacement also is required. The mortality rate can approach 50% if mental status changes are present at the time of diagnosis.

10. **What are the classic presenting symptoms of new-onset diabetes?**
    Polyuria, polydipsia, and polyphagia (pee a lot, drink a lot, and eat a lot). You also should be suspicious if patients present with candidal infections (e.g., thrush or vaginal yeast infection),

lose weight (as a result of excessive urination), or have blurry vision. Prolonged hyperglycemia causes the lenses in the eyes to swell, and the patient may become myopic. Older patients may even claim that they no longer need their reading glasses (i.e., presbyopia is temporarily corrected by lens swelling).

11. **What are the common long-term complications of diabetes mellitus?**
   - **Atherosclerosis, coronary artery disease, myocardial infarction.** Diabetics often have "silent" heart attacks (no chest pain because of autonomic neuropathy).
   - **Retinopathy.** Diabetes is the leading cause of blindness in the United States for persons under the age of 50 years.
   - **Nephropathy.** Diabetes is the number-one cause of end-stage renal disease requiring hemodialysis (roughly 30% of cases; hypertension is a close second) (Fig. 7-1).

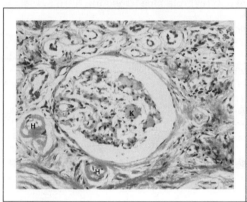

Figure 7-1. Nodular diabetic glomerulosclerosis. The micrograph shows a characteristic acellular Kimmelstiel-Wilson nodule (K) in a glomerulus. Hyalinization of arterioles (H) is also present, which can be seen in hypertension but characteristically affects both efferent and afferent arterioles (versus only afferent arterioles in hypertension). (From Stevens A, et al.: Wheater's Basic Histopathology, 4th ed. New York, Churchill Livingstone, 2002, p 175, with permission.)

   - **Peripheral vascular disease.** Diabetes is a leading cause of limb amputation and may lead to claudication, strokes, and impotence.
   - **Peripheral neuropathy.** This complication causes "silent" heart attacks, numbness in the feet, and other findings (see question 12).
   - **Increased risk of infection.** White blood cells do not function as well in a hyperglycemic environment. Couple this dysfunction with an inability to sense pain and clogged arteries that cannot deliver white cells to the site of an early infection—and you have a recipe for disaster.
     All of these complications can be delayed or even prevented by good glucose control.

12. **What problems may result from diabetic peripheral neuropathy?**
   - **Gastroparesis.** Because the stomach does not empty well, patients experience early satiety and vomiting. Treat with motility enhancers, such as **metoclopramide.**
   - **Charcot joints.** Joints are deformed secondary to lack of sensation. Patients may break a bone and not feel it.
   - **Impotence.** The causes are neuropathy and atherosclerosis.
   - **Cranial nerve palsies** (especially of cranial nerves III, IV, and VI). Patients present with diplopia and extraocular muscle paralysis, which should resolve within 8 weeks without treatment.
   - **Orthostatic hypotension.** This problem occurs even when the patient is well hydrated, because the arteries do not "clamp down" when the patient stands up and the heart rate fails to increase.

■ **Pressure ulcers in the feet.** As with Charcot joints, lack of sensation leads to overuse or failure to rest an injured or tired foot because it is numb and the patient is unaware. All diabetics with foot numbness should wear socks and comfortably fitting shoes and inspect their feet regularly. Most cases of foot gangrene in diabetics begin as a simple callous or blister.

13. **Describe the treatment for diabetic retinopathy.**
If the retinopathy is proliferative (neovascularization or new, irregular vessel formation), the treatment is **panretinal laser photocoagulation.** A laser beam is used to burn tiny spots around the periphery of the retina, sparing the central retina, to prevent progression to blindness. Focal (limited) laser photocoagulation generally is done for nonproliferative retinopathy only if it produces symptoms (from macular edema). All diabetics should be seen annually by an ophthalmologist to monitor retinal changes.

14. **How do you adjust the dosage of neutral protamine Hagedorn (NPH) or regular insulin for high glucose levels?**
Regular insulin starts to work in 45 minutes; its action peaks around 3 to 4 hours after injection; and the duration of action is 6 to 8 hours. NPH insulin takes 1 to 1.5 hours until onset of action; its action peaks at 6 to 8 hours; and the total duration of action is about 12 to 20 hours. For insulin adjustments, therefore, the following guidelines apply:
■ If the patient has high (low) glucose at 7 AM, increase (decrease) NPH insulin at dinner the night before.
■ If the patient has high (low) noon glucose, increase (decrease) the morning dose of regular insulin.
■ If the patient has high (low) glucose at 5 PM, increase (decrease) the morning dose of NPH insulin.
■ If the patient has high (low) glucose at 9 PM, increase (decrease) the dinner-time dose of regular insulin.

15. **Define the Somogyi effect and the dawn phenomenon.**
The **Somogyi effect** is the body's reaction to hypoglycemia. If too much NPH insulin is given at dinner time, the glucose level at 3 AM on the next morning will be low (hypoglycemia). The body reacts to hypoglycemia by releasing stress hormones, which cause a high glucose level at 7 AM. The treatment is to decrease evening (NPH) insulin. The **dawn phenomenon** is hyperglycemia caused by normal secretion of growth hormone early in the morning. The glucose level is high at 7 AM and normal or high at 3 AM (no hypoglycemia). The treatment is to increase evening (NPH) insulin.

16. **How do you manage diabetic patients who are not allowed to eat because they are scheduled for surgery?**
Generally, one-third to one-half of the normal dose of insulin is given. Glucose is monitored closely intra- and postoperatively by the anesthesiologist. Regular intravenous insulin can be given to control glucose levels.

17. **What is the deal with beta blockers, hypoglycemia, and diabetics?**
If you give a beta blocker to a diabetic patient, you will mask the classic symptoms of hypoglycemia (tachycardia, diaphoresis), which are caused by catecholamine release. You must weigh the risk-to-benefit ratio of using beta blockers in diabetics (as in all patients). If a diabetic patient is having or has had a previous myocardial infarction, the benefits outweigh the risks of treatment.

18. **What are the best oral agents to use in type 1 diabetes?**
None. Patients with type 1 diabetes require insulin. Currently available oral agents do not work for type 1 diabetics.

19. **What is the first treatment for type 2 diabetes?**

Weight loss, because it may reduce glucose levels by reducing insulin resistance. However, medications are usually needed, and oral agents are tried first, typically beginning with metformin. Other agents include insulin secretagogues (glipizide, glimepiride, nateglinide, glyburide, repaglinide), thiazolidinediones (rosiglitazone, pioglitazone), alpha-glucosidase inhibitors (acarbose, miglitol), incretin mimetics (exenatide), incretin enhancers (saxagliptin, sitagliptin), and amylin analogues (pramlintide). Many type 2 diabetics eventually require insulin, and insulin may be required early if the blood glucose or hemoglobin A1C levels are significantly elevated.

CHAPTER 8

EAR, NOSE, AND THROAT SURGERY

1. **What is the most common cause of lower motor neuron facial nerve paralysis? How does it present?**
   The most common cause is Bell palsy. Look for sudden unilateral onset, usually after an upper respiratory infection. The cause is thought to be a reactivation of latent herpes simplex I infection in most cases. Patients may have *hyperacusis,* in which everything sounds loud because the stapedius muscle in the ear is paralyzed. In severe cases, patients may be unable to close the affected eye; if so, use drops to protect the eye. Most cases resolve spontaneously in about 1 month, although some have permanent sequelae. Oral prednisone and antiviral treatment for herpes (e.g., valacyclovir, acyclovir) may improve outcome and lessen duration of symptoms.

2. **What are the other causes of lower motor neuron facial nerve paralysis?**
   - Herpes infection (Ramsay Hunt syndrome), which commonly involves the eighth nerve. Look for vesicles on the pinna and inside the ear; encephalitis or meningitis may be present.
   - Lyme disease (one of the most common causes of bilateral facial nerve palsy)
   - Stroke
   - Middle ear or mastoid infections
   - Meningitis
   - Temporal bone fracture (look for Battle sign and/or bleeding from the ear)
   - Tumor, classically an acoustic schwannoma (i.e. neuroma) of the cerebellopontine angle (Fig. 8-1)
   Order a computed tomography (CT) or magnetic resonance (MR) scan of the head if the cause is not apparent or if the history or physical exam raises suspicion—especially in the presence of additional neurologic signs.

3. **What are the common causes of hearing loss?**
   The most common cause is **aging** (presbyacusis); prescribe a hearing aid, if needed.
   The history may suggest other causes:
   - Prolonged or intense exposure to loud noise (e.g., work-related)
   - Congenital TORCH infection (**t**oxoplasmosis, **o**thers, **r**ubella, **c**ytomegalovirus, **h**erpes virus)
   - Ménière disease (accompanied by severe vertigo, tinnitus, nausea and vomiting; treat with anticholinergics and antihistamines [meclizine]; surgery may be used for refractory cases)
   - Drugs (e.g., aminoglycosides, aspirin, quinine, loop diuretics, cisplatin)
   - Tumor (classically acoustic neuroma)
   - Labyrinthitis (may be viral or follow or extend from meningitis or otitis media)
   - Miscellaneous causes (diabetes, hypothyroidism, multiple sclerosis, sarcoidosis, pseudotumor cerebri).

4. **What is the usual cause of sudden deafness?**
   Sudden deafness (developing over a few hours) most often is due to a viral cause (endolymphatic labyrinthitis from mumps, measles, influenza, chickenpox, or adenovirus).

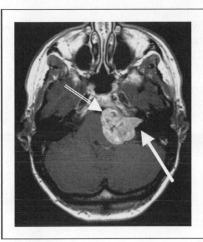

Figure 8-1. Acoustic neuroma. On this T1-weighted MR image, a large acoustic neuroma widens the left internal auditory canal (*solid arrow*) and compresses the brain stem (*hollow arrow*). (From Goldman L, Ausiello D: Cecil Medicine, 23rd ed. Philadelphia, Saunders, 2008, Fig. 419-9.)

Hearing usually returns within 2 weeks, but the loss may be permanent. No treatment has proved effective, but empirical steroids often are used. Trauma with temporal bone fracture is another cause of sudden hearing loss. Treatment is supportive.

5. **What is the most common cause of acquired hearing loss in children?**
   Bacterial meningitis. All children should receive formal hearing testing after a bout of meningitis.

6. **What are the common causes of vertigo?**
   Vertigo can result from the same eighth cranial nerve lesions that cause hearing loss (Meniere disease, tumor, infection, multiple sclerosis). Another common cause is benign positional (paroxysmal) vertigo, which is induced by certain head positions, may be accompanied by nystagmus, and is not associated with hearing loss. This condition often resolves spontaneously; no treatment is required.

7. **How is a deviated nasal septum treated in patients with recurrent sinusitis?**
   Surgical correction.

8. **What are the three common causes of rhinitis?**
   Viral, allergic, and bacterial.

9. **How do you recognize and treat viral rhinitis?**
   Viral rhinitis (the common cold) may be due to rhinovirus (the most common cause), influenza, parainfluenza, coxsackie virus, adenovirus, respiratory syncytial virus, coronavirus, or echovirus. Treatment is symptomatic. Vasoconstrictors such as phenylephrine can be used for short-term symptomatic relief, but they may cause rebound congestion when discontinued.

10. **How do you recognize and treat allergic rhinitis?**
    Allergic rhinitis (hay fever) is associated with seasonal flare-ups, boggy and bluish turbinates, onset before 20 years of age, nasal polyps, sneezing, pruritus, conjunctivitis, wheezing or asthma, eczema, positive family history, eosinophils in nasal mucous, and elevated serum IgE. Skin tests may identify an allergen. Treat with avoidance of known antigens (e.g., pollen). Antihistamines, cromolyn, and/or nasal steroids may be used for more severe symptoms. Desensitization also is an option.

11. **What causes bacterial rhinitis? How is it treated?**
    Group A streptococci, pneumococci, or staphylococci are the most common culprits. Look for coexisting sore throat, fever, and tonsillar exudate. Do streptococcal throat cultures and treat with antibiotics, if appropriate.

12. **What causes nosebleeds?**
    The most common cause of nosebleed is trauma; for example, nose-picking is a common cause in children. Also watch out for the following causes:
    - Local tumor (nasopharyngeal angiofibroma; seen in adolescent boys with no history of trauma or blood dyscrasia; signs include recurrent nosebleeds and/or obstruction)
    - Leukemia (from pancytopenia; typically in children with associated fever and anemia)
    - Other causes of thrombocytopenia (e.g., idiopathic thrombocytopenic purpura, hemolytic uremic syndrome)

13. **True or false: A neck mass is more likely to be benign in a child than in an adult.**
    True. Roughly 75% of neck masses are benign in children, whereas 75% are malignant in patients over 40 years old.

14. **What are the common causes of a neck mass?**
    In children, watch for thyroglossal duct cysts, which have a *midline* location and elevate with tongue protrusion; branchial cleft cysts, which are *lateral* in location and often become infected; cystic hygroma, a benign tumor also known as lymphangioma that is associated with Turner syndrome and treated with surgical resection; and cervical lymphadenitis. Cervical lymphadenitis usually is due to streptococcal pharyngitis, Epstein-Barr virus (common in the second and third decades), cat-scratch disease, or mycobacterial infection (scrofula). In terms of malignancy in children, leukemia or lymphoma may present with cervical lymphadenopathy.
    In **adults**, suspect malignancy, either lymphadenopathy from a primary tumor (lymphoma) or metastatic neoplasm (usually squamous cell carcinoma). The mass also may represent the tumor itself (especially with thyroid cancer).

15. **Describe the work-up for an unknown cancer in the neck.**
    The work-up includes random biopsy of the nasopharynx, palatine tonsils, and base of the tongue as well as laryngoscopy, bronchoscopy, and esophagoscopy (with biopsies of any suspicious lesions). This approach is known as "triple endoscopy with triple biopsy."

16. **What is the scientific name for "swimmer's ear"? What causes it?**
    Otitis externa (inflammation of the outer ear), which most often is due to infection with *Pseudomonas aeruginosa*. Patients have pain with manipulation of the auricle and erythematous, swollen skin in the auditory canal. Foul-smelling discharge and conductive hearing loss also may be present. Treat with topical antibiotics (e.g., neomycin, polymyxin B) and possibly topical steroids to reduce swelling.

17. **What causes otitis media? How do you recognize it?**
    Otitis media (inflammation of the middle ear) is an extremely common pediatric infection, most often due to infection with *Streptococcus pneumoniae, Haemophilus influenzae,* or *Moraxella catarrhalis*. Patients have no pain with manipulation of the auricle; positive symptoms include earache, fever, erythematous and bulging tympanic membranes (the light reflex and landmarks are difficult to see with otoscopy), and nausea and vomiting.

18. **What are the complications of otitis media? How are they avoided?**
    Complications include tympanic membrane perforation (bloody or purulent discharge), mastoiditis (fluctuance and inflammation over the mastoid process roughly 2 weeks after the

onset of otitis media), labyrinthitis, palsies of cranial nerves VII and VIII, meningitis, cerebral abscess, dural sinus thrombosis, and chronic otitis media (due to permanent perforation of the tympanic membrane). Patients with chronic otitis media may develop cholesteatomas with marginal perforations that require surgical excision.

Otitis media generally is treated with antibiotics to avoid these complications (e.g., amoxicillin, second-generation cephalosporin such as cefuroxime, or a macrolide).

19. What is the problem with recurrent otitis media? How is it treated?
Recurrent otitis media is a common pediatric problem (along with prolonged secretory otitis, a result of incompletely resolved otitis media) and can cause hearing loss with resultant developmental problems (speech, cognitive functions). Treat with prophylactic antibiotics or tympanostomy tubes. Adenoidectomy is controversial but may help in some cases; it is thought to help prevent blockage of the eustachian tubes.

20. What causes infectious myringitis? How do you recognize and treat it?
Infectious myringitis, also known as bullous myringitis, is an inflammation of the tympanic membranes that can be diagnosed when otoscopy reveals vesicles on the tympanic membrane. Infectious myringitis classically is caused by *Mycoplasma* species, but *Streptococcus pneumoniae* or viruses also may be the culprit. Treat with erythromycin or clarithromycin to cover *Mycoplasma* species and *S. pneumoniae.*

21. What are the common bacterial causes of sinusitis? How is this condition recognized clinically?
Sinusitis is often due to *S. pneumoniae, H. influenzae,* or other streptococcal or staphylococcal species. Look for tenderness over the affected sinuses, headache, and purulent nasal discharge (yellow or green). Associated symptoms are headache and/or toothache (maxillary sinusitis). Radiographs or CT are used to confirm the diagnosis and show opacification of the sinus, classically with an air-fluid level in acute sinusitis; CT scans are preferred to evaluate chronic sinusitis or suspected extension of infection outside the sinus (watch for high fever and chills). Treat with antibiotics (amoxicillin, trimethoprim-sulfamethoxazole, a 2nd or 3rd generation cephalosporin, a macrolide, or amoxicillin clavulanate for 10 to 14 days or for up to 6 weeks in chronic cases). Culture usually is not necessary unless the patient fails to respond to antibiotics. Operative intervention (drainage procedure, sinus obliteration) may be required for resistant cases.

22. By what age are the frontal sinuses well-developed in children?
The frontal sinuses may not be well developed until the age of 10 years.

23. Define otosclerosis. How is it treated?
In otosclerosis, the otic bones become fixed together and impede hearing. It is the most common cause of progressive conductive hearing loss in adults, whereas presbyacusis is the most common cause of sensorineural hearing loss in adults. Treat with a hearing aid or surgery.

24. What causes parotid gland swelling?
The classic cause is mumps. The best treatment for mumps and the complication of infertility is prevention through immunization. Parotid gland swelling also may be due to neoplasms, of which pleomorphic adenoma is the most common type; Sjögren syndrome; sialolithiasis (a stone in the parotid duct); and sarcoidosis. Alcoholism can cause parotid gland hypertrophy as well. Remember too that the parotid gland contains lymph nodes within its parenchyma (unique in this regard), which can become enlarged in a number of conditions, as with lymph nodes elsewhere.

25. **How do you recognize a nasal fracture? What complication may result?**
    A nasal fracture can be seen on radiographs or CT scan. Watch for a septal hematoma, which must be removed surgically to prevent pressure-induced septal necrosis.

26. **What is the Weber test used to evaluate? How is it performed and interpreted?**
    The Weber test compares bone conduction in the two ears. A vibrating tuning fork is placed on the forehead, and the patient is asked where the vibrating sound is heard best. The normal response is to hear the vibration in the middle (or equally in both ears). In patients with conductive hearing loss, the sound is heard best in the affected ear, whereas in patients with sensorineural hearing loss, the sound is heard best in the unaffected ear.

27. **What is the Rinne test used to evaluate? How is it performed and interpreted?**
    The Rinne test compares air conduction with bone conduction. A vibrating tuning fork is placed on the tip of the mastoid process. When the patient can no longer hear the sound, the tuning fork is removed from the mastoid and placed next to the auditory meatus of the external ear and the patient is asked if the sound can be heard.

    Because air conduction normally is greater than bone conduction, patients can hear the tuning fork when it is placed next to the auditory meatus (air conduction) even after they can no longer hear it vibrating on the mastoid (bone conduction). In patients with conductive hearing loss, bone conduction is greater than air conduction; thus they cannot hear the tuning fork when it is placed next to the external auditory meatus. In patients with sensorineural hearing loss, both air and bone conduction are impaired, but the normal ratio (air conduction > bone conduction) is maintained. Thus, they still hear the tuning fork next to the ear after they can no longer hear it on the mastoid.

CHAPTER 9

EMERGENCY MEDICINE

1. **What are the three causes of burns? How should all burns be managed initially?**

   Burns may be thermal, chemical, or electrical. Initial management of all burns includes lots of intravenous fluids (first choice: lactated Ringer solution; back-up choice: normal saline), removal of all clothes and other smoldering items on the body, copious irrigation of chemical burns, and, of course, the ABCs (airway, breathing, circulation). You should have a low threshold for intubation. In the setting of burns related to a fire, give 100% oxygen until significant carboxyhemoglobin from carbon monoxide inhalation is ruled out.

2. **What are the important sequelae of electrical burns?**

   Because most of the tissue destruction due to electrical burns is internal, sequelae include muscle necrosis, myoglobinuria, acidosis, and renal failure. Use large amounts of intravenous hydration to prevent renal shutdown. The immediate life-threatening risk with electricity exposure and burns (including lightning and a child who puts his or her finger in an electrical outlet) is cardiac arrhythmias. Get an electrocardiogram (EKG).

3. **How are chemical burns managed? Which is worse—acid or alkali burns?**

   All chemical burns should be treated with copious irrigation from the nearest source (e.g., tap water), because the sooner you dilute the chemical, the less damage will be done. Alkali burns are worse than acidic burns, because alkaline substances penetrate more deeply.

4. **What is burned skin prone to develop?**

   Burned skin is much more prone to infection, usually by *Staphylococcus aureus* or *Pseudomonas aeruginosa.* With pseudomonal infection, look for a fruity smell and/or blue-green appearance. Prophylactic antibiotics are given topically only. Give a tetanus booster to all burn patients unless they have recently received one (within the past 5 years).

5. **How is burn severity classified? Describe the management of each class.**

   Burn depth terminology no longer includes the use of "first-, second-, and third-degree" burns. Burn severity is now classified as superficial, superficial partial thickness, deep partial thickness, and full thickness burns.

   Superficial burns are erythematous without blister formation, involve only the epidermis, and pain is localized.

   Superficial partial thickness burns are painful, warm, and moist with blister formation and involve the epidermis and superficial papillary dermis.

   Deep partial thickness burns reveal skin that is mottled, waxy, and white in appearance with ruptured blisters. Pain sensation is absent, but pressure sensation is intact.

   Full thickness burns involve both the epidermis and dermis, and have a white to gray leathery appearance and do not blanch with pressure.

6. **Define hypothermia. How is it managed? What are the complications?**

   Hypothermia is defined as a body temperature $< 95°F$ ($35°C$), usually accompanied by mental status changes and generalized neurologic deficits. If the patient is conscious, you can use slow rewarming with blankets. If the patient is unconscious, consider gastric and bladder lavage with warm water as well as warm intravenous fluids.

Monitor the EKG for arrhythmias, which are common in hypothermic patients. You may see the classic **J wave**—a small, positive deflection following the QRS complex (Fig. 9-1). Also monitor electrolytes, renal function, and acid-base status.

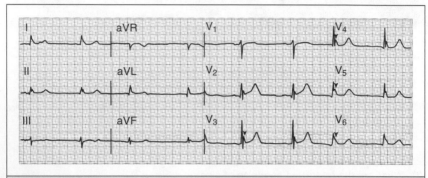

Figure 9-1. Systemic hypothermia resulting in prominent sinus bradycardia. The arrowheads (V₃ through V₆) point to the characteristic convex J waves, termed Osborn waves. (From Libby P, et al.: Braunwald's Heart Disease: A Textbook of Cardiovascular Medicine, 8th ed. Philadelphia, Saunders, 2008, Fig. 12-53.)

7. **Distinguish between frostnip and frostbite. How are they managed?**
   In **frostnip,** a mild form of cold injury, the affected skin is cold and painful. In **frostbite,** a more severe form of cold injury, the skin is cold and numb. Treat both with warming of the affected areas, using warm water (not scalding hot) and generalized warming (e.g., blankets).

8. **True or false: You should not give up resuscitation efforts until the patient is fully warmed in the setting of hypothermic cardiac arrest.**
   True. An old saying in medicine claims that the patient is not considered dead "until warm and dead." Hypothermia can slow body function to a remarkable degree, and there are case reports of resuscitation hours after initial attempts in the field once the body was warmed.

9. **Define hyperthermia. What causes it? How is it managed?**
   Hyperthermia is defined as a body temperature greater than 104°F. The three primary causes are infections, medications, and heat stroke. If heat stroke is the cause, look for a history of prolonged heat exposure and a high temperature (> 104°F), without clues to other culprits. Treat with immediate cooling (e.g., wet blankets, ice, cold water). The immediate threats to life are convulsions (treat with diazepam) and cardiovascular collapse. Always rule out infection and medications (especially those with anticholinergic activity such as antihistamines, antipsychotics, and antidepressants) as the cause.

10. **What are the two classic examples of hyperthermia due to medication?**
    Malignant hyperthermia is an idiosyncratic, genetically related reaction to general anesthesia, usually caused by succinylcholine or halothane exposure. Treat with dantrolene.

    Neuroleptic malignant syndrome is thought to be related to malignant hyperthermia and is an idiosyncratic, genetically related reaction to an antipsychotic. Look for extremely high levels of creatine phosphokinase and mental status changes in a patient taking antipsychotics.

The first step is stop the medication. The second step is supportive treatment, especially with lots of intravenous fluids to prevent renal shutdown due to rhabdomyolysis. The third step, if necessary, is to treat with dantrolene.

Drug fevers are idiosyncratic reactions to a medication that usually was started within the past week. They rarely cause fever above 104°F, but cases have been reported.

11. **How are patients managed after a near-drowning episode?**

Some (not all) believe that fresh water is worse than salt water, because fresh water, if aspirated, can cause hypervolemia, electrolyte disturbances, and hemolysis. Intubate patients after a near-drowning episode if they are unconscious, and monitor arterial blood gases if they are conscious. Patients who drown in cold water often do better than those who drown in warm water because of decreased metabolic needs. Death is usually due to hypoxia and/or cardiac arrest.

CHAPTER 10

ENDOCRINOLOGY

1. What are the common symptoms and signs of hyperthyroidism?

Symptoms: nervousness, anxiety, irritability, insomnia, heat intolerance, sweating, palpitations, tremors, weight loss with increased appetite, fatigue, weakness, emotional lability, and diarrhea.

Signs: enlarged thyroid gland, warm skin, thyroid "stare"/lid lag, exophthalmos, proptosis, ophthalmoplegia (Graves disease), pretibial myxedema (Graves disease), tremor, tachycardia, and atrial fibrillation. Check thyroid-stimulating hormone (TSH) when patients present with new-onset atrial fibrillation.

2. What are the most common causes of hyperthyroidism?

The most common cause is **Graves disease,** which is characterized by a diffusely enlarged thyroid gland, positive thyroid-stimulating immunoglobulins and antibodies, exophthalmos, proptosis, ophthalmoplegia, and pretibial myxedema. In elderly patients, look for toxic multinodular goiter (individual lumps instead of diffuse enlargement of the gland and "hot" nodules on thyroid nuclear scan). Other causes include adenoma (single lump that is "hot" on nuclear scan), subacute thyroiditis (viral infection with **tender, painful** thyroid gland), and factitious hyperthyroidism (in which the patient takes thyroid hormone). Rare, exotic causes include amiodarone (which can cause hypo- or hyperthyroidism), TSH-producing pituitary tumor, thyroid carcinoma, and struma ovarii (an ovarian teratoma that secretes thyroid hormone).

3. Describe the classic laboratory pattern of hyperthyroidism.

The TSH level is low (unless the patient has a TSH-secreting tumor), whereas triiodothyronine (T_3) and thyroxine (T_4) are increased.

4. How is hyperthyroidism treated?

Short-term (stabilizing) treatment: Propylthiouracil (PTU) and methimazole/carbimazole can be used as suppressive agents. Beta blockers are used in the setting of thyroid storm (severe hyperthyroid state—an emergency). Iodine can also suppress the thyroid gland but is rarely used for this purpose clinically.

Definitive (curative) treatment: Radioactive iodine ablation of the thyroid gland is typically used. Surgery is preferred in pregnant patients. Hypothyroidism may result from either treatment; if so, it is treated with thyroid hormone replacement (for life).

5. What are the symptoms and signs of hypothyroidism?

Symptoms: weakness, lethargy, fatigue, cold intolerance, weight gain with anorexia, constipation, loss of hair, hoarseness, menstrual irregularity (menorrhagia is classic), myalgias and arthralgias, memory impairment, and dementia. Always rule out hypothyroidism as a cause of dementia.

Signs: bradycardia; dry, coarse, cold, and pale skin; periorbital and peripheral edema; coarse, thin hair; thick tongue; slow speech; decreased reflexes; hypertension; carpal tunnel syndrome and paresthesias; vitiligo, pernicious anemia, and diabetes (remember the autoimmune association between these three conditions and Hashimoto disease); and coma (severe disease).

In children, cretinism may occur (mental, motor, and growth retardation).

6. **What are the common causes of hypothyroidism?**
   The most common known cause is Hashimoto thyroiditis. Women of reproductive age outnumber men by 8:1. Histology reveals lymphocytes in the thyroid gland as well as antithyroid and antimicrosomal antibodies. Other autoimmune diseases may coexist. The associated goiter is nontender. The second most common cause is iatrogenic after treatment of hyperthyroidism. Other less common causes include iodine deficiency, amiodarone, lithium, and secondary hypothyroidism due to pituitary or hypothalamic failure (look for decreased TSH), such as with Sheehan syndrome.

7. **Describe the laboratory findings in hypothyroidism.**
   Elevated TSH (unless due to secondary causes), decreased T_3 and T_4, antithyroid and antimicrosomal antibodies (if due to Hashimoto thyroiditis), hypercholesterolemia, and anemia (which may be due to chronic disease or coexisting pernicious anemia).

8. **Why is free T_4 (or free T_4 index) better than total T_4 for measuring thyroid hormone activity?**
   Free T_4 (free T_4 index) measures the active form of thyroid hormone. Many conditions cause a change in the amount of thyroid-binding globulin (TBG), thus changing total T_4 levels in the absence of hypo- or hyperthyroidism. Common examples include pregnancy, estrogen therapy, and oral contraceptive pills, all of which increase TBG. Nephrotic syndrome, cirrhosis, and corticosteroid treatment all decrease TBG. T_3 resin uptake is an older test that is not worth the effort to learn for Step 2, but if you are asked, it should rise or fall in the same way as free T_4. Although an oversimplification, this principle should serve you well on the exam.

9. **How is hypothyroidism treated?**
   With T_4 or thyroxine. T_3 should not be used. In elderly patients, it is important to "start low and go slow," because overtreatment can be dangerous.

10. **What is euthyroid sick syndrome?**
    Any patient with any illness may have temporary derangements in thyroid function tests that resemble hypothyroidism. TSH ranges from normal to mildly elevated, and serum T_4 ranges from normal to mildly decreased. Clinical circumstances and physical findings are the best guides to whether the patient has true hypothyroidism. In patients with euthyroid sick syndrome, simply treat the underlying illness. If the diagnosis is in doubt, either remeasure thyroid tests after the patient recovers (preferred) or try an empirical dose of levothyroxine (if the patient does not respond to treatment of the underlying illness).

11. **What are the symptoms and signs of Cushing syndrome (Increased corticosteroids)?**
    Symptoms: weight gain, changes in appearance, easy bruising, acne, hirsutism, emotional lability, depression, psychosis, weakness, menstrual changes, sexual dysfunction, insomnia, and memory loss.
    Signs: buffalo hump, truncal and central obesity with wasting of extremities, round plethoric facies, purplish skin striae, acne, hirsutism, weakness (especially of the proximal muscles), hypertension, depression, psychosis, peripheral edema, poor wound healing, glucose intolerance or diabetes, osteoporosis, and hypokalemic metabolic alkalosis (due to mineralocorticoid effects of certain corticosteroids). Growth may be stunted in children.

12. **What causes Cushing syndrome?**
    The most common cause is iatrogenic, since steroids are prescribed for many different disorders. The second most common cause is Cushing disease (a pituitary adenoma that secretes adrenocorticotropic hormone [ACTH]), which causes roughly 60% of noniatrogenic

cases. Women of reproductive age outnumber men by 5:1. Other causes include ectopic ACTH production (classically by small cell lung cancer, which is more common in men) and adrenal adenomas or carcinomas (more common in children).

13. **How is Cushing syndrome diagnosed?**
The first test is either a 24-hour measurement of free cortisol in urine (free cortisol levels are abnormally elevated) or a dexamethasone suppression test (cortisol levels are not appropriately suppressed several hours after administration of dexamethasone). Random cortisol level is an inappropriate test because of wide inter- and intrapatient variations. **Remember that ACTH is elevated in Cushing disease but decreased with an adrenal adenoma.** If ACTH is increased, a magnetic resonance (MR) scan of the brain should be obtained to look for a pituitary adenoma. If ACTH is decreased and the patient has no history of taking steroids, an abdominal computed tomography (CT) or MR scan should be obtained to look for an adrenal tumor. Primary cancer is usually obvious when ectopic ACTH is the cause (e.g., weight loss, hemoptysis with lung mass on chest radiograph in patients with small cell lung cancer). Treatment is based on the cause and usually involves surgery.

14. **What are the symptoms and signs of hypoadrenalism (Addison disease)?**
Symptoms: anorexia, weight loss, weakness, apathy.
   Signs: hypotension, hyperkalemia, hyponatremia, hyperpigmentation (only if the pituitary is functioning because of melanocyte stimulating hormone), nausea and vomiting, diarrhea, abdominal pain, mild fever, hypoglycemia, acidosis, eosinophilia, and shock.

15. **What is the most common type of hypoadrenalism?**
Secondary (iatrogenic) hypoadrenalism due to steroid treatment. People who are removed from long-term steroid therapy may be unable to secrete an appropriate amount of corticosteroids in response to stress for up to 1 year. Watch out for the classic postoperative patient who crashes (with hypotension, shock, and hyperkalemia) shortly after surgery and has a history of a disease requiring steroid therapy within the past year. You may assess ACTH (usually high) and cortisol levels (inappropriately low) to help make the diagnosis, but do not wait for the results to give steroids. The patient may die. Give prophylactic stress doses of corticosteroids in the setting of an illness, operation, or other stressor to prevent problems.

16. **What are the other causes of hypoadrenalism?**
The most common primary (noniatrogenic) cause is autoimmune (idiopathic) disease. Patients may have other autoimmune diseases, such as hypothyroidism, pernicious anemia, vitiligo, diabetes, or hypoparathyroidism. Other causes include metastatic cancer (especially lung cancer), infection (tuberculosis, fungal infections, opportunistic infections in AIDS and other immunosuppressed states), ketoconazole, and pituitary/hypothalamic failure.

17. **How is hypoadrenalism diagnosed?**
An ACTH stimulation test can be done. Plasma cortisol is measured, ACTH is administered, and cortisol is remeasured in 1 hour. The cortisol level should rise appropriately, usually 18 μg/dL or doubling of the baseline, depending on the baseline value. An inappropriate response to ACTH means hypoadrenalism. Do not withhold treatment to make a diagnosis if the patient is crashing.

18. **Define hirsutism. What causes it?**
Hirsutism is a male hair growth pattern in women or pre-pubescent children (Fig. 10-1). The most common cause is familial, genetic, or idiopathic hirsutism, but on the boards watch for **polycystic ovary syndrome** (Stein-Leventhal syndrome), Cushing syndrome, and drugs

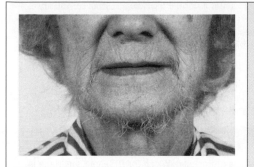

Figure 10-1. Hirsutism. This finding is usually benign and due to ethnic/familial predilections, polycystic ovarian syndrome, corticosteroid excess, menopause or medications. However, new-onset hirsutism can be a sign of a testosterone-secreting ovarian neoplasm; accompanying signs of virilization should be present in this setting. (From du Vivier A: Atlas of Clinical Dermatology, 3rd ed. New York, Churchill Livingstone, 2002, p 629, with permission.)

(minoxidil, phenytoin, cyclosporine). These disorders do not produce virilization. If virilization (clitoral enlargement, deepening of the voice, temporal balding) accompanies the hirsutism, an androgen-secreting ovarian tumor (e.g., Sertoli-Leydig cell tumor or arrhenoblastoma) or adrenal source (congenital adrenal hyperplasia, Cushing syndrome, or adrenal tumor) is likely.

19. **What causes virilization in children?**
In female neonates, congenital adrenal hyperplasia is a likely cause of virilization. The classic example is a female infant born with ambiguous genitalia. However, the patient also may be a male child with precocious puberty. At least 90% of cases are due to **21-hydroxylase deficiency.** Because 21-hydroxylase is involved in the production of both aldosterone and cortisol, children develop signs of hypoadrenalism, with salt-wasting, hypotension, hyperkalemia, hyponatremia, hypoglycemia, acidosis, and nausea and vomiting. Abnormally high levels of serum 17-hydroxyprogesterone or urinary 17-ketosteroids (dehydroepiandrosterone [DHEA], DHEA sulfate, and androsterone), along with decreased free cortisol in the serum, clinch the diagnosis. Give corticosteroids to prevent death. In older children, worry about a testosterone-secreting gonadal neoplasm.

20. **What are the symptoms and signs of hyperparathyroidism?**
The same as those for hypercalcemia ("bones, stones, groans, and psychiatric overtones"; see question 24). In primary cases, serum calcium is high, phosphorus is normal to low, and parathyroid hormone (PTH) is increased. In secondary cases, calcium is low.

21. **What causes hyperparathyroidism?**
Ninety percent of primary cases are due to a parathyroid adenoma, which can usually be confirmed with a nuclear medicine scan (Fig. 10-2). Other causes include parathyroid hyperplasia and parathyroid carcinoma. Secondary cases include low calcium levels (e.g., from

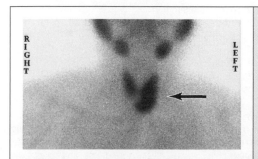

Figure 10-2. Parathyroid adenomas are almost always solitary lesions. This technetium-99m-sestamibi radionuclide scan demonstrates an area of increased uptake corresponding to the left inferior parathyroid gland *(arrow)*. This patient had a parathyroid adenoma. (From Kumar V, Abbas A, Fausto N: Robbins and Cotran: Pathologic Basis of Disease, 7th ed. Philadelphia, Saunders, 2005, Fig. 24-24.)

renal failure), to which an increase in PTH is a normal physiologic response. Tertiary hyperparathyroidism occurs when PTH has been elevated for too long (secondary to long-standing hypocalcemia) and continues to be oversecreted even when calcium is normalized with treatment. Translation: Put all patients with renal failure on calcium supplements to prevent this complication.

22. What are the signs and symptoms of hypoparathyroidism?
The same as those for hypocalcemia (tetany, prolonged QT interval on EKG; see question 26). Calcium is low, phosphorus is high, and PTH is low.

23. What causes hypoparathyroidism?
The most common cause is accidental removal or damage after thyroid surgery. Watch for tetany after thyroid surgery. Rare causes are genetic. Watch for **DiGeorge syndrome** in children with congenital absence of parathyroid glands, tetany in the first 48 hours of life, absent thymus gland, immunodeficiency, cardiac anomalies, and midline facial defects.

24. What are the symptoms and signs of hypercalcemia?
Symptoms: "bones, stones, groans, and psychiatric overtones." In other words: bone resorption with osteomalacia and osteitis fibrosa cystica; kidney stones; abdominal pain secondary to nausea and vomiting, ileus, nephrolithiasis, peptic ulcer disease, constipation, or pancreatitis (all increased with hypercalcemia); and emotional lability, delirium, depression, and/or psychosis.
Signs: shortened QT interval on EKG, weakness, polyuria, bone changes and kidney stones on radiograph, and renal failure.

25. What causes hypercalcemia?
In outpatients, the most common cause is hyperparathyroidism. In hospitalized patients, the most common cause is malignancy. Multiple types of cancer can cause hypercalcemia, but the classic board question involves either multiple myeloma or secretion of PTH-like hormone by a squamous cell carcinoma, especially in the lung. Familial hypocalciuric hypercalcemia is characterized by hypercalcemia with low calcium levels in the urine (opposite of other hypercalcemias). Other causes include vitamin A or D intoxication, sarcoidosis or other granulomatous diseases, and excessive calcium intake (milk-alkali syndrome).

26. What are the symptoms and signs of hypocalcemia?
Symptoms: paresthesias (the classic pattern is perioral or distal extremities), muscle aches, dementia, depression, and psychosis.
Signs: prolonged QT interval on EKG, tetany, **Chvostek sign** (tetany elicited by tapping on the facial nerve to cause facial muscle contraction), **Trousseau sign** (carpopedal spasm caused by inflation of a blood pressure cuff or application of a tourniquet), dementia, depression, psychosis, seizures, and papilledema.

27. What causes hypocalcemia?
■ Hypoparathyroidism (usually after thyroid gland surgery)
■ Pseudohypoparathyroidism (genetic end-organ unresponsiveness to PTH with normal PTH levels, shortened metacarpal bones, short stature, and mental retardation)
■ DiGeorge syndrome
■ Vitamin D deficiency (osteomalacia, rickets)
■ Renal failure of any cause and certain renal tubular problems
■ Acute pancreatitis (one of Ranson criteria)
■ Secondary to hypomagnesemia
Hypoproteinemia of any cause may lead to low levels of total serum calcium, but levels of ionized calcium (the active form) are normal. In any patient with low serum calcium, the first step is to determine whether the serum albumin level is decreased. If it is, no treatment is required and no symptoms will develop.

28. What specific problems are caused by obesity?

Obesity causes an increase in overall mortality (at any age) and increases the risk for insulin resistance and diabetes, hypertension, hypertriglyceridemia, heart disease and coronary artery disease, gallstones, sleep apnea and hypoventilation, osteoarthritis, thromboembolism, varicose veins, and cancer (especially endometrial cancer).

29. Define precocious puberty and pseudoprecocious puberty.

True precocious puberty is defined as activation of the hypothalamic-pituitary axis with sexual maturation before the age of 8 years in females and before the age of 9 years in males. In **pseudoprecocious puberty,** secondary sex characteristics develop prematurely because of high circulating levels of androgen or estrogen.

30. How is precocious puberty different from pseudoprecocious puberty?

True precocious puberty is usually idiopathic but can be caused by central nervous system (CNS) lesions. A general rule of thumb is that true precocious puberty causes testicular or ovarian enlargement, which does not occur with pseudoprecocious puberty (ovarian cysts are not considered true ovarian enlargement). All patients with suspected precocious puberty should have a gonadotropin-releasing hormone (GnRH) stimulation test. If a dose of GnRH produces the typical pubertal response of increased follicle-stimulating hormone (FSH) and luteinizing hormone (LH), true precocious puberty is diagnosed. An MRI of the brain should be obtained to rule out CNS disease (e.g., hamartomas, tumors, cysts, trauma) as the cause.

31. What causes pseudoprecocious puberty?

Pseudoprecocious puberty may be caused by exogenous hormones, adrenal tumors, congenital adrenal hyperplasia (e.g., 21-hydroxylase deficiency), hormone-secreting tumors, or **McCune-Albright syndrome** in females (ovarian cysts, pseudoprecocious puberty, polyostotic fibrous dysplasia of bone and café-au-lait spots) (Fig. 10-3).

32. How is precocious puberty treated?

Because premature puberty causes premature fusion of growth plates in the bone and can cause serious social problems for affected children, treatment is indicated. Treatment of any underlying disorders is indicated for pseudoprecocious puberty. For true idiopathic precocious puberty, treatment with long-acting GnRH agonists is indicated to suppress the pituitary-hypothalamic axis and to delay the onset of puberty until an appropriate age.

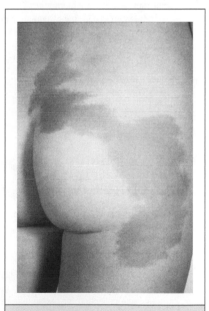

Figure 10-3. McCune-Albright syndrome. The figure demonstrates a large café-au-lait macule. These macules are fewer, larger, and darker compared with those seen in neurofibromatosis, a more classic etiology for this dermatologic finding. (From du Vivier A: Atlas of Clinical Dermatology, 3rd ed. New York, Churchill Livingstone, 2002, p 471, with permission.)

33. **What is the difference between a primary and secondary endocrine disorder?**
In **primary disorders** the problem is in the gland; the hypothalamic-pituitary axis is functioning appropriately. In primary hypothyroidism, for example, the thyroid gland does not function properly for whatever reason, but the pituitary and hypothalamus respond appropriately. Therefore, thyroid hormone is low (as in all cases of hypothyroidism), but TSH and thyroid-releasing hormone (TRH) are high (the appropriate response from the pituitary and hypothalamus to low levels of thyroid hormone).
    In **secondary disorders** the true dysfunction is outside the gland itself. For example, in secondary hypothyroidism, thyroid hormone is low, but TSH and/or TRH is also low (inappropriate in the setting of low thyroid hormone). If the pituitary is destroyed or surgically removed, secondary hypothyroidism results from low TSH; the thyroid gland functions well, but no TSH is available to stimulate it. To confuse the picture, the dysfunction also may be completely outside the endocrine axis (for example, heart failure that causes secondary hyperaldosteronism).
    This concept in endocrine gland dysfunction is quite important. Simple blood tests can localize the problem. You may be able to answer a USMLE question simply by reading through the various values for hormones and hormone-releasing factors and figuring out where in the hypothalamus-pituitary-target gland axis the problem lies.

34. **What are the symptoms and signs of primary hyperaldosteronism (Conn syndrome)? What are the causes?**
Symptoms: weakness and edema.
    Signs: hypertension, hypokalemia, hypernatremia, and edema.
    Conn syndrome is caused by an aldosterone-secreting adrenal neoplasm. Because it is a primary disease, renin levels are low; the rest of endocrine axis responds appropriately to gland dysfunction. Order a CT of the abdomen to look for an adrenal mass. The treatment is surgical removal of the tumor.

35. **What causes secondary hyperaldosteronism?**
Secondary hyperaldosteronism is *much more common* than primary disease. It is due to low perfusion of the kidney, as in congestive heart failure, renal artery stenosis (bruit), dehydration, nephrotic syndrome, and cirrhosis. The key mechanism is that the kidney senses hypoperfusion and secretes renin; therefore, the renin level is high. Treatment of the underlying disorder (if possible) resolves the hyperaldosteronism. Potassium levels may be normal or even high. Of note, hyperkalemia may be the cause of increased aldosterone release just as hypocalcemia causes increased release of parathyroid hormone. Both are normal physiologic responses.

36. **Give the classic clinical description of a pheochromocytoma. How is it diagnosed?**
Look for wild swings in blood pressure (with some measurements dangerously high), tachycardia, postural hypotension, headaches, sweating, flushing, dizziness, mental status changes, and/or a feeling of impending doom (like a panic attack). The screening test is a 24-hour urine collection for metanephrines, homovanillic acid, and/or vanillylmandelic acid (catecholamine breakdown products that are abnormally elevated in the urine). If levels are high, order an abdominal CT scan to look for an adrenal mass (Fig. 10-4). Surgical tumor removal is the treatment of choice after stabilization with alpha and then beta blockers.

37. **Define diabetes insipidus (DI). What are the two types?**
DI is a lack of antidiuretic hormone (ADH or vasopressin) effect in the body. Patients with DI secrete inappropriately dilute urine because of a lack of ADH effect and may urinate up to 25 liters of urine per day, resulting in dehydration and hypernatremia. Such patients die rapidly if

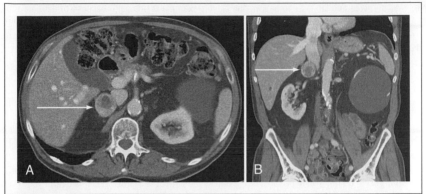

Figure 10-4. A computed tomographic (CT) scan of the abdomen with intravenous contrast agent of a 71-year-old man with an incidentally discovered right adrenal mass. The fractionated plasma free metanephrines were abnormal. **A,** The axial CT image shows a typical 3.8-cm heterogeneously enhancing right adrenal mass just lateral to the inferior vena cava and consistent with pheochromocytoma (*arrow*). **B,** Coronal view shows the location (*arrow*) of the mass superior to the right kidney and inferior and medial to the liver. After α- and β-adrenergic blockade, a pheochromocytoma was removed laparoscopically. (From Kronenberg H, et al.: Williams Textbook of Endocrinology, 11th ed. Philadelphia, Saunders, 2008, Fig. 15-3.)

they are unable to drink water. Normally, when the body is dehydrated, ADH causes urine to become highly concentrated through retention of free water. In DI, the urine remains dilute even though the serum osmolarity is quite high as a result of dehydration. The two types are **central** and **nephrogenic.**

38. **What causes central DI?**
    Central DI is caused by a lack of ADH production by the posterior pituitary. Although it is often idiopathic, look for trauma, neoplasm, or sarcoid/granulomatous disease as the cause. Order a CT or MR scan of the head, if indicated.

39. **What causes nephrogenic DI?**
    Nephrogenic DI is due to kidney unresponsiveness to ADH. Look for medications (e.g., lithium, methoxyflurane, demeclocycline) as the cause.

40. **What diagnostic test can reveal whether DI is central or nephrogenic? How are these conditions treated?**
    Give the patient a dose of antidiuretic hormone (ADH), and measure urine osmolarity. If central DI is the cause, urine osmolarity increases with ADH challenge. In nephrogenic DI, the urine remains inappropriately dilute after the patient is given ADH. Treatment for central DI is ADH replacement (given orally or as a nasal spray). Treatment for nephrogenic DI involves stopping any offending drug and giving a thiazide diuretic; ADH does not help. Although giving a diuretic to a patient with DI seems counterintuitive, it has the paradoxical effect of decreasing urine output.

41. **Define the syndrome of inappropriate antidiuretic hormone secretion (SIADH). How is it diagnosed?**
    The name says it all: ADH is released inappropriately. SIADH is a consideration in patients with hyponatremia and normal volume status (euvolemic). In SIADH, serum osmolarity is low, but urine osmolarity is high (inappropriate urine concentration). Look for the values of all

electrolytes and lab tests to be low (the classic example is uric acid) because of dilution of the serum with free water secondary to inappropriate ADH.

42. **What causes SIADH?**
Central nervous system causes: stroke, hemorrhage, infection, trauma
   Medications: narcotics, oxytocin (watch for pregnant patients), chlorpropamide, antiepileptic agents.
   Trauma: pain is a powerful stimulus for ADH. Watch for the postoperative patient who is receiving fluids (and often narcotics) and has pain to develop SIADH.
   Lung problems: simple pneumonia or ADH-secreting small cell cancer of the lung.

43. **How is SIADH treated?**
   Treat with water restriction. Stop intravenous fluids and restrict oral fluid intake. For Step 2 purposes, do not give hypertonic saline unless the patient has active seizures before your eyes. You may cause brainstem damage or central pontine myelinolysis from too rapid correction of sodium level. **Demeclocycline** is sometimes used to treat SIADH if water restriction fails because it induces nephrogenic diabetes insipidus, which allows the patient to get rid of free water.

CHAPTER 11

ETHICS

1. **True or false: Adult patients of sound mind are allowed to refuse life-saving treatments.**
   True. You should not force blood products, antibiotics, or any other treatments on a patient who does not want them.

2. **What should you do if a child has a life-threatening condition and the parents refuse a simple, curative treatment (e.g., antibiotics for meningitis)?**
   First try to persuade the parents to change their mind; if this fails, attempt get a court order to give the treatment. Do not treat until you have talked to the courts if you can at all avoid it. Even with Jehovah's witnesses who do not want their children to receive a blood transfusion, you should seek the court's assistance in getting the transfusion if it is the only treatment option available.

3. **True or false: People with terminal illnesses can choose to die.**
   True. This is the rationale behind hospice care. Let competent people die if they want to do so. Do not commit active euthanasia, but respect a patient's wishes for passive euthanasia.

4. **What is the difference between active and passive euthanasia?**
   Active euthanasia is the intentional hastening of death, whereas passive euthanasia is withholding treatments and "letting nature take its course."

5. **With whom can you discuss your patient's condition?**
   Only with people who need to know because they are directly involved in the patient's care and with people authorized by the patient (e.g., authorized family members). Do not tell a medical colleague who is uninvolved with the patient's care how that patient is doing, even if the colleague is a friend of yours or the patient.

6. **In what situations are you allowed to breach patient confidentiality?**
   Break confidentiality only in the following situations:
   - The patient asks you to do so.
   - Child abuse is suspected.
   - The courts mandate you to do so.
   - You must fulfill the duty to warn or protect (if a patient says that he is going to kill someone or himself, you have to tell someone, the authorities, or both).
   - The patient has a reportable disease.
   - The patient is a danger to others (e.g., if a patient is blind or has seizures, let the proper authorities know so that they can revoke the patient's license to drive; if the patient is an airplane pilot and is a paranoid, hallucinating schizophrenic, then authorities need to know).

7. **What are the components of informed consent?**
   Informed consent involves giving the patient information about the following:
   - Diagnosis (his or her condition and what it means)
   - Prognosis (the natural course of the condition without treatment)

- Proposed treatment (description of the procedure and what the patient will experience)
- Risks and benefits of the treatment
- Alternative treatments

The patient then must be allowed to make his or her own choice. The documents seen on the wards that patients are made to sign are not technically required or sufficient for informed consent. They are used for medicolegal purposes (i.e., lawsuit paranoia).

8. **What should you do if a patient is incompetent to make decisions?**
Get the family and/or courts to appoint a guardian (surrogate decision-maker or health-care power of attorney).

9. **True or false: A living will should not be respected if the next of kin asks you not to follow it.**
False. Such situations are tricky, but technically (and for the USMLE) living wills or patient-mandated "do-not-resuscitate" orders should be respected and followed if properly documented. The classic boards question involves a patient who says in a living will that if he or she is unable to breathe independently, a ventilator should not be used. Do not put the patient on a ventilator, even if the husband, wife, son, or daughter tells you to do so.

10. **What should you do if a patient is in critical condition or in a coma and has made no advance directive or living will?**
The wishes of the family, next of kin, or health-care power of attorney should be followed. In cases of disagreement among family members, suspicion of ulterior motives, or uncertainty, involve the hospital's ethics committee. As a last resort, go to the courts for help.

11. **What about depression in the context of end-of-life decisions?**
Depression always should be evaluated as a reason for "incompetence." Patients who are suicidal may refuse all treatment, but their refusal should not be respected until the depression is treated.

12. **True or false: In some circumstances, patients can be hospitalized against their will.**
True. Psychiatric patients frequently are hospitalized against their will if they are deemed to be a danger to themselves or others. Patients can be held only for a limited time (1 to 3 days) before they must have a hearing before a court official to determine whether they must remain in custody. These decisions are based on the principle of **beneficence** (the principle of doing good for the patient and avoiding harm).

13. **True or false: Restraints can be used on patients against their will.**
True. Restraints can be used on an incompetent or violent (e.g., delirious, psychotic) patient if needed, but their use should be brief and reevaluated often (at least once every 24 hours). Be aware that the use of restraints in delirious or demented patients rarely helps prevent falls and may cause injury.

14. **When do patients under the age of 18 years not require parental consent for a medical decision?**
In general, people under the age of 18 do not require parental consent if they are emancipated (married, living on their own and financially independent, raising children, or serving in the armed forces); have a sexually transmitted disease, want contraception, or are pregnant; want illicit drug treatment or counseling; or have psychiatric illness. Some states have exceptions to these rules, but for Step 2 purposes, in such situations let minors make their own decisions.

15. **What should you do if a child has a medical emergency and the parents are unavailable for decision-making?**
Treat the child as you see fit; that is, act in the child's best interest.

16. **True or false: It is acceptable to hide a diagnosis from a patient if the family asks you to do so.**
False. Do not hide a diagnosis from a patient (including a child) if the patient wants to know (even if the family asks you to do so). Do not lie to any patient because the family asks you to do so. Conversely, you should not force patients to receive information against their will; if they do not want to know the diagnosis, do not tell them.

17. **What should you do if a patient requires emergency care but the patient cannot communicate and no family members are available?**
Treat the patient as you see fit unless you know that the patient wishes otherwise.

18. **True or false: Withdrawing care and withholding care are the same in the eyes of the law.**
True. It is important to communicate this principle to family members who feel guilty. The simple fact that a patient is on a respirator does not mean that you cannot turn the respirator off.

19. **True or false: In terminally ill, noncurable patients, one of the primary goals is to relieve pain.**
True. Opioids are commonly used, even though they may cause respiratory depression. It is more important to make patients comfortable and pain-free than to worry about respiratory depression in this setting.

CHAPTER 12

GASTROENTEROLOGY

1. **Define gastroesophageal reflux disease (GERD). What causes it?**

   GERD means that stomach acid refluxes into the esophagus. It is due to inappropriate, intermittent relaxation of the lower esophageal sphincter. The incidence is increased greatly in patients with a hiatal hernia (see question 4).

2. **Describe the classic symptoms of GERD. How is it treated?**

   The main complaint is usually "heartburn," often related to eating and lying supine. GERD also may cause abdominal or chest pain. Initial treatment is to elevate the head of the bed and to avoid coffee, alcohol, tobacco, spicy and fatty foods, chocolate, and medications with anticholinergic properties. If this approach fails, antacids, histamine-2 blockers, and proton-pump inhibitors may be tried. Many patients have already tried over-the-counter remedies before presentation, and many physicians begin empiric treatment at the first visit, since "lifestyle modifications" usually fail. Surgery (Nissen fundoplication) is reserved for severe or resistant cases.

3. **What are the sequelae of GERD?**

   Sequelae of GERD include esophagitis, esophageal stricture (which may mimic esophageal cancer), esophageal ulcer, hemorrhage, Barrett's metaplasia, and esophageal adenocarcinoma (Fig. 12-1).

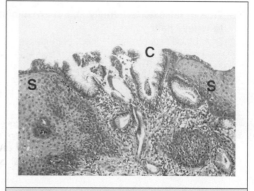

Figure 12-1. Barrett esophagus or metaplasia. Normal native esophageal squamous epithelium (S) is being replaced by gastric-type columnar epithelium (C), whose ability to produce mucous protects the esophagus from the damaging effects of gastric acid. (From Stevens A, et al.: Wheater's Basic Histopathology, 4th ed. New York, Churchill Livingstone, 2002, p 65, with permission.)

4. **What is a hiatal hernia? How is it different from a paraesophageal hernia?**

   A hiatal hernia is a sliding hernia, which means that the whole gastroesophageal junction moves above the diaphragm, pulling the stomach with it. This common and benign finding may predispose to GERD. In a paraesophageal hernia, the gastroesophageal junction stays below the diaphragm, but the stomach herniates through the diaphragm into the thorax. This type of hernia is uncommon but serious; it may become strangulated and should be repaired surgically.

5. **How does peptic ulcer disease (PUD) present?**

   PUD classically presents with chronic, intermittent, epigastric pain (burning, gnawing, or aching) that is localized and often relieved by antacids or milk. Look for epigastric tenderness. Other signs and symptoms include occult blood in the stool and nausea or vomiting. PUD is more common in men. The two types of PUD are gastric and duodenal ulcers.

6. **Explain the classic differences between duodenal and gastric ulcers.**

	Duodenal	Gastric *need to bx to r/o malignancy*
% of cases	75	25
Acid secretion	Normal to high	Normal to low
Main cause	*Helicobacter pylori*	Use of nonsteroidal anti-inflammatory drugs, including aspirin
Peak age	Forties	Fifties
Blood type	O	A
Eating food	Pain gets better, then worse 2–3 hours later	Pain not relieved or made worse

7. **What is the diagnostic study of choice for PUD?**
The gold standard is endoscopy (most sensitive test), but an upper gastrointestinal barium study is cheaper and less invasive. Empirical treatment with medications may be tried in the absence of diagnostic studies if the symptoms are typical. If endoscopy is done, a biopsy of any gastric ulcer is mandatory to exclude malignancy. Duodenal ulcers do not have to be biopsied initially, because malignancy is rare.

8. **What is the most feared complication of PUD? What should you suspect if an ulcer does not respond to treatment?**
The most feared complication of PUD is **perforation.** Look for peritoneal signs, history of PUD, and free air on an abdominal radiograph (Fig. 12-2). Treat with antibiotics and laparotomy with repair of the perforation. If ulcers are severe, atypical (e.g., located in the jejunum), or nonhealing, think about stomach cancer or Zollinger-Ellison syndrome *pancreatic* (gastrinoma; check gastrin level). *tumor* PUD is also a cause of GI bleeding, which can be severe in some cases.

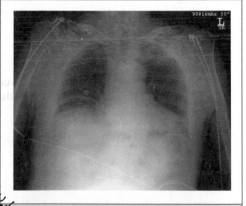

Figure 12-2. This upright chest radiograph of an 80-year-old man with acute onset of severe epigastric pain demonstrates free intra-abdominal air under the right hemidiaphragm. The patient had pneumoperitoneum as a result of a perforated duodenal ulcer. (From Feldman M, Friedman L, Brandt L: Sleisenger and Fordtran's Gastrointestinal and Liver Disease, 8th ed. Philadelphia, Saunders, 2006, Fig. 4-5.)

9. **How is PUD treated initially?**
First, remember that diet changes are not thought to help heal ulcers, although reduced alcohol and tobacco use may speed healing. Start treatment with antacids, histamine-2 receptor blockers, proton-pump inhibitors, and antibiotics to eliminate *Helicobacter pylori*. Many regimens exist, but the most commonly used is triple therapy with a proton pump inhibitor, clarithromycin, and amoxicillin.

10. **List the surgical options for ulcer treatment. What complications may occur?**
    Surgical options may be considered after failure of medical treatment or with complications
    (perforation, bleeding). Commonly performed procedures include antrectomy, vagotomy, and
    Billroth I or II. After surgery (especially with Billroth procedures) watch for dumping syndrome
    (weakness, dizziness, sweating, and nausea or vomiting after eating). Patients also develop
    hypoglycemia 2 to 3 hours after a meal, which causes recurrence of the same symptoms, as well as
    afferent loop syndrome (bilious vomiting after a meal relieves abdominal pain), bacterial
    overgrowth, and vitamin deficiencies (vitamin B_{12} and/or iron, causing anemia).

11. **Define achlorhydria. What causes it?**
    Achlorhydria is an absence of hydrochloric acid (HCl) secretion. It is due most commonly to
    pernicious anemia, in which antiparietal cell antibodies destroy acid-secreting parietal cells
    and thus cause achlorhydria and vitamin B_{12} deficiency. It often is associated with other
    endocrine autoimmune disorders (e.g., hypothyroidism, vitiligo, diabetes, hypoadrenalism).
    Achlorhydria also may be caused by surgical gastric resection.

12. **What are the classic differences between upper and lower gastrointestinal (GI)
    bleeds?**

	Upper GI Bleed	Lower GI Bleed
Location	Proximal to ligament of Treitz	Distal to ligament of Treitz
Common causes	Gastritis, ulcers (Fig. 12-3), varices, esophagitis	Vascular ectasia, diverticulosis, colon cancer, colitis, inflammatory bowel disease, hemorrhoids
Stool	Tarry, black stool (melena)	Bright red blood seen in stool (hematochezia)
NGT aspirate	Positive for blood	Negative for blood
NGT = nasogastric tube.		

*When r/o UGI source - need NG tube c̄ bile
because ⊘ bile doesn't r/o duodenal source.*

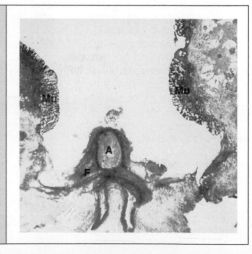

Figure 12-3. Bleeding gastric ulcer. An
eroded artery (A) trapped in the typical
fibrous scar tissue (F) at the base of a
chronic gastric ulcer can result in upper
GI bleeding. Normal gastric mucosa (Mu)
can be seen at the edges of the ulcer
crater. (From Stevens A, et al.: Wheater's
Basic Histopathology, 4th ed. New York,
Churchill Livingstone, 2002, p 140, with
permission.)

13. **How is a GI bleed treated?**
The first step is to *make sure that the patient is stable* (ABCs [airways, breathing, circulation]); intravenous fluids and blood, if needed) before you try to reach a diagnosis. Next, place a nasogastric tube, and test the aspirate for blood to help determine whether the patient has an upper or lower GI bleed. **Endoscopy** is usually the first test performed (upper or lower, depending on symptoms and nasogastric tube aspirate). Endoscopically treatable lesions include ulcers, polyps, vascular ectasias, and varices. EGD (upper)

14. **What radiologic imaging studies can be done to localize a GI bleed? Does surgery have a role?**
Radionuclide (i.e., nuclear medicine) scans can detect slow or intermittent bleeds if a source cannot be found with endoscopy. Angiography can detect more rapid bleeds, and embolization of bleeding vessels can be done during the procedure. Surgery is reserved for severe or resistant bleeds and typically involves resection of the affected bowel (usually colon).

15. **Define diverticulosis. What are its complications?** false diverticula
Diverticulosis is characterized by sac-like mucosal projections through the muscular layer of the colon and/or rectum (Fig. 12-4). It is extremely common, and the incidence increases with age. It is thought to be caused in part by a low-fiber, high-fat diet. Complications include GI bleeding (common cause of painless lower GI bleeds) and diverticulitis (inflammation of a diverticulum), which can lead to abscess, fistula formation, sepsis, or large bowel obstruction.
↳ enterovesicular, enterovaginal usually penetrate near areas where arteries enter the mucosa.

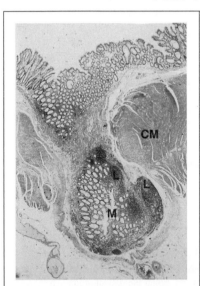

Figure 12-4. Diverticulosis. Herniation of colonic mucosa (M), including mucosal lymphoid tissue (L), occurs through unsupported areas of the inner circular muscle layer (CM, which is characteristically hypertrophied in diverticulosis) that are not supported by the discontinuous outer layer of longitudinal muscle (called teniae coli). (From Stevens A, et al.: Wheater's Basic Histopathology, 4th ed. New York, Churchill Livingstone, 2002, p 153, with permission.)

16. **How do you diagnose and treat diverticulitis? What test should a patient have after a treated episode of diverticulitis?**
Signs and symptoms of diverticulitis include left lower quadrant pain or tenderness, fever, diarrhea or constipation, and increased white blood cell count. The pathophysiology is thought to be similar to appendicitis. Stool or other debris impacts within the diverticulum and causes obstruction, leading to bacterial overgrowth and inflammation. The diagnosis can be confirmed with a CT scan (Fig. 12-5), if needed, which can also help to rule out complications such as

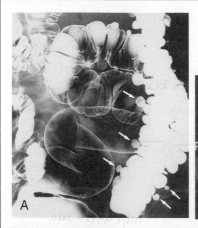
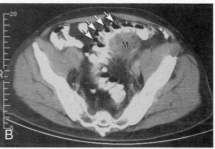

Figure 12-5. Diverticulosis of the colon is seen on this oblique view of the sigmoid colon **(A)** during a double-contrast barium enema showing multiple outpouchings (arrows) that represent diverticula. Diverticula also can be seen in a computed tomography (CT) scan **(B)** as outpouchings (arrows), but a developing focal inflammatory mass (M) also is compatible with a developing abscess. (From Mettler F: Essentials of Radiology, 2nd ed. Philadelphia, Saunders, 2004, Fig. 6-73.)

(Cipro / flagyl)

perforation or abscess. In the absence of complications, the treatment is antibiotics that cover bowel flora (e.g., a fluoroquinolone plus metronidazole) and bowel rest (i.e., no oral intake). Surgery is needed for perforation or abscess.

After a treated episode of diverticulitis, all patients need colon cancer screening with endoscopy or barium enema (colon carcinoma with perforation can mimic diverticulitis clinically and on CT). These studies should be avoided during active diverticulitis, however, due to an increased risk for perforation.

17. **How is diarrhea categorized according to etiology?**
   ■ Systemic*
   ■ Secretory
   ■ Exudative
   ■ Functional
   ■ Osmotic
   ■ Infectious
   ■ Altered intestinal transit
   ■ Malabsorptive

18. **Define osmotic diarrhea. How can an easy diagnosis be made?**
   Osmotic diarrhea is caused by nonabsorbable solutes that remain in the bowel, where they retain water (e.g., lactose or other sugar intolerance). When the patient stops ingesting the offending substance (e.g., avoidance of milk or a trial of not eating), the diarrhea stops—an easy diagnosis.

19. **What causes secretory diarrhea?**
   Secretory diarrhea results when the bowel secretes too much fluid. It is often due to bacterial toxins (cholera, some species of *Escherichia coli*, VIPoma, pancreatic islet cell tumor that

---

*Any illness can cause diarrhea as a systemic symptom, especially in children (e.g., infection).

secretes vasoactive intestinal peptide), or bile acids (after ileal resection). Secretory diarrhea continues when the patient stops eating.

20. **What are the common causes of malabsorptive diarrhea?**

    Celiac sprue (look for dermatitis herpetiformis, and avoid gluten in the diet; Fig. 12-6), Crohn disease, and postgastroenteritis (due to depletion of brush-border enzymes). Malabsorptive diarrhea improves when the patient stops eating.

21. **What are the common clues to infectious diarrhea? What are the common causes?**

    In patients with infectious diarrhea, look for fever and white blood cells in the stool (only with invasive bacteria such as *Shigella, Salmonella, Yersinia,* and *Campylobacter* spp.; not found with toxigenic bacteria). Travel history (Montezuma revenge caused by *E. coli*) is also a tip-off. Hikers and stream-drinkers may have Giardia infection, which presents with

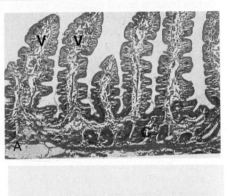

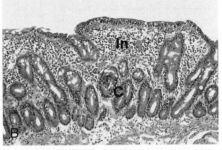

Figure 12-6. Celiac disease. The micrograph **A**, demonstrates normal jejunal mucosa, with villi (V) and short crypts (C). The figure **B**, from a patient with celiac disease, demonstrates infiltration of the mucosa by inflammatory lymphocytes and plasma cells (In), loss of villi/villous atrophy, and hyperplasia/elongation of the crypts (C). The results are a flat, small bowel mucosa and malabsorption. (From Stevens A, et al.: Wheater's Basic Histopathology, 4th ed. New York, Churchill Livingstone, 2002, p 143, with permission.)

steatorrhea (fatty, greasy, malodorous stools that float) due to small bowel involvement and unique protozoal cysts in the stool. Treat with metronidazole. Also watch for *Clostridium difficile* diarrhea in patients with a history of antibiotic use. Test the stool for *C. difficile* toxin, and if the result is positive, treat with metronidazole (vancomycin is a second-line agent if metronidazole is not an option). (Oral)

22. **What causes exudative diarrhea?**

    Exudative diarrhea results from inflammation in the bowel mucosa that causes seepage of fluid. Mucosal inflammation usually is due to inflammatory bowel disease (Crohn disease or ulcerative colitis; see question 27) or cancer. Patients commonly have fever and white blood cells in the stool, as in infectious diarrhea, but lack of pathogenic organisms, chronicity, and nonbowel symptoms are clues.

23. **What are the common causes of diarrhea due to altered intestinal transit?**

    This type of diarrhea is seen after bowel resections, in patients taking medications that interfere with bowel function, and in patients with hyperthyroidism or neuropathy (e.g., diabetic diarrhea). Watch for factitious diarrhea, which is caused by secret laxative abuse.

black colon

24. **Define irritable bowel syndrome. How do you recognize it?**
Irritable bowel syndrome is a common cause of gastrointestinal complaints. Patients may be anxious or neurotic and have a history of diarrhea aggravated by stress; bloating; abdominal pain relieved by defecation; and/or mucous in the stool. Look for psychosocial stressors in the history and normal physical findings and test results. Irritable bowel syndrome is a diagnosis of exclusion; you must do at least basic lab tests, rectal exam, stool exam, and sigmoidoscopy. Because it is so common, however, it is the most likely diagnosis if the question gives no positive findings, especially in young adults (female-to-male ratio = 3:1).

25. **What should you do if a patient has diarrhea?**
In all patients with diarrhea, watch for and treat dehydration and electrolyte disturbances, especially metabolic acidosis and hypokalemia. Diarrhea is a common and preventable cause of death in underdeveloped countries. Do a rectal exam, look for occult blood in stool, and examine the stool for bacteria (Gram stain and culture), ova and parasites, fat content (steatorrhea), and white blood cells.

26. **What should you watch for in children after a bout of diarrhea?**
After bacterial (especially *E. coli* or *Shigella* sp.) diarrhea in children, watch for **hemolytic uremic syndrome,** which is characterized by thrombocytopenia, hemolytic anemia (schistocytes, helmet cells, and fragmented red blood cells on peripheral blood smear), and acute renal failure. Treatment is supportive. Patients may need dialysis and/or transfusions.

27. **Specify the classic differences between Crohn disease and ulcerative colitis.**

	Crohn Disease	Ulcerative Colitis
Place of origin	Distal ileum, proximal colon	Rectum
Thickness of pathology	Transmural	Mucosa/submucosa only
Progression	Irregular (skip-lesions)	Proximal, continuous from rectum; no skipped areas
Location	From mouth to anus	Involves only colon, rarely extends to ileum
Bowel habit changes	Obstruction, abdominal pain	Bloody diarrhea
Classic lesions	Fistulas/abscesses, cobblestoning (Fig. 12-7), string sign on barium x-ray	Pseudopolyps, lead-pipe colon on barium x-ray (Fig. 12-8), toxic megacolon
Colon cancer risk	Slightly increased	Markedly increased
Surgery	No (may make worse)	Yes (proctocolectomy with ileoanal anastomosis)

(surgery always includes the rectum)

28. **Describe the extraintestinal manifestations of inflammatory bowel disease.**
Both forms of inflammatory bowel disease can cause uveitis, arthritis, ankylosing spondylitis, erythema nodosum, erythema multiforme, primary sclerosing cholangitis, failure to thrive or grow in children, toxic megacolon, anemia of chronic disease, and fever. Toxic megacolon is more common in ulcerative colitis; look for markedly distended colon on abdominal radiograph. ＋ signs of sepsis: SRS · HR ⟩90 RR⟩20
T ⟩38 ⟨36
WBC ⟩12,000
⟨4,000
⟩10% bands.

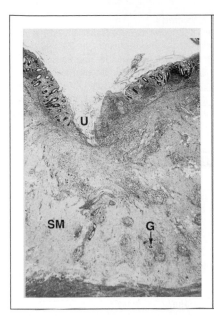

Figure 12-7. Crohn disease. There is gross wall thickening, mainly due to marked edema and inflammation of the submucosa (SM). A typical fissured ulcer (U) and submucosal granuloma (G) are shown. The combination of criss-crossing fissured ulcers and domed areas of mucosal and submucosal edema causes the classic macroscopic "cobblestone" appearance of Crohn disease. (From Stevens A, et al.: Wheater's Basic Histopathology, 4th ed. New York, Churchill Livingstone, 2002, p 146, with permission.)

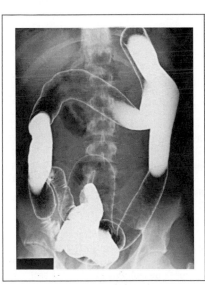

Figure 12-8. A double-contrast barium enema in a patient with long-standing ulcerative colitis demonstrates a marked loss of haustration. The terminal ileum is normal. (From Feldman M, Friedman L, Brandt L: Sleisenger and Fordtran's Gastrointestinal and Liver Disease, 8th ed. Philadelphia, Saunders, 2006, Fig. 109-9.)

29. How is inflammatory bowel disease treated?

Patients are treated with 5-aminosalicylic acid with or without a sulfa drug (e.g., sulfasalazine), when stable. Steroids and other immune modulators (e.g., azathioprine) are used during severe disease flare-ups.

30. **What causes toxic megacolon? How is it treated?**
Toxic megacolon is classically seen with inflammatory bowel disease (especially ulcerative colitis) and infectious (especially *C. difficile*) colitis. It may be precipitated by the use of antidiarrheal medications, which for this reason usually are not given for infectious diarrhea. Most patients have a high fever, leukocytosis, abdominal pain, rebound tenderness, and a dilated segment of colon on abdominal radiograph. Toxic megacolon is an emergency! Start treatment by discontinuing all antidiarrheal medications. Do not allow the patient to eat, place a nasogastric tube, start intravenous fluids, and give antibiotics to cover bowel flora (coverage equivalent to ampicillin, gentamicin, and metronidazole) as well as steroids if the cause is inflammatory bowel disease. Surgery is required if perforation occurs (free air is seen on abdominal radiograph). *amp/gent, flagyl*

31. **List the common findings of acute liver disease.**
- Elevated liver function tests (aspartate aminotransferase [AST], alanine aminotransferase [ALT], bilirubin, alkaline phosphatase, and/or prothrombin time and international normalized ratio [INR])
- Jaundice
- Nausea and vomiting
- Right upper quadrant pain or tenderness
- Hepatomegaly

32. **List the common causes of acute liver disease.**
- Alcohol
- Medications
- Infection (usually hepatitis)
- Reye syndrome
- Biliary tract disease
- Autoimmune disease

33. **What is the classic abnormality on liver function tests in patients with alcoholic hepatitis?**
An elevated AST that is more than twice the value of ALT, although both may be elevated.

34. **What clues suggest hepatitis A? Describe the diagnostic serology.**
Look for outbreaks from a foodborne source. There are no long-term sequelae of infection, although acute liver failure is a remote possibility. IgM antihepatitis A virus (HAV) is positive during jaundice or shortly thereafter. The incubation period for hepatitis A is about 4 weeks, though IgM may be detected by the time symptoms begin.

35. **How is hepatitis B acquired? What is the best treatment?**
Hepatitis B is acquired through needles, sex, or perinatal transmission. Transfused blood is now screened for hepatitis B, but this risk of transmission is still about 1/200,000 according to the American Red Cross. A history of transfusion years ago is still a risk factor (screening by blood banks began in 1972 in the United States). Prevention is the best treatment (vaccination). Interferon alfa-2b, peginterferon alfa-2a, adefovir, dipivoxil, entecavir, telbivudine, or tenofovir can be tried in patients with chronic hepatitis and elevated liver enzymes.

36. **Describe the serology of hepatitis B infection, including the surface, core, and "e" markers.**
The hepatitis B surface antigen (HBsAg) is positive with any unresolved infection (acute or chronic). The hepatitis B "e" antigen (HBeAg) is a marker for infectivity; patients positive for

the hepatitis B "e" antibody (HBeAb) have a low likelihood of spreading disease. The first antibody to appear is the IgM hepatitis B core antibody (HBcAb), which appears during the "window phase" when both HBsAg and hepatitis B surface antibody (HBsAb) are negative. Positive HBsAb means that the patient is immune (as a result of either recovery from infection or vaccination); HBsAb never appears if the patient has chronic hepatitis.

Make sure you know and understand Table 12-1. It is high yield.

TABLE 12-1. SEROLOGIC MARKERS AT DIFFERENT STAGES OF DISEASE

	HBsAg	HBeAg	HBeAb	HBsAb	HBcAb
Incubation	+	+	-	-	-
Acute stage	+	+	-	-	+
Persistent carrier	+	+/-	-/+	-	+
Recovery (immune)	-	-	+	+	+
Immunization	-	-	-	+	-

The presence of HBeAg and anti-HBe depends on degree of infectivity.
Adapted from Cohen J, Powderly WG, Berkley SF, et al.: Infectious diseases, 2nd ed. Edinburgh, Mosby, 2004, p 2015, with permission.

Hep C always to chronic.

37. **What are the possible sequelae of chronic hepatitis B or C?**
Cirrhosis and hepatocellular cancer (only with chronic, not acute, infection).

38. **What should be given to persons acutely exposed to hepatitis B?**
Hepatitis B immunoglobulin and hepatitis B vaccination or hepatitis B vaccination alone have been demonstrated to be effective in preventing transmission after exposure to hepatitis B virus.

39. **Which type of viral hepatitis is the new king of chronic hepatitis?**
Hepatitis C. The hepatitis C virus is the most likely cause of hepatitis after a blood transfusion. Although blood is now screened for hepatitis B and C, the hepatitis C test was developed later (screening in the United States began in 1972 for hepatitis B and 1992 for hepatitis C). Hepatitis C also is more likely than hepatitis B to progress to chronic hepatitis, cirrhosis, and cancer.

40. **Describe the serology and treatment for hepatitis C.**
A positive hepatitis C antibody means that the patient has had an infection in the past but does not mean the infection has been cleared. Many patients become chronic carriers of the virus. A test for hepatitis C virus RNA is available to detect and quantify the virus. Treatment with pegylated interferon alfa and ribavirin is available, though success rates depend on the type of infection. Genotype 1 is the most common in the United States, but treatment success rates are higher with genotypes 2 and 3.

41. **When is hepatitis D seen? Describe the serology.**
Hepatitis D is seen only in patients with hepatitis B. It may become chronic (with hepatitis B coinfection) and is acquired in the same ways as hepatitis B. IgM antibodies to the hepatitis D antigen demonstrate resolution of recent infection. Presence of the hepatitis D antigen, hepatitis D virus RNA, and high levels of IgM antibodies to hepatitis D means chronicity.

42. **How is hepatitis E transmitted? What is special about the infection in pregnant women?**
Hepatitis E is transmitted like hepatitis A (via food and water, no chronic state). It is often fatal in pregnant women (for unknown reasons).

43. **What are the classic causes of drug-induced hepatitis?**
Acetaminophen, isoniazid, and other tuberculosis drugs (e.g., rifampin and pyrazinamide), halothane, HMG CoA-reductase inhibitors, and carbon tetrachloride. The first step in treatment is to stop the drug. *(STATINS)*

44. **When should you suspect idiopathic autoimmune hepatitis? What is the serologic marker?** ANTI-SMOOTH M. ANTIBODY!
Idiopathic autoimmune hepatitis is classically seen in 20- to 40-year-old women with antismooth muscle or antinuclear antibodies and no risk factors or lab markers for other causes of hepatitis. Treat with steroids.

45. **What are the usual causes of chronic liver disease?**
Alcohol, hepatitis, and metabolic diseases. Watch for the stigmata of chronic liver disease: gynecomastia, testicular atrophy, palmar erythema, spider angiomas on skin, and ascites.
(ESTROGEN EFFECT)

46. **Which species of viral hepatitis can lead to chronic liver disease?**
Hepatitis B, C, and D. Hepatitis D can cause infection only in the setting of coexisting hepatitis B (Fig. 12-9).

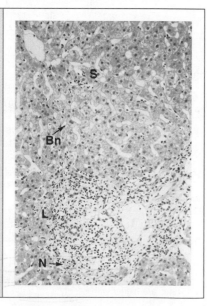

Figure 12-9. Chronic hepatitis. The micrograph shows moderately severe involvement, with inflammation and necrosis (N) that extend out from the portal tract to involve periportal hepatocytes (L). Regeneration of hepatocytes, reflected in binucleate cells (Bn), and areas of "spotty" necrosis (S) in the liver lobule are also present. In the most severe forms of chronic hepatitis, there are confluent bands of inflammation and necrosis that extend between adjacent portal tracts, which is known as bridging necrosis. (From Stevens A, et al.: Wheater's Basic Histopathology, 4th ed. New York, Churchill Livingstone, 2002, p 158, with permission.)

47. **Define hemochromatosis. How do you recognize it?**
Hemochromatosis, in its primary form, is usually autosomal recessive; look for a family history. Nearly 1 in 250 people in the United States are homozygous for this condition, although penetrance and clinical expression are variable. The pathophysiology is incompletely understood but includes excessive iron absorption by the intestine. Excessive iron is deposited in the liver (potentially causing cirrhosis and/or hepatocellular carcinoma), pancreas

Men sx earlier - F lose iron.

(potentially causing diabetes), heart (resulting in dilated cardiomyopathy), skin (causing pigmentation classically known as **bronze diabetes**), and joints (arthritis). Men are symptomatic earlier and more often because women lose iron with menstruation. Treat with phlebotomy. Secondary iron overload can cause secondary hemochromatosis, which is classically due to anemia that results in ineffective erythropoiesis (e.g., thalassemia) and excessive iron intake.

48. **Define Wilson disease. How do you recognize it? How is it treated?**
Wilson disease is an autosomal recessive disease caused by excessive serum copper. Serum **ceruloplasmin** (a copper transport protein) is usually low or absent, but serum copper may be normal. Biopsy shows excessive copper in the liver. Patients classically have liver disease with central nervous system and psychiatric manifestations (due to copper deposits in basal ganglia; another name for this disease is hepatolenticular degeneration) and **Kayser-Fleischer** rings in the eye. Treat with penicillamine (copper chelator).

49. **What are the clues to a diagnosis of alpha$_1$ antitrypsin deficiency?**
The classic description is a young adult who develops cirrhosis and/or emphysema without risk factors for either. Alpha$_1$ antitrypsin deficiency has an autosomal recessive inheritance pattern; look for a positive family history.

50. **What metabolic derangements accompany liver failure?** *Coagulopathy = unable to coagulate.*
Coagulopathy: prolonged prothrombin time. In severe cases, partial thromboplastin time also may be prolonged. Vitamin K does not solve the problem because it cannot be utilized by the damaged liver. Symptomatic patients must be treated with fresh frozen plasma.
Jaundice/hyperbilirubinemia: elevated conjugated and unconjugated bilirubin with hepatic damage (vs. biliary tract disease; see below).
Hypoalbuminemia: the liver synthesizes albumin. *- marker of synthetic fnxn.*
Ascites: due to portal hypertension and/or hypoalbuminemia. Ascites can be detected on physical exam by shifting dullness or a positive fluid wave. A possible complication is **spontaneous bacterial peritonitis** with infected ascitic fluid that can lead to sepsis. Look for fever and/or change in mental status in a patient with known ascites. Do paracentesis, examine the ascitic fluid for elevated white blood cell count (especially neutrophils), and do Gram stain, culture and sensitivity tests, glucose (low with infection), and protein (high with infection). The usual causes are *E. coli, Streptococcus pneumoniae,* and other enteric bugs. Treat with broad-spectrum antibiotics.
Portal hypertension: seen with cirrhosis (chronic liver disease); causes hemorrhoids, varices, and caput medusae (engorged veins on the abdominal wall).
Hyperammonemia: the liver clears ammonia. Treat with decreased protein intake (source of ammonia) and lactulose (prevents absorption of ammonia). The last choice is neomycin, which kills bowel flora that make ammonia.
Hepatic encephalopathy: mostly due to hyperammonemia; often precipitated by protein intake, GI bleed, or infection. Look for asterixis and/or mental status changes.
Hepatorenal syndrome: liver failure may cause kidney failure (idiopathic). *- significant!.*
Hypoglycemia: the liver stores glycogen.
Disseminated intravascular coagulation: activated clotting factors are cleared by the liver.

51. **What signs and symptoms suggest biliary tract obstruction as a cause of jaundice?**
- Markedly elevated alkaline phosphatase
- Elevated conjugated bilirubin. Conjugated bilirubin is more elevated than unconjugated bilirubin because the liver still functions and can conjugate bilirubin, but conjugated bilirubin cannot be excreted because of biliary tract disease.
- Pruritus *- bile salts!.*

- Clay-colored stools
- Dark urine, which is strongly positive for conjugated bilirubin. Unconjugated bilirubin is not excreted in the urine because it is tightly bound to albumin.

52. **What are the commonly tested types of biliary tract obstruction?**
Bile duct obstruction, cholestasis, cholangitis, primary biliary cirrhosis, and primary sclerosing cholangitis. *(anti-mitochondrial ab)*

53. **What are the two major causes of common bile duct obstruction? How are they distinguished?**
The most common cause is obstruction with a gallstone (choledocholithiasis). Look for a history of gallstones or the four Fs (female, forty, fertile, and fat). Ultrasound often images the stone; if not, use magnetic resonance cholangiopancreatography (MRCP) or endoscopic retrograde cholangiopancreatography (ERCP). Treatment is removal of the stone. The second major cause of common bile duct obstruction is cancer. Look for weight loss. Pancreatic cancer is the most common type; look for **Courvoisier sign** (jaundice with a palpably enlarged gallbladder). Sometimes cholangiocarcinoma or bowel cancer blocks the common bile duct.

54. **What are the two common causes of cholestasis?**
Medications (e.g., birth control pills, phenothiazines, androgens) and pregnancy.

55. **What clues suggest a diagnosis of primary biliary cirrhosis?**
This condition usually is seen in middle-aged women with no risk factors for liver or biliary disease. It causes marked pruritus, jaundice, and positive **antimitochondrial antibodies.** The rest of the work-up is negative. Cholestyramine helps with symptoms, but the only treatment is liver transplantation.

56. **Who gets primary sclerosing cholangitis?**
Primary sclerosing cholangitis usually occurs in young adults with inflammatory bowel disease (usually ulcerative colitis). It presents similarly to bacterial cholangitis.

57. **What usually precipitates cholangitis? What is the tip-off to its presence? How is it treated?**
Cholangitis usually is precipitated by a gallstone that blocks the common bile duct with subsequent infection of the bile duct system. The tip-off is the presence of **Charcot triad:** fever, right upper quadrant pain, and jaundice. Treat with antibiotics, and remove gallstones surgically or endoscopically.

58. **What are the classic symptoms of esophageal disease?**
Dysphagia (difficulty in swallowing) and/or odynophagia (painful swallowing). Patients also may have atypical chest pain.

59. **Define achalasia. How is it diagnosed and treated?**
Achalasia is caused by incomplete relaxation of a hypertensive lower esophageal sphincter and loss or derangement of peristalsis. It is usually idiopathic but may be secondary to **Chagas disease** (South America). Patients have intermittent dysphagia for solids and liquids but no heartburn because the lower esophageal sphincter stays tightly closed and does not allow acid reflux. Barium swallow reveals a dilated esophagus with distal "bird-beak" narrowing. The diagnosis often is confirmed with esophageal manometry. Treat with calcium channel blockers, pneumatic balloon dilatation, or botulism toxin injection. Surgery (myotomy) is a last resort. Patients have an increased risk for esophageal carcinoma.

60. **What are the symptoms and signs of esophageal spasm? How is it treated?**
Both diffuse esophageal spasm (Fig. 12-10) and nutcracker esophagus (best thought of as a special variant of esophageal spasm) are characterized by irregular, forceful, and painful esophageal contractions that cause intermittent chest pain. Diagnose with esophageal manometry. Treat with calcium channel blockers and, if needed, surgery (myotomy).

61. **What clues suggest scleroderma as the cause of esophageal complaints?**
Scleroderma may cause aperistalsis due to esophageal fibrosis and atrophy of smooth muscle. The lower esophageal sphincter often becomes incompetent, and many patients have heartburn (opposite of achalasia). Look for positive antinuclear antibody and mask-like facies as well as other autoimmune symptoms. Remember also the **CREST** syndrome, which consist of **c**alcinosis, **R**aynaud phenomenon, **e**sophageal dysmotility, **s**clerodactyly, and **t**elangiectasias.

62. **What do you need to know about the epidemiology of esophageal cancer?**
First, the epidemiology has recently changed, as adenocarcinoma is now more common than squamous cell carcinoma. Squamous cell carcinoma is usually caused by alcohol and tobacco (synergistic effect) and classically is seen in black men over the age of 40 years who smoke and drink alcohol. Patients complain of weight loss and food "sticking" in the chest (solids more than liquids). The tumor is usually in the proximal esophagus. Adenocarcinoma is due to the long standing effects of gastric acid reflux and thus occurs in the distal esophagus.

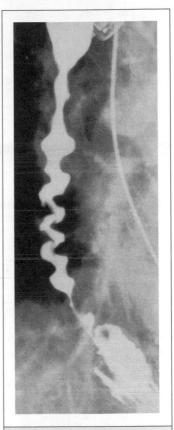

Figure 12-10. Barium esophagogram showing a "corkscrew" esophagus in a patient with diffuse esophageal spasm. The patient had dysphagia and chest pain. Upper endoscopy was normal. (From Feldman M [ed]: Gastroenterology and Hepatology: The Comprehensive Visual Reference. New York, Churchill Livingstone, 1997, with permission.)

63. **What is the relationship between Barrett esophagus and esophageal cancer?**
Barrett esophagus, which usually is caused by long-standing GERD, predisposes to esophageal adenocarcinoma. Barrett esophagus describes a columnar metaplasia of the normally squamous cell esophageal mucosa. Once Barrett esophagus is seen on endoscopy and confirmed with endoscopic biopsy, periodic biopsies must be done to monitor for development of esophageal cancer.

64. **What causes acute pancreatitis?**
More than 80% of cases are due to alcohol or gallstones. Other causes include hypertriglyceridemia, viral infections (mumps, coxsackie virus), trauma, hypercalcemia, peptic ulcer disease, medications (steroids, azathioprine), and, of course, scorpion bites.

65. **What are the signs and symptoms of acute pancreatitis?**
Patients classically have epigastric abdominal pain that radiates to the back, nausea with vomiting that fails to relieve the pain, leukocytosis, and elevated amylase and lipase levels.

Watch for **Grey Turner sign** (blue-black flanks) and **Cullen sign** (blue-black umbilicus), both of which are due to a hemorrhagic pancreatic exudate and indicate severe pancreatitis. Remember that perforated ulcers also are associated with elevated amylase and present similarly. However, patients usually have free air on abdominal radiographs and a history of peptic ulcer disease.

66. **How is acute pancreatitis treated?**
Patients are not allowed to eat, a nasogastric tube often is placed, and intravenous fluids and narcotics are given. For pain control, use meperidine (which has a risk of seizures) or morphine (which causes sphincter of Oddi spasm, though clinical evidence of this is lacking).

67. **What are the complications of acute pancreatitis?** 7 60cm, > 6 wks
Complications include pseudocyst (drain surgically if symptomatic and persistent for several weeks), abscess or infection (treat with antibiotics and drainage if needed), and chronic pancreatitis.

68. **What causes chronic pancreatitis? How is it treated?**
Chronic pancreatitis in the United States is almost always due to alcoholism and usually results from repeated bouts of acute pancreatitis. Gallstones do not cause chronic pancreatitis. Chronic pancreatitis may lead to diabetes, steatorrhea (excessive fat in stool due to lack of pancreatic enzymes), calcification of the pancreas (which may be seen on a plain abdominal radiograph), and fat-soluble vitamin deficiencies (due to malabsorption). The incidence of pancreatic cancer is slightly increased in patients with pancreatitis, although smoking is a greater risk factor than alcohol for pancreatic cancer.
    Treat chronic pancreatitis with alcohol abstinence, oral pancreatic enzyme replacement, and fat-soluble vitamin supplements.

69. **Distinguish between Mallory-Weiss and Boerhaave tears in the esophagus. How are they diagnosed?**
Mallory-Weiss tears are superficial erosions in the esophageal mucosa, whereas Boerhaave tears are full-thickness esophageal ruptures. Both may cause a GI bleed and usually are seen with vomiting and retching (alcoholics and bulimic patients) if they are not iatrogenic (due to endoscopy). Diagnosis usually is made endoscopically (bleeding vessels should be sclerosed) and/or from contrast radiographs. Mallory-Weiss tears usually stop bleeding on their own or with endoscopic treatment, but Boerhaave tears require immediate surgical repair and drainage.

70. **What is the rule about bowel contrast when a GI perforation is suspected?**
For all GI studies, barium is preferred because it provides higher quality images. However, with suspected GI perforation, do not use barium because it can cause chemical peritonitis or mediastinitis when a perforation/leak is present. Instead, use water-soluble contrast (e.g., Gastrografin). Things get tricky in patients with a significant risk for aspiration, because the lungs tolerate barium well but develop chemical pneumonitis from water-soluble contrast. When in doubt, give water-soluble contrast, followed by barium once perforation has been excluded.

71. **Which GI malformations are common in children? How can they be distinguished?**

Name	Presenting Age	Vomit Description	Findings/Key Words
Pyloric stenosis	0–3 mo	Nonbilious, projectile	Males >> females; palpable olive-shaped mass in epigastrium; low Cl/low K metabolic alkalosis

(continued)

Name	Presenting Age	Vomit Description	Findings/Key Words
Intestinal atresia *— multiple air fluid levels.*	0–1 wk	Bilious	"Double-bubble" sign, Down syndrome
TE fistula*	0–2 wk	Food regurgitation	Respiratory compromise with feeding, aspiration pneumonia, inability to pass nasogastric tube into stomach, gastric distention (from air)
Hirschsprung's disease *biopsy the narrowed segment (aganglionic)*	0–1 yr	Feculent	Abdominal distention, obstipation, no nerve ganglia seen on rectal biopsy; males >> females
Anal atresia *VACTERL*	0–1 wk	Late, feculent	Detected on initial exam in nursery; males > females
Choanal atresia	0–1 wk	—	Cyanosis with feeding, relieved by crying; inability to pass nasogastric tube through nose

Cl = chloride; K = potassium; TE = tracheoesophageal.
*The most common variant (85% of cases) has esophageal atresia with a fistula from the bronchus to the distal esophagus. The result is gastric distention, as each breath transmits air to the GI tract. Be able to recognize a sketch of this most common variant.

Treat each of the above conditions with **surgical repair.**

72. **What other pediatric GI conditions are commonly found on the Step 2 boards? How are they distinguished?**

Name	Presenting Age	Vomit Description	Findings/Key Words
Intussusception *Colicky ap* *Eperiods of — curl up into ball + then remission.* *calm.*	3 mo to 2 yrs	Bilious	Currant-jelly stools (<u>blood and mucous</u>), palpable sausage-shaped mass; treat with x-ray air enema (diagnostic and therapeutic)
Necrotizing enterocolitis	0–2 mo	Bilious	Premature baby, fever, rectal bleeding, air in bowel wall, treat with NPO,

Pneumointestinalis. (continued)

Name	Presenting Age	Vomit Description	Findings/Key Words
			orogastric tube, IV fluids, and antibiotics
Meconium ileus	0–1 wk	Feculent, late	Cystic fibrosis manifestation (as is rectal prolapse)
Midgut volvulus	0–2 yrs	Bilious	Sudden onset of pain, distention, rectal bleeding, peritonitis, "bird's beak" on abdominal radiograph; treat with surgery
Meckel's diverticulum	0–2 yrs	Varies	Rule of 2s*; GI ulceration/bleeding; use Meckel scan to detect; treat with surgery
Strangulated hernia	Any age	Bilious	Physical exam detects bowel loops in inguinal canal

NPO = nothing by mouth (no feedings); IV = intravenous.
*Rule of 2s for Meckel diverticulum: 2% of population affected (most common GI tract abnormality; remnant of omphalomesenteric duct), 2 inches long, within 2 feet of ileocolic junction, presents in the first 2 years of life. Meckel diverticulum can cause intussusception, obstruction, or volvulus.

73. **Which GI malformation causes primarily respiratory problems?**
    Diaphragmatic hernia, which is more common in males. Ninety percent are on the left side. The main point to know is that bowel herniates into the thorax through the diaphragmatic defect, compressing the lung and impeding lung development (pulmonary hypoplasia develops). Patients present with respiratory distress and have bowel sounds in the chest and bowel loops in the thorax on chest radiographs (Fig. 12-11). Treat with surgical correction of the diaphragm.

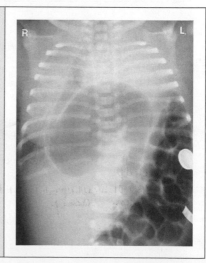

Figure 12-11. Diaphragmatic hernia shown in a newborn with significant respiratory difficulty. An anteroposterior (AP) view of the chest and abdomen demonstrates opacification of the left hemithorax, with bowel loops pushing up into the opacified left hemithorax. This condition carries a high fatality rate and should be recognized immediately. (From Mettler F: Essentials of Radiology, 2nd ed. Philadelphia, Saunders, 2004, Fig. 9-13.)

74. **How are omphalocele and gastroschisis differentiated?**

An **omphalocele** is in the midline, the sac contains multiple abdominal organs, the umbilical ring is absent, and other anomalies are common. **Gastroschisis** is to the right of the midline, only small bowel is exposed (no true hernia sac), the umbilical ring is present, and other anomalies are rare.

75. **What is Henoch-Schönlein purpura? Why is it mentioned in the GI section?**

Henoch-Schönlein purpura is a vasculitis that may present with GI bleeding and abdominal pain. Look for a history of upper respiratory infection, characteristic rash on lower extremities and buttocks, swelling in hands and feet, arthritis, and/or hematuria and proteinuria. Treat supportively.

76. **What is the most common cause of diarrhea in children?**

As a primary cause, probably viral gastroenteritis (Norwalk virus). Remember, however, that diarrhea often is a nonspecific sign of any systemic illness.

77. **True or false: Children may develop inflammatory bowel disease and irritable bowel syndrome.**

True. GI complaints may be due to anxiety or psychiatric problems. Watch for separation anxiety, children who do not want to go to school, depression, and child abuse. Abdominal pain may be the result of inflammatory bowel disease or irritable bowel syndrome. Diarrhea, fever, bloody stools, anemia, joint pains, and poor growth are more concerning for inflammatory bowel disease.

78. **What is the first step in evaluating neonatal jaundice? Why is jaundice of concern in a neonate?**

The first step is to determine whether the jaundice is physiologic or pathologic. Measure total, direct, and indirect bilirubin. The main concern is **kernicterus,** which is due to high levels of unconjugated bilirubin with subsequent deposit in the basal ganglia. Look for poor feeding, seizures, flaccidity, opisthotonos, and apnea in the setting of severe jaundice.

79. **What causes physiologic jaundice of the newborn? Who gets it?**

Fifty percent of normal infants have physiologic jaundice, and it is even more common in premature infants. Bilirubin is mostly unconjugated because of incomplete maturation of liver function. In full-term infants, bilirubin is less than 12 mg/dl , peaks at day 2 to 4, and returns to normal by 2 weeks. In premature infants, bilirubin is less than 15 mg/dL, peaks at 3 to 5 days, and may be elevated for up to 3 weeks.

80. **How is pathologic jaundice recognized? What are the causes?**

In pathologic jaundice, bilirubin levels go higher than those mentioned above and continue to rise or fail to decrease appropriately. *Any* **jaundice present at birth is pathologic.** Causes include the following:

Breast milk jaundice: breast-fed infants with peak bilirubin levels of 10 to 20 mg/dL at 2 to 3 weeks of age. Treat with temporary cessation of breast feeding (switch to bottle) until jaundice resolves.

Illness: infection or sepsis, hypothyroidism, liver insult, cystic fibrosis, and other illnesses may prolong neonatal jaundice and lower the threshold for kernicterus. The youngest, sickest infants are at greatest risk for hyperbilirubinemia and kernicterus.

Hemolysis: from Rhesus (Rh) incompatibility or congenital red cell diseases that cause hemolysis in the neonatal period. Look for anemia, peripheral smear abnormalities, positive family history, and higher levels of unconjugated bilirubin.

Metabolic disorders: Crigler-Najjar syndrome causes severe unconjugated hyperbilirubinemia, whereas Gilbert's syndrome causes a mild form. Rotor and Dubin-Johnson syndromes cause conjugated hyperbilirubinemia.

Biliary atresia: full-term infants with clay- or gray-colored stools and high levels of conjugated bilirubin. Treat with surgery.

Medications: avoid sulfa drugs in neonates; they displace bilirubin from albumin and may precipitate kernicterus.

81. **How is pathologic jaundice treated?**

    Unconjugated hyperbilirubinemia that persists, rises above 15 mg/dL, or rises rapidly is treated with **phototherapy** to convert unconjugated bilirubin to a water-soluble form that can be excreted. A last resort is exchange transfusion, but don't even think about it unless the level of unconjugated bilirubin is greater than 20 mg/dL.

82. **What should you do if an infant is born to a mother with active hepatitis B?**

    An infant born to a mother with active hepatitis B should receive the first immunization shot and hepatitis B immune globulin at birth.

CHAPTER 13

GENERAL SURGERY

1. **Define the acute abdomen. What physical exam signs suggest its presence?**
   Acute abdomen generally refers to an inflamed peritoneum (peritonitis), which is often
   due to a surgically correctable problem. Patients with an acute abdomen often receive a
   laparotomy and/or laparoscopy because it signifies a potentially life-threatening
   condition. The best physical exam confirmations of peritonitis are **rebound tenderness** and
   involuntary guarding. Rebound tenderness is elicited by letting go quickly after deep
   palpation of the abdomen; acute pain occurs in the area of palpation (with generalized
   peritonitis) or at the location of localized inflammation (e.g., Rovsing sign in appendicitis).
   Involuntary guarding describes abdominal wall muscle spasm that cannot be controlled.
   Voluntary guarding (person reflexively or willfully tenses their abdomen during
   attempted palpation) and tenderness to palpations are softer signs often present in
   benign diseases.

2. **What should you do if you are not sure whether a stable patient has an acute
   abdomen?**
   When you are in doubt and the patient is stable, use minimal as needed pain medications (to avoid
   masking symptoms before you have a diagnosis), perform serial abdominal exams and consider
   CT scan. If the patient becomes unstable, proceed to laparoscopy and/or laparotomy.

3. **Name a few causes of peritonitis that do not require laparotomy or
   laparoscopy.**
   Pancreatitis, many cases of diverticulitis, and spontaneous bacterial peritonitis.

4. **Specify which conditions are associated with pain and peritonitis in the listed
   abdominal areas.**

Area	Organ (Conditions)
Upper right quadrant	Gallbladder/biliary (cholecystitis, cholangitis) or liver (abscess)
Upper left quadrant	Spleen (rupture with blunt trauma)
Lower right quadrant	Appendix (appendicitis), pelvic inflammatory disease (PID)
Left lower quadrant	Sigmoid colon (diverticulitis), pelvic inflammatory disease (PID)
Epigastric area	Stomach (peptic ulcer) or pancreas (pancreatitis)

5. **What are the classic symptoms and signs of gallstone disease?**
   Classic gallstone symptoms include postprandial, colicky pain in the right upper quadrant
   with bloating and/or nausea and vomiting. The pain usually begins 15 to 60 minutes after a
   meal (especially a fatty meal). Look for **Murphy sign** (palpation of the right upper quadrant
   under the rib cage causes arrest of inspiration due to pain) as the main physical exam finding
   for cholecystitis.

6. **What are the six Fs of cholecystitis? How are the demographics of patients with pigment stones different from those with cholesterol stones?**

   The first five Fs summarize the demographics of people with cholesterol gallstones: fat, forty, fertile, female, and flatulent; the sixth F is febrile, which indicates that such patients have now developed acute cholecystitis. Patients with pigment (i.e., calcium bilirubinate) stones are classically young patients with hemolytic anemia (e.g., sickle cell disease, hereditary spherocytosis).

7. **How is a clinical suspicion of cholecystitis confirmed and treated?**

   Ultrasound is the best first imaging study for suspected gallbladder disease (Fig. 13-1). It may show gallstones, a thin layer of fluid around the gallbladder, and/or a thickened gallbladder wall. A more specific ultrasonographic Murphy sign using direct visualization of the gallbladder can be obtained (variant anatomy and significant obesity can create uncertainty). A nuclear hepatobiliary scintigraphic study (e.g., hepato-iminodiacetic acid [HIDA] scan) clinches the diagnosis with nonvisualization of the gallbladder (Fig. 13-2). The treatment is cholecystectomy; a laparoscopic approach is generally preferred over an open procedure.

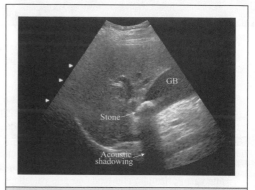

Figure 13-1. Typical ultrasonographic appearance of cholelithiasis. A gallstone is present within the lumen of the gallbladder (GB), casting an acoustic shadow. If the patient is repositioned, the stones will move, thereby excluding the possibility of a gallbladder polyp. (From Feldman M, Friedman L, Brandt L: Sleisenger and Fordtran's Gastrointestinal and Liver Disease, 8th ed. Philadelphia, Saunders, 2006, Fig. 62-6A.)

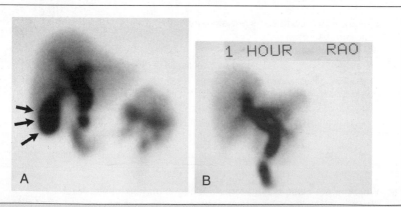

Figure 13-2. A, Normal HIDA scan. The gallbladder has filled with radionuclide *(arrows).* **B,** Acute cholecystitis. The common duct and a portion of the duodenum have filled with radionuclide, but the gallbladder does not fill despite the administration of morphine. (From Katz DS, Math KR, Groskin SA, eds: Radiology Secrets. Philadelphia, Hanley & Belfus, 1998, p 145, with permission.)

8. **Define cholangitis. How does it differ from cholecystitis? How is it treated?**
   Cholangitis is an inflammation of the bile ducts, whereas cholecystitis is an inflammation of the gallbladder. Cholangitis is classically due to biliary obstruction with subsequent bile stasis and infection. Choledocholithiasis (a gallstone in the common bile duct) and malignancy are common causes of obstruction. Autoimmune cholangitis (e.g., sclerosing cholangitis) and primary infection (e.g., *Clonorchis sinensis* and other parasite infections common in some parts of Asia) are other causes. Cholangitis classically presents with **Charcot triad:** (1) right upper quadrant pain, (2) fever or shaking chills, and (3) jaundice. Patients may have a history of gallstones. Start broad-spectrum antibiotics to cover bowel flora (e.g., piperacillin with tazobactam), then manage more definitively depending on the circumstances (e.g., cholecystectomy with evacuation of any common duct stones for gallstone disease, biliary stent placement for unresectable malignant obstruction).

9. **Describe the classic presentation of appendicitis. How is it treated?**
   Appendicitis classically presents in 10- to 30-year-olds with a history of crampy, poorly localized periumbilical pain followed by nausea and vomiting. Then the pain localizes to the right lower quadrant, and peritoneal signs develop with worsening of nausea and vomiting. It is said that a patient who is hungry and asking for food does not have appendicitis (called the "hamburger" sign). A classic clue to the diagnosis is **Rovsing sign:** when you palpate a different quadrant and then quickly release your hand, the patient feels pain at McBurney point (two-thirds of the way from the umbilicus to the anterior superior iliac spine). McBurney point is the area of maximal tenderness in the right lower quadrant and the site where a typical appendectomy incision (the treatment of choice) is made. CT is increasingly used to confirm the diagnosis before surgery in stable patients (Fig. 13-3).

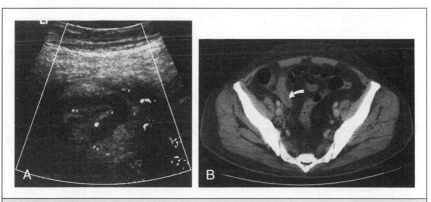

Figure 13-3. Appendicitis. **A,** Ultrasound shows a thickened hypoechoic tubular blind-ended structure in the right iliac fossa. The surrounding fat is hyperechoic. **B,** CT scan shows the thickened inflamed appendix (*arrow*). (Courtesy of Dr A. McLean, St Bartholomew's Hospital, London.)

10. **What is the cause of left lower quadrant pain and fever in a patient over 50 years old until proved otherwise? How is it treated?**
    Diverticulitis. Treat medically with broad-spectrum antibiotics, avoidance of eating, and a nasogastric tube if nausea and vomiting are present. For disease that recurs or is refractory to medical therapy, consider sigmoid colon resection.

11. **What tests should and should not be done to confirm possible cases of diverticulitis? What test does every patient need after a treated episode of diverticulitis?**

    Colonoscopy should not be performed in the acute setting, because colon rupture may occur; barium enema is also avoided for the same reason. However, one of these tests should be done in every patient after treatment to exclude colon carcinoma. Order a CT scan, if necessary, to confirm a diagnosis of diverticulitis (Fig. 13-4).

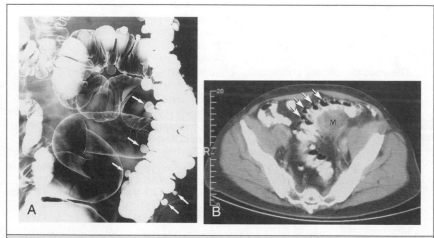

Figure 13-4. Diverticulosis of the colon is seen on this oblique view of the sigmoid colon (**A**) during a double-contrast barium enema showing multiple outpouchings (*arrows*) that represent diverticula. Diverticula also can be seen in a computed tomography (CT) scan (**B**) as outpouchings (*arrows*), but a developing focal inflammatory mass (M) also is compatible with a developing abscess. (From Mettler F: Essentials of Radiology, 2nd ed. Philadelphia, Saunders, 2004, Fig. 6-73.)

12. **Describe the typical history, physical exam and lab findings of pancreatitis. How is it treated?**

    Look for epigastric pain that radiates to the back in an alcohol abuser or a patient with a history of (or risk factors for) gallstones. Serum amylase and/or lipase should be elevated. If these values are not given, order them! Other common signs include decreased bowel sounds, localized ileus ("sentinel" loop of bowel on abdominal radiograph) and nausea, vomiting, and/or anorexia.

    Treat pancreatitis supportively; narcotics are often needed for pain control; meperidine, which has a risk of seizures, has traditionally been favored over morphine because of the concern about sphincter of Oddi spasm, though clinical evidence of this is lacking. Fentanyl is another option. Do not feed the patient initially; place a nasogastric tube as needed for nausea and vomiting; and give intravenous fluids as well as other needed supportive care. Watch for the complications of pseudocyst and pancreatic abscess, both of which can be diagnosed by CT scan and may require surgical intervention.

13. **Describe the usual history of a perforated ulcer. How is it treated?**

    Patients often have no history of alcohol abuse or gallstones (pancreatitis risk factors). Abdominal radiographs classically show free air under the diaphragm, and a history of peptic ulcer disease often is included in the patient description. Remember that a perforated bowel can cause an increased amylase level. Treat with surgery.

14. **What are the hallmarks of small bowel obstruction? How is it treated?**

Small bowel obstruction commonly causes bilious vomiting (early symptom), abdominal distention, constipation, hyperactive bowel sounds (high-pitched, rushing sounds), and usually poorly localized abdominal pain. Radiographs show multiple air-fluid levels. Patients often have a history of previous surgery.

Start treatment by withholding food, placing a nasogastric tube, and giving intravenous fluids. If the obstruction does not resolve or if peritoneal signs develop, laparotomy is usually needed. CT scanning can confirm an uncertain diagnosis in stable patients and may reveal the underlying cause of obstruction.

15. **What are the common causes of a small bowel obstruction?**

In adults, the most common cause is **adhesions,** which usually develop from prior surgery. Incarcerated hernias and Crohn disease are other common causes. Other causes include Meckel diverticulum and intussusception (both typically seen in children).

16. **Describe the signs and symptoms of large bowel obstruction. What causes it? How is it treated?**

Large bowel obstruction usually presents with gradually increasing abdominal pain, abdominal distention, constipation, and feculent vomiting (late symptom). In older adults, the most common causes are diverticulitis, colon cancer, and volvulus. In children, watch for Hirschsprung disease. Treat early by withholding food and placing a nasogastric tube for nausea and vomiting. Sigmoid volvulus (Figs. 13-5 and 13-6) often can be decompressed with an endoscope. Other causes or refractory cases require surgery to relieve the obstruction.

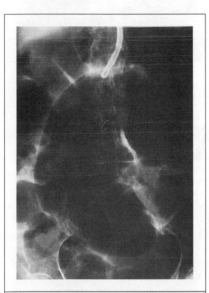

Figure 13-5. This plain film of the abdomen shows a large, dilated loop which is characteristic of sigmoid volvulus. (From Marx J, Hockberger R, Walls R: Rosen's Emergency Medicine: Concepts and Clinical Practice, 6th ed. Philadelphia, Mosby, 2006, Fig. 94-2.)

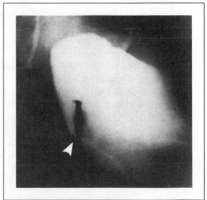

Figure 13-6. This barium enema shows the characteristic "bird's beak" sign of volvulus. (From Marx J, Hockberger R, Walls R: Rosen's Emergency Medicine: Concepts and Clinical Practice, 6th ed. Philadelphia, Mosby, 2006, Fig. 94-3.)

17. **List and differentiate the three common types of groin hernias.**
    1. **Indirect hernias** are the most common type in both sexes and all age groups. The hernia sac travels through the inner and outer inguinal rings (protrusion begins lateral to the inferior epigastric vessels) and into the scrotum or labia because of a patent processus vaginalis (congenital defect).
    2. **Direct hernias** (no sac) protrude medial to the inferior epigastric vessels because of weakness in the abdominal musculature of Hesselbach's triangle.
    3. **Femoral hernias** are more common in women. The hernia (no sac) goes through the femoral ring onto the anterior thigh (located below the inguinal ring).

    Of the three types, femoral hernias are the most susceptible to incarceration and strangulation. All three types are treated with elective surgical repair if symptomatic.

18. **Define incarcerated and strangulated hernias.**
    Incarceration occurs when a herniated organ is trapped and becomes swollen and edematous. Incarcerated hernias are the most common cause of small bowel obstruction in patients who have had no previous abdominal surgery and the second most common cause in patients who have had previous abdominal surgery (Fig. 13-7). Treatment is prompt surgery.

    Strangulation occurs after incarceration when the entrapment becomes so severe that the blood supply is cut off. Strangulation can lead to necrosis and is a surgical emergency. Patients may present with symptoms of small bowel obstruction and shock.

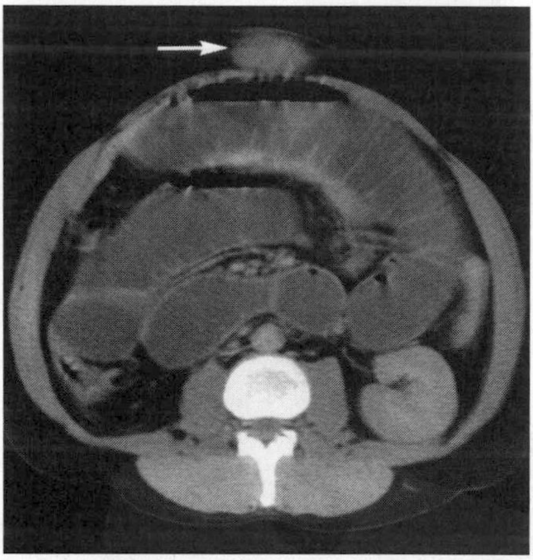

Figure 13-7. Small intestinal obstruction. A section through the mid-abdomen from a CT scan shows dilated, mainly fluid-filled, small intestinal loops. The obstruction was due to an incarcerated paraumbilical hernia, the edge of which can be identified (*arrow*). (From Adam A, et al.: Grainger & Allison's Diagnostic Radiology, 5th ed. Edinburgh, Churchill Livingstone, 2008, Fig. 32-37.)

19. **True or false: Generally, patients should not eat or drink for 8 or more hours before surgery.**
    True. This protocol reduces the chance of aspiration and subsequent pneumonia.

20. **What is the best test (other than a good history) for preoperative evaluation of pulmonary function?**
    Spirometry, which gives functional vital capacity, forced expiratory volumes, and maximal voluntary ventilation. A good history (e.g., activity level, exercise tolerance) is also useful.

21. **What measures help to prevent intraoperative and postoperative deep venous thrombosis and pulmonary embolus?**
    Compressive/elastic stockings, early ambulation, and/or low-dose heparins (unfractionated or low molecular weight).

22. **What is the most common cause of fever in the first 24 hours after surgery?**
Atelectasis. Prevent and treat atelectasis with early ambulation, chest physiotherapy/percussion, incentive spirometry, and proper pain control. Both too much pain and too many narcotics (both can decrease respiratory effort) increase the risk of atelectasis.

23. **What are the other common causes of postoperative fever?**
The five Ws—**w**ater, **w**ind, **w**alk, **w**ound, and **w**eird drugs—summarize the common causes of postoperative fever. Water stands for urinary tract infection, wind for atelectasis and pneumonia, walk for deep venous thrombosis, wound for surgical wound infection, and weird drugs for drug fever. In patients with daily fever spikes that do not respond to antibiotics, think about an intraabdominal abscess. Order a CT scan to locate, then drain the abscess if one is present.

24. **Define fascial or wound dehiscence. How do you recognize it?**
Fascial or wound dehiscence occurs when the surgical wound opens spontaneously, usually 5 to 10 days postoperatively. Look for leakage of serosanguineous fluid from the wound, particularly after the patient coughs or strains. Frequently the wound is infected. Surgical reclosure of the wound and treatment of infection are required.

25. **Explain the ABCDEs of trauma. How are they used?**
The ABCDEs of trauma are **a**irway, **b**reathing, **c**irculation, **d**isability, and **e**xposure. They are the keys to the initial management of trauma patients. Follow them in order if simultaneous management is not possible. For example, if a patient is bleeding to death and has a blocked airway, address airway management first.

26. **What is the difference between airway and breathing in trauma protocol?**
Airway means provision, protection, and maintenance of an adequate airway at all times. If the patient can answer questions, the airway is fine. You can use an oropharyngeal airway in uncomplicated cases and give supplemental oxygen. When you are in doubt or the patient's airway is blocked, intubate. If intubation fails, do a cricothyroidotomy.

   Breathing is similar to airway, but even patients with an open airway may not be breathing spontaneously. The end result is the same. When you are in doubt or the patient is not breathing, intubate. If intubation fails, do a cricothyroidotomy.

27. **Explain circulation, disability, and exposure.**
Circulation refers to circulating blood volume. For practical purposes, it means that if the patient seems hypovolemic (tachycardic, bleeding, weak pulse, pale, diaphoretic, capillary refill more than 2 seconds), give intravenous fluids and/or blood products. Initially you should start two large-bore intravenous lines and give a bolus of 10 to 20 mL/kg (roughly 1 L) of lactated Ringer solution or normal saline. Then reassess the patient after the bolus for improvement. Repeat the bolus, if needed.

   Disability refers to the need to check neurologic function. In practical terms, this need translates into doing a Glasgow coma scale assessment.

   Exposure reminds you to expose and examine the entire body. In other words, remove all of the patient's clothes and "put a finger in every orifice" so that you do not miss any occult injuries.

28. **What imaging films are routinely ordered for most patients with at least moderately severe trauma?**
Cervical spine, chest, and pelvic radiographs.

29. **What is the imaging study of choice for head trauma?**
Noncontrast CT (better than magnetic resonance imaging for acute trauma).

30. **How do you manage a patient with blunt abdominal trauma?**

In patients with blunt abdominal trauma, the initial findings determine the appropriate course of action. If the patient is awake and stable and your examination is "benign," observe the patient and repeat the abdominal exam later. If the patient is hemodynamically unstable (hypotension and/or shock that does not respond to fluid challenge), proceed directly to laparotomy. Patients between these two extremes typically get a CT scan with oral and IV contrast for further evaluation (Fig. 13-8).

31. **How is penetrating abdominal trauma managed?**

In patients with penetrating abdominal trauma (i.e., gunshot, stab wound), the type of injury and the initial findings determine the course of action. With any gunshot wound that may have violated the peritoneal cavity, proceed directly to laparotomy. With a wound from a sharp instrument, management is more controversial. Either proceed directly to laparotomy (your best choice if the patient is unstable) or perform CT scan if the patient is stable. With nonoperative management, perform serial abdominal exams.

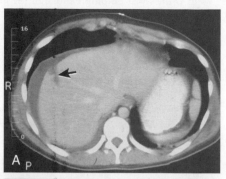

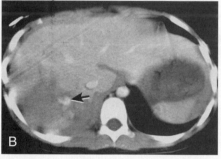

Figure 13-8. Small and large hepatic lacerations. **A,** A computed tomography (CT) scan was obtained through the upper abdomen in this patient after a motor vehicle accident. A small area of low density (*arrow*) is seen in the lateral portion of the right lobe, and blood surrounds the liver. **B,** A CT scan in another patient after a motor vehicle accident shows a much larger area of lacerated liver in the posterior aspect of the right lobe. A central area of increased density (the white area at the *tip of the arrow*) indicates acute hemorrhaging at the time of the scan. (From Mettler F: Essentials of Radiology, 2nd ed. Philadelphia, Saunders, 2004, Fig. 6-47.)

32. **Which six thoracic injuries can be rapidly fatal?**
    1. Airway obstruction
    2. Open pneumothorax
    3. Tension pneumothorax
    4. Cardiac tamponade
    5. Massive hemothorax
    6. Flail chest

    You may be asked to recognize and/or treat any of these six conditions on the USMLE.

33. **How do you recognize and treat airway obstruction?**
Patients with airway obstruction have no audible breath sounds, cannot answer questions even if awake, and may be gurgling. Treat with intubation. If intubation fails, do a cricothyroidotomy (or a tracheostomy in the operating room if time allows).

34. **How do you recognize and treat an open pneumothorax?**
An open pneumothorax presents with an open defect in the chest wall and decreased or absent breath sounds on the affected side. This condition causes poor ventilation and oxygenation. Treat with intubation, positive-pressure ventilation, and closure of the defect in the chest wall. To close the defect, use gauze and tape it on three sides only. This approach allows excessive pressure to escape so that you do not convert an open pneumothorax into a tension pneumothorax.

35. **How do you recognize and treat a tension pneumothorax?**
A tension pneumothorax may occur after blunt or penetrating trauma to the chest. Air forced into the pleural space cannot escape and collapses the affected lung, then shifts the mediastinum and trachea to the opposite side of the chest (Fig. 13-9). Findings include absent breath sounds on the affected side and a hypertympanic percussion sound. Hypotension and/or distended neck veins may result from impaired cardiac filling. Treat with needle thoracentesis, followed by insertion of a chest tube.

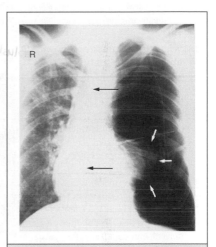

Figure 13-9. Tension pneumothorax. On a posteroanterior chest x-ray, the left hemithorax is very dark or lucent because the left lung has collapsed completely (*white arrows*). The tension pneumothorax can be identified because the mediastinal contents, including the heart, are shifted toward the right, and the left hemidiaphragm is flattened and depressed. (From Mettler F: Essentials of Radiology, 2nd ed. Philadelphia, Saunders, 2004, Fig. 3-72.)

36. **Describe the usual presentation of cardiac tamponade. How is it diagnosed and treated?**
Cardiac tamponade classically is associated with penetrating trauma to the left chest. Patients have hypotension (due to impaired cardiac filling), distended neck veins, muffled heart sounds, **pulsus paradoxus** (exaggerated fall in blood pressure on inspiration), and normal breath sounds. If the patient is unstable, treat with pericardiocentesis; put a catheter through the skin and into the pericardial sac and aspirate blood and fluid. If the patient is stable, you can first do an echocardiogram to confirm the diagnosis.

37. **Define massive hemothorax. How is it diagnosed and treated?**
Massive hemothorax is defined as a loss of more than 1 liter of blood into the thoracic cavity. Patients have decreased (not absent) breath sounds in the affected area, dull note on percussion, hypotension, collapsed neck veins (from blood leaving the vascular tree), and tachycardia. Placement of a chest tube allows the blood to come out. Give intravenous fluids and/or blood before you place the chest tube if the diagnosis is known in advance. If the bleeding stops after the initial outflow, order a chest radiograph or CT scan to check for remaining blood or pathology. Treat supportively. Treatment is emergent thoracotomy if the bleeding does not stop.

prevent empyema c̄ stagnant blood.

38. How do you recognize and treat flail chest?

Flail chest occurs when several adjacent ribs are broken in multiple places, causing the affected part of the chest wall to move paradoxically during respiration (inward during inspiration, outward during expiration). Almost all patients have an associated pulmonary contusion, which, combined with pain, may make respiration inadequate. When you are in doubt or the patient is not doing well, intubate and give positive pressure ventilation.

39. What is the most common cause of immediate death after an automobile accident or a fall from a great height?

Aortic rupture. Look for a widened mediastinum on chest radiograph and an appropriate history of trauma. Order a CT scan or angiogram if a contained aortic rupture (of those who survive to be admitted to the hospital, 50% will die in the first 24 hours) is suspected. Aortic laceration, traumatic aortic injury and traumatic pseudoaneurysm all pretty much describe the phenomenon seen in initial survivors: an aortic rupture contained by a hematoma or an inadequate amount of surrounding tissue (e.g., adventitia only). Treat with immediate surgical repair.

40. What do you need to know about splenic rupture?

Blushing on spleen CT.

The spleen is the most commonly injured organ in blunt trauma (Fig. 13-10). Patients with splenic rupture, the most severe form of injury, have a history of blunt abdominal trauma, hypotension, tachycardia, shock, and/or **Kehr sign** (referred pain in the left shoulder). Patients with Epstein-Barr virus infection or infectious mononucleosis and splenomegaly should avoid contact sports to prevent rupture. Make sure patients needing splenectomy have received the pneumococcal, meningococcal, and *H. influenzae* (i.e., encapsulated bugs) vaccines.

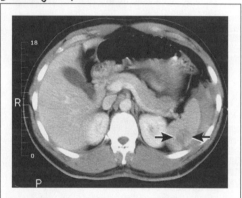

Figure 13-10. Splenic laceration. This computed tomography (CT) scan done on a patient after a motor vehicle accident shows a dark area near the posterior aspect of the spleen (*arrows*), which is the laceration. Note also the blood surrounding the spleen. (From Mettler F: Essentials of Radiology, 2nd ed. Philadelphia, Saunders, 2004, Fig. 6-60.)

41. What clues suggest a diagnosis of diaphragmatic rupture? How is it treated?

Diaphragm rupture usually occurs after blunt trauma and on the left side (because the liver protects the right side of the diaphragm). You may hear bowel sounds when listening to the chest or see bowel that has herniated into the chest on chest radiograph. Treatment is surgical repair of the diaphragm.

42. What are the three zones of the neck? How is trauma in each of the different zones managed?

Zone I is the base of the neck from 2 cm above the clavicles to the level of the clavicles.

Zone II is the midcervical region from 2 cm above the clavicle to the angle of the mandible.

Zone III is the top of the neck from the angle of the mandible to the base of the skull.

With zone I and III injuries, you generally should order an arteriogram before going to the operating room. With zone II injuries, proceed to the operating room for surgical exploration without an arteriogram. In patients with obvious bleeding or a rapidly expanding hematoma in the neck, proceed directly to operating room, no matter where the injury is.

43. **How should a choking victim be managed?**
Always leave choking patients alone if they are speaking, coughing, or breathing. If they stop doing all of these, perform the Heimlich maneuver.

44. **What should you do if a tooth is knocked out?**
Put the tooth back in place with no cleaning (or only saline to rinse it off) and stabilize the tooth in place. The sooner this is done, the better the prognosis for salvage of the tooth.

CHAPTER 14

GENETICS

1. Specify how the following disorders are *usually* transmitted genetically. The choices are autosomal dominant or recessive, X-linked recessive, chromosomal disorder or polygenic disorder.

Disorder	Inheritance Pattern
von Willebrand disease	Autosomal dominant
Neurofibromatosis	Autosomal dominant
MEN I/II syndrome	Autosomal dominant
Achondroplasia	Autosomal dominant
Sphingolipidoses (Tay-Sachs disease, Gaucher disease)	Autosomal recessive
Fabry disease*	X-linked recessive
Mucopolysaccharidoses (e.g., Hurler disease)	Autosomal recessive
Hunter disease†	X-linked recessive
Glycogen storage diseases (e.g., McArdle disease)	Autosomal recessive
Cystic fibrosis	Autosomal recessive
Marfan syndrome	Autosomal dominant
Huntington disease	Autosomal dominant
Pyloric stenosis	Polygenic disorder
Cleft lip/palate	Polygenic disorder
Type II diabetes	Polygenic disorder
Down syndrome	Chromosomal disorder (trisomy 21)
Familial hypercholesterolemia	Autosomal dominant
Galactosemia	Autosomal recessive
Amino acid disorders (e.g., phenylketonuria)	Autosomal recessive
Edward syndrome	Chromosomal disorder (trisomy 18)
Sickle cell disease	Autosomal recessive
Hemophilia	X-linked recessive
Glucose-6-phosphatase deficiency	X-linked recessive
Patau syndrome	Chromosomal disorder (trisomy 13)
Lesch-Nyhan syndrome	X-linked recessive
Obesity	Polygenic disorder

(continued)

Disorder	Inheritance Pattern
Neural tube defects	Polygenic disorder
Turner syndrome	Chromosomal disorder (XO)
Schizophrenia	Polygenic disorder
Duchenne muscular dystrophy	X-linked recessive
Wiskott-Aldrich syndrome	X-linked recessive
Bruton agammaglobulinemia	X-linked recessive
Fragile X syndrome	X-linked recessive
Children's polycystic kidney disease	Autosomal recessive
Wilson disease	Autosomal recessive
Bipolar disorder	Polygenic disorder
Ischemic heart disease	Polygenic disorder
Alcoholism	Polygenic disorder
Hemochromatosis	Autosomal recessive
Adrenogenital syndrome (e.g., 21-hydroxylase deficiency)	Autosomal recessive
Familial polyposis coli	Autosomal dominant
Adult polycystic kidney disease	Autosomal dominant
Hereditary spherocytosis	Autosomal dominant
Tuberous sclerosis	Autosomal dominant
Myotonic dystrophy	Autosomal dominant

MEN = multiple endocrine neoplasia.
*Fabry disease is the exception to the rule that the sphingolipidosis disorders are autosomal recessive.
†Hunter disease is the exception to the rule that the mucolipopolysaccharidase disorders are autosomal recessive.

2. **What is the likelihood that a mother with an autosomal dominant condition will pass the condition to the child if the father does not have the disease?**
50%. The father is not a carrier (because autosomal dominant diseases express themselves in carriers), and it is reasonable to assume that the mother has one copy of the diseased gene and one normal gene (unless told otherwise). It is exceedingly rare to find two diseased genes.

3. **Genetic testing reveals that both mother and father are carriers of a diseased gene for an autosomal recessive condition but do not have the condition themselves. What are the odds that their first child will develop the condition or be an asymptomatic carrier?**
The child has a 25% risk of developing the condition, a 50% risk of being an asymptomatic carrier, and a 25% chance of not inheriting the diseased gene at all.

4. **The father has an X-linked recessive disorder. What are the chances that he will pass the disease to his son or daughter if the mother does not have the diseased gene?**
There is no chance that he will pass the condition to his son; he will give his son a Y chromosome. On the other hand, there is a 100% chance he will pass the diseased gene to his

daughter, but because it is X-linked recessive, she has no chance of developing the condition. She will get a diseased X chromosome from the father and a healthy X chromosome from the mother.

5. **The mother is a carrier for an X-linked recessive disorder and the father is healthy. What are the odds that a son or daughter will develop the disease?**
There is a 50% chance for a son and no chance for a daughter. However, there is a 50% chance that the daughter will become a carrier.

6. **How do you recognize Down syndrome?**
Down syndrome (trisomy 21) is the most common known cause of mental retardation in the United States. The biggest risk factor is maternal age (1 in 1500 offspring of 16-year-old mothers and 1 in 25 offspring of 45-year-old mothers). At birth look for hypotonia, transverse palmar crease, and characteristic facies. Congenital cardiac defects (especially ventricular septal defects) are common, and affected persons have an increased risk for leukemia, duodenal atresia, and early Alzheimer disease.

7. **What is the second most common known cause of inherited mental retardation?**
Fragile X syndrome (X-linked recessive). Affected males often have large testicles.

8. **How do you recognize Edward syndrome?**
Edward syndrome (trisomy 18) affects females more than males. Characteristics include mental retardation, small size for age, a small head with hypoplastic mandible and low-set ears, and clenched fist with the index finger overlapping the third and fourth fingers (almost pathognomonic).

9. **What is Patau syndrome?**
Patau syndrome (trisomy 13) presents with mental retardation, apnea, deafness, holoprosencephaly (fusion of cerebral hemispheres), myelomeningocele, cardiovascular abnormalities, and rocker-bottom feet.

10. **How do you recognize Turner syndrome?**
Patients with Turner syndrome (females with XO instead of XX) have nuchal (neck) lymphedema at birth, short stature, webbed neck, widely spaced nipples, amenorrhea, and lack of breast development (due to primary ovarian failure). Coarctation of the aorta is common, and you may see horse-shoe kidneys or cystic hygroma. A buccal smear classically reveals absent Barr bodies.

11. **Describe Klinefelter syndrome.**
Patients with Klinefelter syndrome (males who are XXY instead of XY) are tall with small testes (less than 2 cm in length), gynecomastia, sterility, and a slightly decreased IQ (on average). The classic case on the Step 2 exam is a man who presents with complaints of infertility.

12. **What is the hallmark of cri du chat syndrome?**
Cri du chat (French for cry of the cat) syndrome is due to a deletion on the short arm of chromosome 5. Look for a high-pitched cry that sounds like the cry of a cat along with severe mental retardation.

13. **What presentation suggests galactosemia?**
Congenital cataracts and neonatal sepsis with vomiting after breast-feeding. Patients should avoid galactose- and lactose-containing foods.

14. **Describe the clinical findings in tuberous sclerosis.**

This autosomal dominant disorder presents with hypopigmented skin macules, seizures, mental retardation, central nervous system hamartomas (tubers), and an increased risk for cardiac rhabdomyomas and renal tumors known as angiomyolipomas. Look for a positive family history.

15. **What causes Lesch-Nyhan syndrome? What classic behavior do patients exhibit?**

This syndrome is due to a deficiency of hypoxanthine-guanine phosphoribosyltransferase (HGPRT), which causes congenital hyperuricemia. Patients have mental retardation and self-mutilating behavior. The classic example is the patient who bites off his or her own fingers.

16. **What causes Marfan syndrome? How do you recognize it?**

Marfan syndrome is an autosomal dominant connective tissue disorder caused by abnormal microfibrillin protein and associated with ocular, skeletal, and cardiovascular problems. Look for a positive family history. Patients are tall and have arachnodactyly (long, thin fingers), hyperextensible joints, mitral valve prolapse, dislocation of the lens of the eye, and a high risk for thoracic aortic dissection.

CHAPTER 15

GERIATRICS

1. **What age group constitutes the most rapidly growing segment of the population?**
Persons over the age of 85.

2. **True or false: An 80-year-old person needs more calories than a 30-year-old person.**
False. An 80-year-old person has half the lean body mass of a 30-year-old person and thus needs fewer calories. The basal metabolic rate is based on lean body mass. Elderly patients, however, need more sodium, vitamin B_{12}, vitamin D (and/or calcium), folate, and nonheme iron than younger patients.

3. **True or false: Hearing and vision changes are a normal part of aging.**
True. **Presbyopia** (hardening of the lens that decreases the ability to accommodate) becomes almost universal after age 50; thus the common need for reading glasses after age 50. **Presbyacusis,** the loss of ability to discriminate between sounds, also is part of the normal process of aging.

4. **True or false: Brain atrophy is a normal part of aging.**
True. Decreased brain weight, enlarged ventricles and sulci, and a slightly decreased ability to learn new material are normal parts of aging.

5. **Describe the normal changes in male sexual function that occur with aging.**
   - Increased refractory period (after ejaculation, it takes longer before he can have another erection)
   - Increased amount of time to achieve an erection
   - Delayed ejaculation (an elderly man may ejaculate only 1 of every 3 times that he has sex)

6. **Describe the normal changes in female sexual function that occur with aging.**
   - Decreased lubrication (women not on hormone replacement therapy may use estrogen cream or water-soluble lubricants)
   - Dyspareunia due to atrophy of clitoral, labial, and vaginal tissues (treated with estrogen cream)
   - Delayed orgasm

7. **True or false: Impotence and lack of sexual desire are normal in elderly people.**
False. Impotence in men and lack of sexual desire in either sex are not normal and should be investigated. Look for psychiatric disorders (e.g., depression) as well as physical causes, such as medications (antihypertensives are notorious culprits), vascular disease (watch for atherosclerosis risk factors), and neurologic disease (especially in diabetics).

8. **What is the best prophylaxis for pressure ulcers in an immobilized patient?**
Frequent turning and the use of special air mattresses.

9. **Describe the normal changes in sleep habits in elderly people.**
Elderly persons require less sleep, sleep less deeply, wake up more frequently during the night, and awaken earlier in the morning. It also takes longer for elderly persons to fall asleep (longer sleep latency), and they have less stage 3 and 4 and rapid eye movement sleep.

10. **Define pseudodementia. How do you recognize it on the Step 2 exam?**
Depression in the elderly can resemble dementia. Look for a history that would trigger depression (e.g., loss of a spouse, terminal or debilitating disease) and other symptoms of depression (e.g., frequent crying, suicidal thoughts).

11. **True or false: Roughly 2% of the population is over the age of 65.**
False. Approximately 15% of people are over the age of 65, and this number is increasing.

12. **True or false: Almost 50% of patients over the age of 65 suffer from some type of dementia.**
False. Roughly 15% of people over the age of 65 suffer from dementia. The most common causes, in decreasing order of frequency, are Alzheimer disease (gradually progressive, with neurofibrillary tangles), multiinfarct dementia (stepwise, with risk factors for stroke), and other disorders (e.g., HIV, Pick disease). Test for reversible causes of dementia such as hypothyroidism, depression, and vitamin B_{12} deficiency.

13. **True or false: Only 5% of people over the age of 65 live in nursing homes.**
True. Watch for the boards to try to push you into old-fashioned stereotypes of the elderly. Not all old people are demented and living in nursing homes.

CHAPTER 16

GYNECOLOGY

1. **What is the most common cause of preventable infertility in the United States?**
   Pelvic inflammatory disease (PID).

2. **What is the most likely cause of infertility in a normally menstruating woman under the age of 30?**
   PID.

3. **What is PID? How do you recognize it on the Step 2 exam?**
   PID is typically due to an ascending sexually-transmitted infection of the upper female genital tract that may involve the endometrial cavity (endometritis), fallopian tubes (salpingitis), ovaries (oophoritis), parametrial tissues/ligaments (parametritis), and/or peritoneal cavity (peritonitis). Look for a female aged 13 to 35 years with the following symptoms: (1) abdominal pain, (2) adnexal tenderness, *and* (3) **cervical motion tenderness.** All three criteria must technically be present. In addition, one or more of the following should be present: elevated erythrocyte sedimentation rate/C-reactive protein level, leukocytosis, fever, or purulent cervical discharge.

4. **How is PID treated? What are the common sequelae?**
   Treat PID with more than one antibiotic (e.g., cefoxitin/ceftriaxone and doxycycline for outpatients; clindamycin and gentamicin for inpatients) to cover multiple organisms, especially *Neisseria gonorrhoeae* and *Chlamydia trachomatis* (the most common organisms). Also consider Escherichia coli, anaerobes, and, with a history of intrauterine device use, *Actinomyces israelii.*

   Common sequelae include infertility due to scarring of the fallopian tubes and progression to tuboovarian abscess (palpable on exam, may respond to antibiotics alone) that may rupture. Treat rupture with emergent laparotomy and excision of the affected tube (unilateral disease) or total abdominal hysterectomy and bilateral salpingo-oophorectomy for bilateral disease.

5. **Define endometriosis. What are the symptoms and signs?**
   Endometriosis is defined as endometrial glands outside the uterus (ectopic). Patients are usually nulliparous and over 30 with the following symptoms: **dysmenorrhea** (painful menstruation), **dyspareunia** (painful intercourse), **dyschezia** (painful defecation), and/or perimenstrual spotting. The most common site for the ectopic endometrial glands is the ovaries; look for tender adnexa in an afebrile patient. Other sites include the broad (uterosacral) ligament and peritoneal surface. Nodularities on the broad ligament are classic findings on physical exam; the classic sequela is a retroverted uterus.

6. **How is endometriosis diagnosed and treated?**
   The gold standard of diagnosis is laparoscopy with visualization of the endometriosis. Treat first with birth control pills (if acceptable to patient); danazol and gonadotropin-releasing

hormone agonists are second-line agents. Surgery and cautery can be used to destroy the endometriomas, a procedure that often improves fertility. In an older patient, consider hysterectomy and bilateral salpingo-oophorectomy for severe symptoms.

7. **What is the most likely cause of infertility in a menstruating woman over the age of 30 without a history of PID?**
Endometriosis.

8. **Cover the right-hand columns and specify the findings and treatment for the following vaginal infections:**

Bug	Findings	Treatment
Candida sp.	"Cottage cheese," pseudohyphae on KOH preparation, history of diabetes, antibiotic treatment, or pregnancy	Topical or oral antifungal
T. vaginalis	Bugs can be seen swimming under microscope; pale green, frothy, watery discharge; "strawberry" cervix	Metronidazole
G. vaginalis	Malodorous discharge; fishy smell on KOH preparation, clue cells	Metronidazole
Human papillomavirus	Venereal warts, koilocytosis on Pap smear	Many (acid, cryo therapy, laser, podophyllin)
Herpes virus	Multiple shallow, painful ulcers; recurrence and resolution	Acyclovir
Syphilis (stage I)	Painless chancre, spirochete on dark-field microscopy	Penicillin
Syphilis (stage II)	Condyloma lata, maculopapular rash on palms, serology	Penicillin
C. trachomatis	Most common STD; dysuria, positive culture and antibody tests	Doxycycline or azithromycin*
Neisseria gonorrhoeae	Mucopurulent cervicitis; gram-negative bug on Gram stain	Ceftriaxone or fluoro quinolone*
Molluscum	Characteristic appearance of lesions, intracellular inclusions	Curette, cryotherapy, or electrocauterization/ coagulation
Pediculosis	"Crabs;" look for itching; lice can be seen on pubic hairs	Permethrin cream (or malathion)

KOH = potassium hydroxide; STD = sexually transmitted disease.
*Chlamydia can be treated with erythromycin if the patient is pregnant. If compliance is an issue (alcoholic, drug abusing, homeless, or unreliable patient), give azithromycin, 1 g orally in a single dose, so that you can watch the patient take it. Patients with gonorrhea should be treated for presumed chlamydial coinfection (but the opposite is not true).

9. **True or false: With all of the infections listed in the previous table, you should seek out and treat the patient's sexual partners.**

   False. *Candida* and *Gardnerella* species are not typically sexually transmitted diseases; they are usually caused by disturbances in the normal vaginal flora. You should treat the patient's sexual partners and give counseling (e.g., condoms) for the other infections, which are sexually transmitted.

10. **True or false: Patients with gonorrhea usually are treated for presumed chlamydial infection.**

    True. A common current treatment strategy is to give both ceftriaxone (for gonorrhea) and doxycycline (for chlamydia) together to patients with gonorrhea. The reverse is not true; do *not* automatically give gonorrhea treatment to patients with chlamydial infection.

11. **Define adenomyosis. How does it classically present? What is the treatment?**

    Adenomyosis is defined as endometrial glands within the uterine musculature (Fig. 16-1). Patients are usually over 40 with dysmenorrhea and menorrhagia and have a large, boggy uterus on physical exam. Do dilation and curettage first to rule out endometrial cancer. Consider hysterectomy to relieve severe symptoms; gonadotropin-releasing hormone agonists also may relieve symptoms.

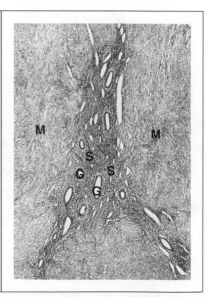

Figure 16-1. Adenomyosis. Islands of ectopic endometrial glands (G) and stroma (S) are present within the myometrium (M), often at a considerable distance from the normal endometrium. Because the ectopic endometrium reflects outgrowth of the basal endometrial layer, the ectopic tissue is not responsive to hormones in the normal manner. Thus, cyclic shedding during menstruation and evidence of bleeding are typically absent, unlike endometriosis, which contains hormone-responsive tissue. (From Stevens A, et al.: Wheater's Basic Histopathology, 4th ed. New York, Churchill Livingstone, 2002, p 207, with permission.)

12. **What are fibroids? How common are they? How often do they become malignant?**

    Fibroids (i.e., leiomyomas) are benign uterine tumors (Fig. 16-2). They are the most common tumors in women and the most common indication for hysterectomy (when they grow too large or cause symptoms). Up to 40% of women have fibroids by age 40. Malignant transformation is quite rare (<1%).

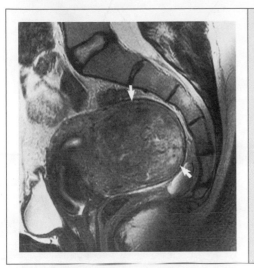

Figure 16-2. This T2-weighted sagittal MRI shows a subserosal leiomyoma (*arrows*) that distends the posterior aspect of the uterus, displacing the endometrium. (From Adam A, et al.: Grainger & Allison's Diagnostic Radiology, 5th ed. Edinburgh, Churchill Livingstone, 2008, Fig. 54-12.)

13. **Explain the relationship between uterine leiomyomas and hormones. How do leiomyomas present? What is the treatment?**

   Leiomyomas of the uterus are estrogen-dependent. Therefore, you may see rapid growth during pregnancy or use of oral contraceptive pills and regression after menopause. Leiomyomas may cause infertility, pain, and menorrhagia or metrorrhagia. Anemia due to leiomyoma is an indication for hysterectomy. Rare patients present with a polyp protruding through cervix. Dilation and curettage are needed to rule out endometrial cancer in women who present after the age of 35.

   Treatment is usually surgical (the levonorgestrel-releasing intrauterine device is seeing more widespread use, though randomized trials are lacking). Myomectomy can sometimes maintain or even restore fertility; the alternative is hysterectomy.

14. **What is the first test to order in any woman of reproductive age with abnormal uterine bleeding?**

   A pregnancy test.

15. **Define dysfunctional uterine bleeding (DUB). When is it physiologic?**

   DUB is defined as abnormal uterine bleeding not associated with a tumor, inflammation, or pregnancy. It is the most common cause of abnormal uterine bleeding and is a diagnosis of exclusion. More than 70% of cases are associated with anovulatory cycles (unopposed estrogen). The age of the patient is important because after menarche and immediately before menopause, DUB is extremely common and, in fact, is considered physiologic. Most other women have polycystic ovary syndrome (PCOS), the most common nonphysiologic cause of DUB.

16. **Why is dilation and curettage done in women over 35 with DUB? What other test should be ordered in all women with DUB (regardless of age)?**

   To rule out endometrial cancer. Hemoglobin and hematocrit (or complete blood count) should be ordered on all women with DUB to make sure that the patient is not anemic from excessive blood loss.

17. What causes DUB other than PCOS? How is DUB treated?

Causes of DUB include infections, endocrine disorders (thyroid, adrenal, pituitary/prolactin), coagulation defects, and estrogen-producing neoplasms. In the absence of treatable pathology, treat first with nonsteroidal anti-inflammatory drugs (NSAIDs), which are first-line agents for DUB and dysmenorrhea. Oral contraceptive pills are also a first-line agent for menorrhagia and DUB if the patient does not desire pregnancy and menstrual cycles are irregular. Monotherapy with progesterone is used for severe bleeding.

18. Define PCOS. How do you recognize it?

PCOS is an endocrine imbalance characterized by androgen excess as well as a ratio of leuteinizing hormone (LH) to follicle-stimulating hormone (FSH) greater than 2:1. Patients also frequently develop enlarged ovaries with multiple peripherally-oriented cysts, which can be seen on ultrasound (Figs. 16-3 and 16-4). On the Step 2 exam, watch for an overweight woman who has hirsutism, amenorrhea, and/or infertility.

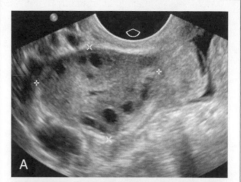
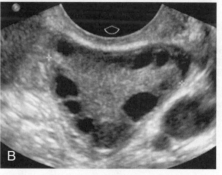

Figure 16-3. Polycystic ovaries. Sagittal (**A**) and transverse (**B**) transvaginal ultrasound of the left ovary depicting enlarged ovaries with multiple subcentimeter peripherally placed follicles and echogenic central stroma. (From Adam A, et al.: Grainger & Allison's Diagnostic Radiology, 5th ed. Edinburgh, Churchill Livingstone, 2008, Fig. 54-22.)

19. What is the most likely cause for infertility in a woman under 30 with abnormal menstruation?

PCOS.

20. How is PCOS treated? With what risk is it associated?

Treat with oral contraceptive pills or cyclic progesterone. If the patient desires pregnancy, you can use **clomiphene** to induce ovulation. Chronic unopposed estrogen (i.e., not enough progesterone; hence, infrequent menses) increases the risk of **endometrial cancer** in affected

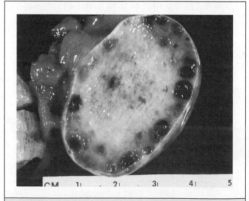

Figure 16-4. This sagittal section of a polycystic ovary demonstrates a large number of follicular cysts and thickened stroma. (From Katz V, et al.: Comprehensive Gynecology, 5th ed. Philadelphia, Mosby, 2007, Fig. 40-7.)

patients. Spironolactone can be used to treat hirsutism associated with PCOS. Metformin sometimes is used to treat the insulin resistance associated with PCOS and to help restore ovulation. However, metformin is not FDA-approved for this use, and oral contraceptive pills or cyclic progesterone are the preferred agents for endometrial protection.

21. **Is infertility usually a male or a female problem?**
Two-thirds of cases are due to a female problem, one-third to a male problem.

22. **Assuming that the history and physical exam offer no clues, what is the first step in evaluating a couple for infertility?**
Semen analysis, which is cheap, easy, and noninvasive.

23. **List the relevant characteristics of normal semen.**
Ejaculate volume   > 1 mL
Sperm concentration   > 20 million/mL
Initial forward motility > 50% of sperm
Normal morphology   > 60% of sperm

24. **What is the next step after semen evaluation?**
Documentation of ovulation. The history may suggest an ovulatory problem (irregular menstrual cycle length, duration, or amount of flow; lack of premenstrual syndrome symptoms). Basal body temperature, luteal phase progesterone levels, and/or endometrial biopsy can be done to check for ovulation.

25. **What radiologic test is commonly used to examine the fallopian tubes and uterus? What points in the history may lead you to suspect a uterine or tube problem?**
The hysterosalpingogram is commonly used to examine the uterus and tubes. The history may suggest a tubal problem (PID, previous ectopic pregnancy) or a uterine problem (previous dilation and curettage that caused intrauterine synechiae, history of fibroids, or symptoms of endometriosis).

26. **What test is the last resort in the work-up for infertility?**
Laparoscopy can be done as a last resort or with a history suggestive of endometriosis. Lysis of adhesions and destruction of endometriosis lesions often restore fertility.

27. **Which two medications can be used to try to restore female fertility? In what situations are they effective?**
Medical therapy usually consists of clomiphene citrate to induce ovulation, but this approach requires adequate production of estrogen. If the woman is hypoestrogenic, use human menopausal gonadotropin (hMG), which is a combination of FSH and LH. If medications fail, in vitro fertilization can be attempted.

28. **What is the main risk associated with medical induction of ovulation?**
Multiple-gestation pregnancies.

29. **Distinguish between primary and secondary amenorrhea.**
A patient with primary amenorrhea has never menstruated or had a menstrual period, whereas a patient with secondary amenorrhea used to menstruate but has stopped.

30. **Until proved otherwise, what is the cause of secondary amenorrhea in a previously menstruating woman of reproductive age?**
Pregnancy. Always order a human chorionic gonadotropin (hCG) test to rule out pregnancy as the first step in your evaluation of secondary amenorrhea.

31. True or false: Excessive exercise may cause amenorrhea.
True. It is not uncommon to find amenorrhea (or hypomenorrhea) in hard-training athletes. It results from an exercise-induced depression of gonadotropin-releasing hormone.

32. What are other common causes of secondary amenorrhea?
- PCOS
- Anorexia (amenorrhea is required for diagnosis of anorexia)
- Endocrine disorders (headaches, galactorrhea, and visual field defects may indicate a pituitary tumor)
- Antipsychotics (due to increased prolactin)
- Previous chemotherapy (causes premature ovarian failure and menopause)
  Although not considered secondary amenorrhea, **menopause** should be kept in mind as a cause for cessation of menstruation.

33. After ruling out pregnancy, if the cause of secondary amenorrhea is not obvious from the history and physical exam, what is the next step in your evaluation?
Administer progesterone to assess the patient's estrogen status. If vaginal bleeding develops within 2 weeks of administering progesterone, the patient has sufficient estrogen. In this case, check the LH level. If it is high, consider PCOS. If it is low or normal, check the levels of prolactin and thyroid-stimulating hormone (TSH). The high TSH level in hypothyroidism causes high prolactin levels. If the prolactin is high with a normal TSH level, order a magnetic resonance (MR) scan of the brain to rule out pituitary prolactinoma. If the prolactin level is normal, look for low levels of gonadotropin-releasing hormone, which may be induced by drugs, stress, or exercise. In these patients, clomiphene can be used in an attempt to facilitate pregnancy.

34. What if the patient fails to have vaginal bleeding after receiving progesterone?
If the patient has no vaginal bleeding, estrogen levels are inadequate. Check the FSH level next. If it is elevated, premature ovarian failure is the problem; check for autoimmune disorders, karyotype abnormalities, and a history of chemotherapy. If the FSH level is low or normal, the problem may be a brain tumor (e.g., craniopharyngioma). Order an MR scan of the brain. Clomiphene is ineffective in these patients.

35. True or false: Pregnancy can present as primary amenorrhea.
True. Always assess the hCG level in the evaluation of any type of amenorrhea.

36. At what age can primary amenorrhea be diagnosed? What is the first step in evaluation?
A diagnosis of primary amenorrhea is made when a girl has not menstruated by the age of 16. Patients also should be evaluated in the absence of secondary sexual characteristics by age 14 or in the absence of menstruation within 2 years of developing secondary sex characteristics. The first step is to rule out pregnancy.

37. In a patient older than 14 with no secondary sexual characteristics or development, what is the most likely cause of amenorrhea?
The most likely cause in this setting is a congenital problem. In a phenotypically normal female with normal breast development but no axillary or pubic hair, think of **androgen insensitivity syndrome.** In such patients the uterus is absent. In the presence of normal breast development and a uterus, the first step is to assess prolactin level to rule out pituitary adenoma. If the prolactin level is high, order an MRI. If it is normal, administer progesterone and follow the same procedure as in the evaluation of secondary amenorrhea.

38. **When in doubt, what is the best way to evaluate any type of amenorrhea?**
First, order a pregnancy test. If it is negative, administer progesterone. Further testing depends on the results of the progesterone challenge (bleeding or no bleeding). A TSH level and/or prolactin level should also be ordered, especially with symptoms of hypothyroidism or pituitary tumor.

39. **When does menopause occur? What are the symptoms and signs?**
The average age of menopause is around 51 years. Patients have irregular cycles or amenorrhea, hot flashes and mood swings, and an elevated FSH level. Patients also may complain of dysuria, dyspareunia, incontinence, and/or vaginal itching, burning, or soreness. Vaginal symptoms often are due to atrophic vaginitis; look for vaginal mucosa to be thin, dry, and atrophic with increased parabasal cells on cytology. Topical estrogen improves vaginal symptoms, but other symptoms require oral therapy.

40. **What is the current state of hormone replacement therapy?**
Hormone replacement therapy is currently recommended short-term for the management of moderate-to-severe vasomotor flushing. Long-term use for the prevention of disease (such as osteoporosis or cardiovascular disease) is no longer recommended based on the results of the Women's Health Initiative and the HERS trial.

41. **When a woman presents with a nipple discharge, what historical points are important?**
A history of using oral contraceptive pills, hormone therapies, antipsychotic medications or symptoms suggestive of hypothyroidism, which can all cause nipple discharge. The color of the discharge and whether the discharge is unilateral or bilateral is also very important. For example, if a nipple discharge is bilateral and non-bloody, it is not due to breast cancer, but it may be due a prolactinoma (check prolactin level) or endocrine disorder (check a thyroid stimulating hormone level). Alternatively, when a nipple discharge is unilateral and bloody (nipple discharge secondary to carcinoma generally contains hemoglobin), and/or associated with a mass, this should raise concern about possible breast cancer. Do a biopsy of any mass if present.

42. **What are the most likely causes of a breast mass in a woman under the age of 35?**
Fibrocystic disease (Fig. 16-5): bilateral, multiple, cystic lesions that are tender to the touch, especially premenstrually. This is the most common of all breast diseases. Generally, no work-up is needed other than routine follow-up. Oral contraceptive pills, progesterone, or danazol may help to relieve symptoms.

Fibroadenoma: a painless, discrete, sharply circumscribed, unilateral, rubbery, mobile mass. This is the most common benign tumor of the female breast. Patients may be observed for one or more menstrual cycles in the absence of symptoms. Because

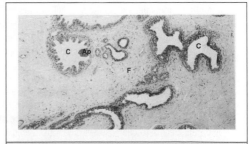

Figure 16-5. Fibrocystic change of the breast. Typical features are shown in the micrograph, including cystic dilatation of ducts (C) with apocrine metaplasia (Ap) and areas of fibrosis (F). This fibrosis can give rise to clinically palpable masses that may have irregular outlines. This condition is benign and considered a physiological variant in the absence of atypical or significant hyperplasia. (From Stevens A, et al.: Wheater's Basic Histopathology, 4th ed. New York, Churchill Livingstone, 2002, p 217, with permission.)

tumors are estrogen-dependent, pregnancy and oral contraceptive pills may stimulate growth, whereas menopause causes regression. Excision is curative but not required except for cosmetic reasons.

Mastitis/abscess: typically in the first few months postpartum, lactating women may develop a painful, swollen, erythematous breast(s). The nipple may be cracked or fissured. The patient should be treated with analgesics (e.g., acetaminophen, ibuprofen) and instructed to continue breast feeding with the affected breast(s) even though it is painful (use a breast pump to empty the breast if needed) to prevent further milk duct blockage and abscess formation. An anti-staphylococcal antibiotic (e.g., dicloxacillin) should be given for more than mild symptoms. Methicillin resistant staphylococcus aureus (MRSA) is becoming an increasingly important pathogen in mastitis. Use trimethoprim-sulfamethoxazole or clindamycin if MRSA is a concern or is cultured. If a fluctuant mass develops or there is no response to antibiotics within a few days, an abscess is likely present and must be drained.

Fat necrosis: patients have a history of trauma in the area of the mass.

43. **True or false: Mammography should be done for any suspicious breast lesion in a woman under age 30.**
False. Mammography is usually not done in women under age 30 because breast tissue is often too dense to discern a mass. If you are suspicious of breast cancer, which is very rare in this age group, proceed to ultrasound imaging or directly to biopsy.

44. **What are the likely causes of a breast mass in a woman over the age of 35?**
Fibrocystic disease: as mentioned previously, but aspiration of cyst fluid and baseline mammography are recommended. If the cyst fluid is non-bloody and the mass resolves after aspiration, the patient needs only reassurance and follow up (with a baseline mammogram). If the fluid is bloody or the cyst recurs quickly, do a biopsy to rule out cancer.

Fibroadenoma: get a baseline mammogram. Observe briefly if the mass is small and seems benign clinically *and* if the woman is premenopausal and has no risk factors for breast cancer. Otherwise, do a biopsy. Phyllodes tumors (minority are malignant) may masquerade as a fibroadenoma.

Fat necrosis: as mentioned previously.

Mastitis/abscess: as mentioned previously.

Breast cancer: on the Step 2 exam, you may not get the classic presentation of nipple retraction and/or peau d'orange in a nulliparous woman with a strong family history. In a woman 35 years old or over, you will never be faulted for doing a biopsy of any mass. In the absence of a classic benign presentation (e.g., trauma to the breast with fat necrosis or bilateral masses with premenstrual syndrome mastalgia), always consider biopsy. Also get a baseline mammography.

45. **True or false: If a patient is postmenopausal or over age 50 and develops a new breast mass, you should assume cancer "until proven otherwise."**
True. The risk of breast cancer begins to increase sharply, and the incidence of benign disorders begins to decrease sharply. Most benign disorders are caused by reproductive hormones that women in this age group lack.

46. **True or false: Mammography is best used as a tool to evaluate a palpable breast mass.**
False. Mammography is best used as a tool to detect nonpalpable breast masses (as a screening tool). A suspicious lesion found on mammography should be biopsied, even if it seems benign or is inapparent on physical exam. Additionally, a clinically suspicious mass should be biopsied unless imaging demonstrates unequivocally benign findings (e.g., a cyst).

47. **What causes pelvic relaxation or vaginal prolapse? What are the symptoms and signs?**
Pelvic relaxation is due to a weakening of pelvic supporting ligaments. Look for a history of several vaginal deliveries, feeling of heaviness or fullness in the pelvis, backache, worsening of symptoms with standing, and resolution of symptoms with lying down.

48. **What types of pelvic relaxation are seen clinically? How are they treated?**
Cystocele: the bladder bulges into the *upper anterior vaginal wall*. Common symptoms include urinary urgency, frequency, and/or incontinence.
Rectocele: the rectum bulges into the *lower posterior vaginal wall*. Watch for difficulty with defecation.
Enterocele: loops of bowel bulge into the *upper posterior vaginal wall*.
Urethrocele: the urethra bulges into the *lower anterior vaginal wall*. Common symptoms include urinary urgency, frequency, and/or incontinence.
Conservative treatment for all types of pelvic relaxation involves pelvic strengthening exercises and/or a pessary (artificial device to provide support). Surgery is used for refractory or severe cases or patient desire.

49. **Other than abstinence, what are the most effective forms of birth control (when used properly)?**
The most effective forms of birth control are sterilization (e.g., tubal ligation or vasectomy), implants (etonogestrel implant) or an intrauterine device followed by injectable hormone depot preparations, then birth control pills/patch and a hormonal vaginal ring.

50. **Which forms of birth control prevent sexually transmitted diseases?**
Abstinence and condoms.

51. **What are the major problems with intrauterine devices?**
They increase the risk of ectopic pregnancies and PID (watch for *Actinomyces* species to be the cause). For these reasons, they are most appropriate for older, monogamous women.

52. **What is the classic cause of ambiguous genitalia on the Step 2 exam?**
Adrenogenital syndrome, also known as congenital adrenal hyperplasia. Ninety percent of cases are caused by **21-hydroxylase deficiency.** Patients are female because affected males experience precocious sexual development. Patients with 21-hydroxylase deficiency have salt-wasting (low sodium), hyperkalemia, hypotension, and elevated 17-hydroxyprogesterone. Treat with steroids and intravenous fluids immediately to prevent death.

53. **What should you tell the parents of a child with ambiguous genitalia?**
Tell the parents the truth: you do not know the child's gender. No patient with ambiguous genitalia should be assigned a sex until the work-up is complete. A karyotype must be done.

54. **What is indicated by a "bunch of grapes" protruding from a pediatric vagina?**
Sarcoma botryoides, a malignant tumor (a type of embryonal rhabdomyosarcoma).

55. **Define precocious puberty. What causes it? How should it be treated?**
By definition, precocious puberty occurs in girls less than 8 years old or boys less than 9 years old. Premature or precocious puberty is usually idiopathic, but it may be caused by a hormone-secreting tumor or central nervous system disorder, both of which must be ruled out. Treat the underlying cause. If the condition is idiopathic, treat with a gonadotropin-releasing hormone analog to prevent premature epiphyseal closure and arrest or reverse puberty until an appropriate age.

56. **What causes vaginitis or discharge in prepubescent girls?**

Most cases are nonspecific or physiologic, but look for a vaginal foreign body, sexual abuse (especially if a sexually transmitted disease is present), or candidal infection. A candidal infection may be a presentation of diabetes; check the serum glucose level and/or the urine for glycosuria.

57. **How do you recognize and treat an imperforate hymen?**

Imperforate hymen classically presents at menarche with hematocolpos (blood in the vagina) that cannot escape; thus, the hymen bulges outward. Treatment is surgical opening of the hymen.

58. **What is the usual cause of vaginal bleeding in neonates? How is it treated?**

Vaginal bleeding in neonates is usually physiologic and due to maternal estrogen withdrawal. No treatment is needed because the bleeding resolves on its own.

59. **Which women are candidates for hormone replacement therapy?**

Hormone replacement therapy (i.e., estrogen with or without progesterone) is now controversial and probably best used only as a means of symptom relief. Observation during therapy is necessary, because estrogen and progesterone are not harmless. Every woman should make the decision on her own after weighing the risks and benefits. See questions 40 and 60 for more details.

60. **What are the known benefits of estrogen therapy?**

- Decreased osteoporosis and decreased fractures
- Reduced hot flashes and genitourinary symptoms of menopause (dryness, urgency, atrophy-induced incontinence, frequency)
- Decreased risk of colorectal cancer (according to the Women's Health Initiative, when combined estrogen and progesterone therapy is used)

61. **What are the known risks of estrogen therapy?**

- Increased risk of endometrial cancer (eliminated by coadministration of progesterone)
- Small increase in risk of coronary heart disease with combined estrogen and progesterone therapy, though the risk is not increased in women who are less than 10 years postmenopausal or 50 to 59 years of age
- Increased risk of venous thromboembolism
- Increased risk of breast cancer (according to the Women's Health Initiative when combined estrogen and progesterone therapy is used. There was a slightly decreased risk of breast cancer with estrogen only, though this decrease was not statistically significant)
- Increased risk of stroke (according to the Women's Health Initiative, with either estrogen only or combined estrogen and progesterone therapy)
- Increased risk of gallbladder disease

62. **What are the most common side effects of estrogen therapy?**

- Endometrial bleeding
- Bloating
- Breast tenderness
- Headaches
- Nausea

63. **What are the absolute contraindications to estrogen therapy?**

- Unexplained vaginal bleeding
- Active liver disease
- History of thromboembolism

- Coronary artery disease
- History of endometrial or breast cancer
- Pregnancy

64. **What are the relative contraindications to estrogen therapy?**
- Seizure disorder
- Hypertension
- Uterine leiomyomas
- Familial hyperlipidemia
- Migraine headaches
- Thrombophlebitis
- Endometriosis
- Gallbladder disease

65. **What test is often done before starting estrogen therapy?**
Women classically get an endometrial biopsy, ultrasound or dilation and curettage at the onset of treatment to rule out hyperplasia and/or cancer and an evaluation of any unexplained bleeding, even while on therapy, unless they have had a normal evaluation within the past 6 months.

66. **True or false: Women without a uterus do not need to take progesterone with estrogen.**
True. The main reason for giving progesterone with hormone replacement therapy is to eliminate the increased risk of endometrial cancer that accompanies unopposed estrogen therapy. If a woman has no uterus, then she has no need for progesterone.

67. **What are the absolute contraindications to oral contraceptive pills?**
- Venous thromboembolism, current or past (deep venous thrombosis or pulmonary embolism)
- Cerebrovascular disease (stroke)
- Coronary artery disease
- Complicated valvular heart disease
- Diabetes with complications
- Breast cancer
- Pregnancy
- Lactation (fewer than 6 weeks postpartum)
- Liver disease
- Headaches with focal neurologic symptoms
- Major surgery with prolonged immobilization
- Age greater than 35 years and smoking greater than or equal to 15 cigarettes per day
- Hypertension (blood pressure greater than 160/100 mm Hg or with concomitant vascular disease)

68. **What are the relative contraindications to oral contraceptive pills?**
- Postpartum fewer than 21 days
- Lactation (6 weeks to 6 months)
- Undiagnosed vaginal or uterine bleeding
- Age greater than 35 years and smoking less than 15 cigarettes per day
- History of breast cancer but no recurrence in past 5 years
- Interacting drugs (certain anticonvulsants, rifampin)
- Gallbladder disease
- Headaches without aura, age greater than or equal to 35 years
- Hypertension (well-controlled or blood pressure 140–159/90–99 mm Hg)

69. **What is the relationship between oral contraceptive pills and hypertension?**
Oral contraceptive pills are one of the most common causes of secondary hypertension. Any patient taking birth control pills who is noted have an increased blood pressure should discontinue the pills, then have their blood pressure rechecked at a later date.

70. **What do you need to know about oral contraceptive pills and surgery?**
Because of the risks of thromboembolism, oral contraceptive pills should be stopped 1 month before elective surgery and not restarted until 1 month after surgery.

71. **What are the side effects of oral contraceptive pills?**
The side effects include glucose intolerance (check for diabetes mellitus annually in women at high risk), depression, edema (bloating), weight gain, cholelithiasis, **benign liver adenomas,** melasma ("the mask of pregnancy"), nausea, vomiting, headache, hypertension, and drug interactions. Drugs such as rifampin and antiepileptics may induce metabolism of oral contraceptive pills and reduce their effectiveness.

72. **What is the relationship between oral contraceptive pills and breast and cervical cancer?**
Oral contraceptive pills have little, if any, effect on the risk of developing breast cancer. Cervical neoplasia may be increased in users of birth control pills, but this effect also may be due to the confounding factor of increased sexual relations or number of partners. Nonetheless, users of birth control pills should have regular Pap smears.

73. **What is the relationship between oral contraceptive pills and ovarian and endometrial cancer?**
Oral contraceptive pills have been shown to reduce the incidence of ovarian cancer by 50%; they also reduce the incidence of endometrial cancer.

74. **What are the other beneficial effects of oral contraceptive pills?**
They decrease the incidence of menorrhagia, dysmenorrhea, benign breast disease, functional ovarian cysts (often prescribed for the previous four effects), premenstrual tension, iron-deficiency anemia, ectopic pregnancy, and salpingitis.

CHAPTER 17

HEMATOLOGY

1. **Define anemia.**
   Hemoglobin less than 12 mg/dL in women or less than 14 mg/dL in men.

2. **What are the symptoms and signs of anemia?**
   Symptoms: fatigue, dyspnea on exertion, light-headedness, dizziness, syncope, palpitations, angina, and claudication.
   Signs: tachycardia, pallor (especially of the sclera and mucous membranes), systolic ejection murmurs (from high flow), and signs of the underlying cause (e.g., jaundice and/or pigment **gallstones** (Fig. 17-1) in hemolytic anemia, positive stool guaiac with a gastrointestinal [GI] bleed).

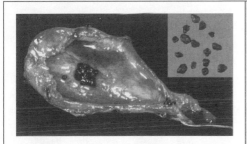

Figure 17-1. Pigment gallstones within the gallbladder, a marker for hemolytic anemia, are typically easily distinguished from cholesterol stones by their gross appearance. (From Hoffbrand AV, Pettit JE: Color Atlas of Clinical Hematology, 3rd ed. St. Louis, Mosby, 2000, p 72, with permission.)

3. **What are the important elements of the history when anemia is present?**
   Important points include medications, blood loss (e.g., trauma, surgery, melena, hematemesis, menorrhagia), chronic diseases (anemia of chronic disease), family history (e.g., hemophilia, thalassemia, sickle cell disease, glucose-6-phosphatase deficiency), and alcoholism (which may lead to iron, folate, and B$_{12}$ deficiencies as well as GI bleeds).

4. **What medications can cause anemia? How?**
   Many medications can cause anemia through various mechanisms. Methyldopa, penicillins, and sulfa drugs can cause red blood cell (RBC) antibodies with subsequent hemolysis; chloroquine and sulfa drugs cause hemolysis in patients with glucose-6-phosphatase deficiency; phenytoin causes megaloblastic anemia through interference with folate metabolism; and chloramphenicol, cancer drugs, and zidovudine cause aplastic anemia and bone marrow suppression. Other drugs also are implicated, but this list should get you through the USMLE exam.

5. **What test should be ordered first to help determine the cause of anemia?**
   The complete blood count with red blood cell indices. First and foremost, the hemoglobin must be below normal. The mean corpuscular volume (MCV) tells you whether the anemia is microcytic (MCV < 80), normocytic (MCV = 80–100), or macrocytic (MCV > 100).

6. **What test should be ordered next?**

Peripheral blood smear. There are many "classic" findings that can help make the diagnoses:

- Sickled cells (sickle cell disease)
- Hypersegmented neutrophils (folate/B$_{12}$ deficiency)
- Hypochromic and microcytic RBCs (iron deficiency)
- Basophilic stippling (lead poisoning)
- Heinz bodies (glucose-6-phosphatase deficiency)
- "Bite cells" (classically, glucose-6-phosphatase deficiency; other hemolytic anemias)
- Howell-Jolly bodies (asplenia)
- Teardrop-shaped RBCs (myelofibrosis)
- Schistocytes, helmet cells, and fragmented RBCs (intravascular hemolysis)
- Spherocytes and elliptocytes (hereditary spherocytosis and elliptocytosis [Fig. 17-2])
- Acanthocytes and spur cells (abetalipoproteinemia)
- Target cells (thalassemia, liver disease)
- Echinocytes, including "burr" cells and acanthocytes (uremia)
- Polychromasia (from **reticulocytosis** [Fig. 17-3]; should alert you to possibility of hemolysis)

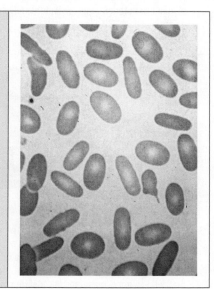

Figure 17-2. Hereditary elliptocytosis. Blood film reveals characteristic elliptical red blood cells. (From Hoffbrand AV, Pettit JE: Color Atlas of Clinical Hematology, 3rd ed. St. Louis, Mosby, 2000, p 75, with permission.)

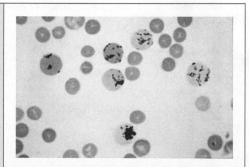

Figure 17-3. Reticulocytosis. Reticulocytes, so named because their precipitated RNA results in visible reticular intracellular material on peripheral smears, cause the laboratory finding known as polychromasia. Classically seen in the setting of hemolysis or blood loss, reticulocytosis indicates an appropriate/physiologic bone marrow response to anemia. (From Hoffbrand AV, Pettit JE: Color Atlas of Clinical Hematology, 3rd ed. St. Louis, Mosby, 2000, p 72, with permission.)

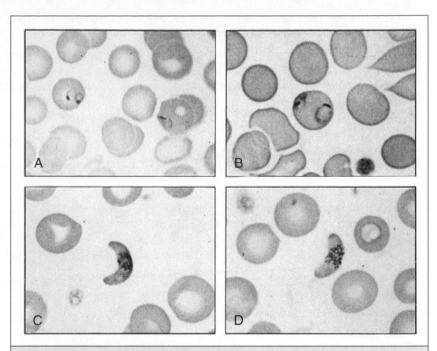

Figure 17-4. Malaria. Peripheral blood film examples of various stages of *P. falciparum*. Figures **A** and **B** demonstrate small ring forms, while figures **C** and **D** reveal crescentic gametocytes with centrally placed chromatin. (From Hoffbrand AV, Pettit JE: Color Atlas of Clinical Hematology, 3rd ed. St. Louis, Mosby, 2000, p 315, with permission.)

- Rouleaux formation (multiple myeloma)
- Parasites inside red blood cells (malaria [Fig. 17-4], babesiosis)
- Iron inclusions in red blood cells of the bone marrow (sideroblastic anemia)

7. **What are reticulocytes? Why is a reticulocyte count routinely ordered in an anemia work-up?**
   Reticulocytes are immature red blood cells. If their count is abnormally decreased in the setting of anemia, the marrow is not responding properly and is the problem. A high reticulocyte count should make you think of hemolysis or blood loss as the cause (the marrow is responding properly and is not the problem).

8. **Which test comes next?**
   At this point, it depends. If you have a complete history and results of the other three tests, most possibilities will be eliminated and you can order a confirmatory test. If the answer is still not clear, consider a bone marrow biopsy. For the Step 2 exam biopsy is unlikely to be necessary unless malignancy is the cause of the anemia.

9. **What are the classic causes of microcytic, normocytic, and macrocytic anemia? Which of these tends to have an inappropriately low reticulocyte count?**

Microcytic	Normocytic
With normal or elevated reticulocyte count Thalassemia/hemoglobinopathy (e.g., sickle cell disease)	*With normal or elevated reticulocyte count* Acute blood loss Hemolytic (multiple causes) Medications (antibody-causing)

With low reticulocyte count
Lead poisoning
Sideroblastic anemia
Anemia of chronic disease (some cases)
Iron deficiency
	With low reticulocyte count
	Cancer/dysplasia (e.g., myelophthisic,
	  acute leukemia)
	Anemia of chronic disease (some cases)
	Aplastic anemia/medications causing bone
	  marrow suppression
	Endocrine failure (thyroid, pituitary)
	Renal failure

Macrocytic (all types have low reticulocyte count)
Folate deficiency Vitamin B_{12} deficiency Medications (methotrexate, phenytoin) Alcohol abuse (interferes with folate use) Cirrhosis, liver disease

10. **What clues point to hemolysis as the cause for anemia?**
   - Elevated lactate dehydrogenase (LDH)
   - Elevated bilirubin (unconjugated as well as conjugated if the liver is functioning)
   - Jaundice
   - Low or absent haptoglobin (intravascular hemolysis only)
   - Urobilinogen, bilirubin, and hemoglobin in urine (only conjugated bilirubin shows up in the urine, and hemoglobin shows up in the urine only when haptoglobin has been saturated, as in brisk intravascular hemolysis)
   - Pigmented gallstones or history of cholecystectomy (usually at a young age)

11. **What is the most common cause of anemia in the United States?**
   Iron deficiency anemia.

12. **Why do people get iron deficiency?**
   Iron deficiency is common in women of reproductive age because of menstrual blood loss. In all patients over age 40 (men and especially postmenopausal women), it is important to rule out colon cancer as a cause of chronic, asymptomatic blood loss. Increased requirements also may lead to iron deficiency in children and pregnant or breast-feeding women. Give iron-containing formula or iron supplements to all infants except full-term infants who are exclusively breast-fed. Start iron supplementation (iron-fortified cereal or daily iron supplement) at 4 to 6 months for full-term infants and at 2 months for preterm infants.

Giving cow's milk before 1 year of age may lead to anemia by causing GI bleeding, so avoidance of cow's milk in the first year is essential. Iron supplements also are commonly given during pregnancy and lactation (because of the increased demand).

13. **What are the classic laboratory abnormalities in iron deficiency anemia? What weird cravings may occur with iron deficiency?**
Look for low iron and low ferritin levels, elevated total iron-binding capacity (TIBC; also known as transferrin), and low TIBC saturation. Rare patients may develop a craving for ice or dirt (**pica**).

14. **What is Plummer-Vinson syndrome?**
A triad of unknown etiology: esophageal web resulting in dysphagia; iron deficiency anemia; and glossitis.

15. **How is iron deficiency treated?**
First you must determine the cause. In a menstruating woman, a presumptive diagnosis of menstrual blood loss is often made. In patients over 40 years, be sure to test the stool for occult blood and strongly consider colonoscopy to detect occult colon cancer. Postmenopausal vaginal bleeding may also cause anemia and warrants screening for gynecologic cancer. Treat with iron supplements for 3 to 6 months in uncomplicated cases to replete body iron stores.

16. **What causes folate deficiency? In what patient populations is it commonly seen?**
Folate deficiency is commonly seen in alcoholics (poor intake) and pregnant women (increased need). All women of reproductive age should take folate supplements to prevent neural tube defects in their offspring. Rare causes of folate deficiency include poor diet (e.g., tea and toast), methotrexate, prolonged therapy with trimethoprim-sulfamethoxazole, anticonvulsant therapy (especially phenytoin), and malabsorption. Look for macrocytes and **hypersegmented neutrophils** (either one should make you think of the diagnosis) with no neurologic symptoms or signs and low folate levels in serum or red blood cells. Treat with oral folate.

17. **What is the most common cause of vitamin B_{12} deficiency?**
Pernicious anemia. This megaloblastic anemia is caused by **antiparietal cell antibodies.** Remember the physiology of B_{12} absorption with intrinsic factor secretion by parietal cells and absorption of the B_{12}—intrinsic factor complex in the ileum. Achlorhydria (no stomach acid secretion and elevated stomach pH) and antibodies to parietal cells are generally present in pernicious anemia.

18. **What else may cause vitamin B_{12} deficiency? How is B_{12} deficiency diagnosed?**
Gastrectomy, terminal ileum resection or disease (e.g., Crohn disease), strict vegan diet, chronic pancreatitis, and the infamous *Diphyllobothrium latum* (fish tapeworm) infection. The peripheral smear looks the same as in folate deficiency (macrocytes, hypersegmented neutrophils), but patients have **neurologic deficiencies** (e.g., loss of sensation and position sense, paresthesias, ataxia, spasticity, hyperreflexia, positive Babinski sign, dementia). Diagnosis is clinched by a low serum B_{12} level. A Schilling test usually determines the etiology.

19. **How is vitamin B_{12} deficiency treated?**
Vitamin B_{12} supplements are given. The usual replacement is via parenteral (intramuscular) injection, because most patients cannot absorb the vitamin through the gut. Supplementation may be required for life.

20. **How is thalassemia differentiated from iron deficiency?**
    Both cause microcytic, hypochromic anemia, but thalassemia must be differentiated from
    iron deficiency because iron levels are normal in thalassemia. Iron supplementation is
    contraindicated in patients with thalassemia because it may cause iron overload. Look for
    elevations in hemoglobin A2 or hemoglobin F (beta thalassemia only); target cells, nucleated
    red blood cells, and diffuse basophilia on peripheral smears; skull radiograph with "crew-cut"
    appearance; extramedullary hematopoiesis (Fig. 17-5); splenomegaly; and positive family
    history. Thalassemia is more common in blacks, Mediterraneans, and Asians.

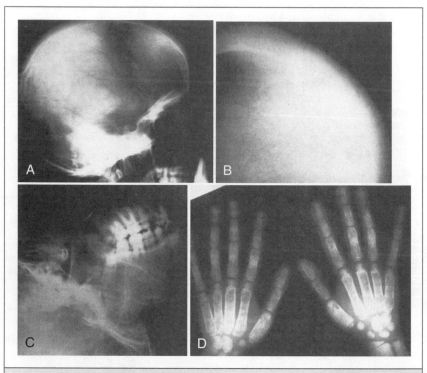

Figure 17-5. Bony abnormalities in a patient with severe β-thalassemia. **A** and **B**, "Hair-on-end"
appearance of the skull, which is especially obvious in the close-up view shown in B. **C**, Distortion of the
maxillary bones and poor development of the sinus cavities due to opaque masses of extramedullary
erythropoiesis. **D**, Squaring and convexity abnormalities of the hands. (From Pearson HA, Benz EJ Jr:
Thalassemia syndromes. In Miller DR, Baehner RL, McMillan CW [eds.]: Smith's Blood Diseases of
Infancy and Childhood, 5th ed. St. Louis, CV Mosby, 1984, p 439.)

21. **What diagnostic test confirms a diagnosis of thalassemia? How is it treated?**
    Diagnosis is made by hemoglobin electrophoresis. There are four gene loci for the alpha chain
    of hemoglobin but only two for the beta chain. Patients with alpha thalassemia are
    symptomatic at birth or die in utero (fetal hydrops), whereas patients with beta thalassemia are
    not symptomatic until 6 months of age.
    No treatment is required for minor thalassemia. Patients are often asymptomatic because
    they are used to living with a lower level of hemoglobin. Thalassemia major is more dramatic
    and severe. Treat with transfusions, as needed, and iron chelation therapy to prevent
    secondary hemochromatosis.

22. **What two clues on the Step 2 exam often point to a diagnosis of sickle cell disease?**
Peripheral smear and race. Eight percent of African Americans are heterozygous for sickle cell trait. Know what sickled red blood cells look like. Patients usually have a high percentage of reticulocytes (8–20%).

23. **What are the clinical manifestations and complications of sickle cell disease?**
■ Aplastic crises (due to parvovirus B19 infection)
■ Bone pain (due to infarcts; the classic example is avascular necrosis of the femoral head)
■ Dactylitis (also known as hand-foot syndrome, seen in children)
■ Renal papillary necrosis
■ Splenic sequestration crisis
■ Autosplenectomy (increased infections with encapsulated bugs such as *Pneumococcus, Haemophilus,* and *Neisseria* species)
■ Acute chest syndrome (mimics pneumonia)
■ Pigment cholelithiasis
■ Priapism
■ Stroke

24. **How is sickle cell disease diagnosed and treated?**
Diagnosis is made by hemoglobin electrophoresis. Screening is done at birth, but symptoms usually do not appear until around 6 months of age because of the lack of adult hemoglobin production. Treat with prophylactic penicillin until at least 5 years of age and perhaps longer, beginning as soon as the diagnosis is made. Proper vaccination includes the pneumococcal, meningococcal, and *H. influenzae* vaccines (given to all children anyway), as well as yearly influenza vaccination. Other strategies include folate supplementation, early treatment of infections, and proper hydration.
A sickle cell crisis involves severe pain in various sites due to red blood cell sickling. Treat with oxygen, lots of intravenous fluids, and analgesics (do not be afraid to use narcotics). Consider transfusions if symptoms and/or findings are severe.

25. **What findings help you in the setting of acute blood loss as a cause of anemia?**
The important point is that immediately after blood loss the hemoglobin may be normal; it takes at least 3 to 4 hours, often more, for reequilibration. Look for obvious bleeding, pale, cold skin, tachycardia, and hypotension (signs of hypovolemic shock). Transfuse if indicated, even with a normal hemoglobin in the acute setting. Consider internal hemorrhage in the setting of trauma and abdominal aortic aneurysm in patients with a pulsatile abdominal mass.

26. **What are the commonly tested causes of autoimmune hemolytic anemia?**
■ Lupus erythematosus (or medications that cause lupus-like syndromes, such as procainamide, hydralazine, and isoniazid) and other autoimmune disorders
■ Drugs (the classic example is methyldopa, but penicillins, cephalosporins, sulfa drugs, and quinidine also have been implicated)
■ Leukemia or lymphoma
■ Infection (the classic examples are mycoplasmosis, Epstein-Barr virus, and syphilis)

27. **What lab test is often positive in patients with autoimmune anemia?**
The **Coombs test** is positive in most autoimmune anemias. You also may see spherocytes on peripheral smear because of incomplete macrophage destruction (extravascular hemolysis) of red blood cells.

28. **What clues point to lead poisoning as a cause of anemia?**

Lead poisoning causes a hypochromic, microcytic anemia, almost always in a child. With acute lead poisoning, look for vomiting, ataxia, colicky abdominal pain, irritability (aggressive behavior, behavioral regression), and encephalopathy, cerebral edema, or seizures. Usually, however, poisoning is chronic and low-level with minimal nonspecific symptoms. Watch for basophilic stippling on peripheral smear, elevated free erythrocyte protoporphyrin or lead level, and consider risk factors for lead exposure (a child who eats paint chips or lives in an old, run-down building).

29. **True or false: Children with risk factors should be screened for lead poisoning.**

True. Screening all asymptomatic children with a serum lead level at 1 and 2 years old regardless of risk is becoming controversial. In children with risk factors, screening is very important because chronic low-level exposure may lead to permanent neurologic sequelae. Screening should start at 6 months in children with risk factors, such as pica (especially paint chips and dust in old buildings that may have lead paint), residence in an old or neglected building, and/or residence near or family members who work at a lead-smelting or battery-recycling plant. Screen and measure symptomatic exposure with serum lead levels (normal value: less than 10 μg/dL).

30. **How is lead poisoning treated?**

Treat initially with decreased exposure (best strategy) as well as lead chelation therapy, if needed. Use succimer in children and dimercaprol in adults; in severe cases, use dimercaprol plus ethylenediamine tetraacetic acid (EDTA) for children or adults.

31. **How can sideroblastic anemia be recognized on the Step 2 exam? Should the presence of sideroblastic anemia raise concern about other conditions?**

The typical description is a microcytic, hypochromic anemia with increased or normal iron, ferritin, and total iron-binding capacity (transferrin). This description should immediately steer you away from iron deficiency. Look for polychromatophilic stippling and the classic "ringed sideroblast" in the bone marrow (know what it looks like). Sideroblastic anemia may be related to myelodysplasia or future blood dyscrasia. Although probably you will not be asked about management, treatment is supportive. In rare cases the anemia responds to **pyridoxine**. Do not give iron.

32. **How do you recognize anemia of chronic disease?**

First, look for the presence of a disease that causes chronic inflammation (e.g., rheumatoid arthritis, lupus erythematosus, cancer, tuberculosis). The anemia is either normocytic or microcytic. Serum iron is low, but so is total iron-binding capacity. Thus, the percent saturation may be near normal. Serum ferritin is elevated (because ferritin is an acute-phase reactant, the level should be increased). Treat the underlying disorder to correct the anemia. Do not give iron.

33. **Describe the hallmarks of spherocytosis.**

This normochromic, normocytic anemia is associated with spherocytes on peripheral smear, positive family history (autosomal dominant), splenomegaly, positive osmotic fragility test, and an increased **mean corpuscular hemoglobin concentration** (the only occasion on which this red blood cell index is useful for the Step 2 exam). Treatment often involves splenectomy. Spherocytes also may be seen in extravascular hemolysis, but the osmotic fragility test is normal.

34. **Why do chronic renal disease patients develop anemia? How do you treat it?**

All patients with chronic renal failure develop a normocytic, normochromic anemia with decreased reticulocyte count due to decreased erythropoietin production. Give erythropoietin to correct the anemia.

35. **What clues point to a diagnosis of aplastic anemia?**
Although aplastic anemia may be idiopathic, on the Step 2 exam watch for chemotherapy, radiation, malignancy affecting the bone marrow (especially leukemias), benzene, and implicated medications (e.g., chloramphenicol, carbamazepine, phenylbutazone, sulfa drugs, zidovudine, gold). Decreased white blood cells and platelets accompany the anemia. Treat first by stopping any possible causative medication; then try antithymocyte globulin, colony-stimulating factors (such as erythropoietin, sargramostim, and filgrastim, pegfilgrastim), or bone marrow transplant.

36. **Define myelophthisic anemia. What clues on the peripheral smear suggest its presence?**
Myelophthisic anemia is due to a space-occupying lesion in the bone marrow. The common causes are malignant invasion that destroys bone marrow (most common) and myelodysplasia or myelofibrosis. On the peripheral smear, look for marked anisocytosis (different size), poikilocytosis (different shape), nucleated red blood cells, giant and/or bizarre-looking platelets, and **teardrop-shaped** red blood cells. A bone marrow biopsy may reveal no cells ("dry tap" if the marrow is fibrotic) or malignant-looking cells.

37. **How do you recognize glucose-6-phosphatase deficiency on the USMLE?**
This genetic disorder is X-linked recessive, affecting males. It is most common in blacks and Mediterraneans. Look for sudden hemolysis or anemia after exposure to fava beans or certain drugs (antimalarials, salicylates, sulfa drugs) or after infection. You may see **Heinz bodies** and "bite cells" on peripheral smear. The diagnosis is made with a red blood cell enzyme assay, which should not be done immediately after hemolysis because of the potential for a false-negative result. All of the older red blood cells already have been destroyed, and the younger red blood cells are not affected in most patients. Treat with avoidance of precipitating foods and medications; discontinue the triggering medication first.

38. **Name some other causes of anemia.**
   - Endocrine failure (especially pituitary and thyroid; look for endocrine symptoms)
   - Mechanical heart valves (hemolyzed red blood cells)
   - Disseminated intravascular coagulation, thrombotic thrombocytopenic purpura (Fig. 17-6), and hemolytic uremic syndrome (look for schistocytes and red blood cell fragments on smear and other appropriate findings)
   - Other hemoglobinopathies (the hemoglobin C and E varieties are fairly common)
   - Paroxysmal nocturnal or cold hemoglobinuria
   - *Clostridium perfringens* infection, malaria, and babesiosis (cause intravascular hemolysis and fever)
   - Hypersplenism (associated with splenomegaly and often with low platelets and white blood cells)

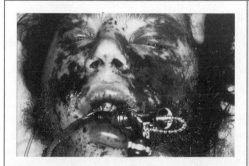

Figure 17-6. Thrombotic thrombocytopenic purpura (TTP). Widespread confluent and necrotic ecchymoses of the facial skin are seen in this man with severe TTP. (From Hoffbrand AV, Pettit JE: Color Atlas of Clinical Hematology, 3rd ed. St. Louis, Mosby, 2000, p 275, with permission.)

39. **When is transfusion indicated for anemia (at what hemoglobin level)?**
Always transfuse on clinical grounds; observe the symptoms. In other words, treat the patient, not the lab value. There is no such thing as a "trigger value" for transfusion. Having said this, hemoglobin levels less than 7 or 8 g/dL in the acute setting make most clinicians nervous.

40. **What are the indications for the use of various blood products?**
Whole blood: used only for rapid, massive blood loss or exchange transfusions (poisoning, thrombotic thrombocytopenic purpura).
Packed red blood cells: used for routine transfusions.
Washed red blood cells: free of traces of plasma, white cells, and platelets; good for IgA deficiency as well as allergic or previously sensitized patients.
Platelets: given for symptomatic thrombocytopenia (usually less than 10,000/μL).
Granulocytes: used on rare occasions for neutropenia.
Fresh frozen plasma (FFP): contains all clotting factors; used for bleeding diathesis when you cannot wait for vitamin K to take effect (e.g., disseminated intravascular coagulation, severe warfarin poisoning) or when vitamin K will not work (liver failure).
Cryoprecipitate: contains fibrinogen and factor 8; used in hemophilia, von Willebrand disease, and disseminated intravascular coagulation.

41. **What is the most common cause of a blood transfusion reaction? What blood type can be given in an emergency to avoid a reaction?**
The most common cause of a blood transfusion reaction is lab error. Type O negative blood can be used to avoid a reaction when you cannot wait for blood typing or when the blood bank does not have the patient's blood type.

42. **Describe the signs and symptoms of a blood transfusion reaction.**
Look for **febrile reaction** (e.g., chills, fever, headache, back pain) from antibodies to white blood cells; **hemolytic reaction** (e.g., anxiety or discomfort, dyspnea, chest pain, shock, jaundice) from antibodies to red blood cells; or **allergic reaction** (e.g., urticaria, edema, dizziness, dyspnea, wheezing, and anaphylaxis) to an unknown component in donor serum. Oliguria may be an associated finding.

43. **What should you do if you suspect a transfusion reaction?**
The first step is to *stop the transfusion.* If oliguria is present, treat with intravenous fluids and diuresis (mannitol or furosemide).

44. **What are the other risks of transfusion?**
There is a small but real risk of infection (usually viral infections such as hepatitis B and C, human immunodeficiency virus, and cytomegalovirus) and hyperkalemia (from hemolysis). With large transfusions (greater than 5 units of packed red blood cells), bleeding diathesis may result from dilutional thrombocytopenia and citrate (a blood preservative and calcium chelator that prevents clotting). Look for oozing from puncture or IV sites.

45. **What are the most common causes of disseminated intravascular coagulation (DIC)?**
The most common cause is pregnancy and obstetric complications (roughly 50% of cases), followed by malignancy (33%), sepsis, and trauma (especially head trauma, prostate surgery, and snake bites).

46. **How do I recognize and treat DIC in a classic at-risk patient?**
DIC usually manifests with bleeding diathesis but may have thrombotic tendencies. Look for the classic oozing or bleeding from puncture and IV sites; prolonged prothrombin time (PT), partial thromboplastin time (PTT), and bleeding time (BT). DIC is the only disorder on the Step

2 exam that prolongs all three tests. Other clues include positive D-dimer, increased fibrin degradation products, thrombocytopenia, decreased fibrin, and decreased clotting factors (including factor 8, which is normal in hepatic necrosis). Treat the underlying cause (e.g., evacuate the uterus, give antibiotics). You may need to give transfusions with fresh frozen plasma or, in rare cases, heparin (only if thrombosis occurs).

47. **With what conditions is eosinophilia associated?**

- Allergic or atopic diseases (allergic rhinitis, asthma, allergic bronchopulmonary aspergillosis, eczema, urticaria, atopic dermatitis, milk-protein allergy, drug reactions)
- Parasitic infections
- Fungal infections
- HIV infection
- Malignancies (lymphoma, leukemia, lung cancer, gastric cancer, pancreatic cancer, colon cancer, ovarian cancer)
- Connective tissue/autoimmune diseases (Churg-Strauss vasculitis, rheumatoid arthritis, lupus, scleroderma, eosinophilic fasciitis, Dressler syndrome, inflammatory bowel disease)
- Granulomatous disorders (sarcoidosis)
- Skin disorders (psoriasis, pemphigus)
- Immune disorders (Wiskott-Aldrich syndrome, hyper-IgE syndrome, IgA deficiency, thymoma)
- Adrenal insufficiency
- Pulmonary eosinophilia (Löffler syndrome)
- Cirrhosis
- Atheroembolic disease
- Familial eosinophilia
- Eosinophilia-myalgia syndrome (from using L-tryptophan)

48. **With what conditions is basophilia associated?**
Allergies or neoplasm/blood dyscrasia.

49. **True or false: The lupus anticoagulant causes a clotting tendency.**
True. Although the lupus anticoagulant may cause a prolonged partial thromboplastin time, the patient has a tendency toward thrombosis. Look for associated lupus symptoms, positive results on the Venereal Disease Research Laboratory or rapid plasma reagin tests for syphilis, or a history of miscarriages to help you recognize this condition.

50. **What genetic and acquired causes of an increased tendency toward clot-forming may appear on the Step 2 exam?**
The list keeps growing. Watch for factor V Leiden mutation (or activated protein C resistance), prothrombin G20210A mutation, hyperhomocysteinemia, elevated factor VIII level, deficiencies in protein C, protein S, or antithrombin III as genetic causes of an increased tendency toward thrombosis. Acquired causes include antiphospholipid syndrome (lupus anticoagulant and anticardiolipin antibody), hyperhomocysteinemia, pregnancy, cancer, and estrogen-containing medications. Note that hyperhomocysteinemia can be genetic or acquired. All are treated with anticoagulant therapy to prevent deep venous thrombosis and pulmonary embolus. Suspect these conditions if a person under age 35 develops recurrent clots or has no risk factors for clot development.

51. **Which clotting tests measure which portions of the coagulation cascade? Which medications affect these tests?**
PT (prothrombin time) measures the function of the extrinsic clotting pathway (prolonged by warfarin), activated PTT (partial thromboplastin time) measures the function of the intrinsic clotting pathway (prolonged by heparin), and BT (bleeding time) measures platelet function (prolonged by aspirin).

52. **How do specific diseases affect clotting tests? What are the main differential points?**

Disease	PT	PTT	BT	Platelet Count	RBC Count	Other
Von Willebrand disease	Normal	High	High	Normal	Normal	Autosomal dominant (look for family history)
Hemophilia A/B	Normal	High	Normal	Normal	Normal	X-linked recessive, A = low factor 8, B = low factor 9
DIC	High	High	High	Low	Normal/low	Appropriate history, low level of factor 8
Liver failure	High	High	Normal	Normal/low	Normal/low	Jaundice, normal factor 8 level; do not give vitamin K (ineffective); use FFP
Heparin	Normal	High	Normal	Normal/low	Normal	Watch for thrombocytopenia and thrombosis
Warfarin	High	Normal	Normal	Normal	Normal	Vitamin K antagonist (factors 2, 7, 9, and 10)
ITP	Normal	Normal	High	Low	Normal	Watch for preceding URI
TTP	Normal	Normal	High	Low	Low	Hemolysis (smear), CNS symptoms; treat with plasmapheresis; do not give platelets!
Scurvy	Normal	Normal	Normal	Normal	Normal	Fingernail and gum hemorrhages, bone hemorrhages; caused by vitamin C deficiency

PT = prothrombin time; PTT = partial thromboplastin time; BT = bleeding time; RBC = red blood cell; DIC = disseminated intravascular coagulation; ITP = idiopathic thrombocytopenic purpura; TTP = thrombotic thrombocytopenic purpura; FFP = fresh frozen plasma; URI = upper respiratory infection; CNS = central nervous system.

53. **What are the common causes of thrombocytopenia? What kind of bleeding problems are caused by low platelet counts?**
Common causes of thrombocytopenia include purpura (idiopathic or thrombotic), hemolytic uremic syndrome, disseminated intravascular coagulation, HIV, splenic sequestration, heparin

(treat by first stopping heparin), other medications (especially quinidine and sulfa drugs), autoimmune disease, and alcohol. Bleeding from thrombocytopenia is in the form of petechiae, nose bleeds, and easy bruising.

54. **What causes petechiae or "platelet-type" bleeding in the setting of normal platelets?**

Vitamin C deficiency (scurvy) causes bleeding similar to that seen with low platelets (splinter and gum hemorrhages, petechiae); perifollicular and subperiosteal hemorrhages are unique to scurvy. Patients have a poor dietary history (the classic example is hot dogs and soda or tea and toast), myalgias and arthralgias, and capillary fragility (bleeding is due to collagen problems in the vessels). Treat with oral vitamin C.

Other causes include uremia (platelet dysfunction), inherited connective tissue disorders (Ehlers-Danlos syndrome, Marfan syndrome), and chronic corticosteroid use (causes capillary fragility).

CHAPTER 18

HYPERTENSION

1. **How often should you screen for hypertension?**
   Although there is no absolutely correct answer, all people should be screened roughly every 2 years, starting at the age of 3.

2. **Define hypertension.**
   Persistent blood pressure greater than 140/90 mm Hg. Individuals with a systolic blood pressure of 120 to 139 mm Hg or a diastolic pressure of 80 to 89 mm Hg should be considered as prehypertensive. Remember that 145/60 mm Hg is hypertension, as is 115/95 mm Hg (isolated systolic or diastolic hypertension, respectively). Treatment is needed. In grading the severity of hypertension, use the worst number, whether it be diastolic or systolic. See Table 18-1 for the 2003 Joint National Committee (JNC-7) classification.

TABLE 18-1. 2003 JOINT NATIONAL COMMITTEE (JNC-7) HYPERTENSION CLASSIFICATION

Systolic BP* (mm Hg)	Diastolic BP* (mm Hg)	Classification
< 120	< 80	Normal
120–139	80–89	Prehypertension
140–159	90–99	Stage I hypertension
≥ 160	≥ 100	Stage II hypertension

*Classification is based on the worst number (e.g., 168/60 mm Hg is considered stage II hypertension even though diastolic pressure is normal).

3. **What is the "two-measurement" rule in the diagnosis of hypertension?**
   The blood pressure should be measured two times on each of two separate office visits before the diagnosis and pharmacologic treatment of hypertension. However, if asked, institute conservative measures (see question 4) and address associated comorbidities (e.g., obesity, diabetes) after the first abnormal measurement. There are a few important exceptions to the "start conservative and remeasure" strategy, however, and more aggressive approaches are gaining favor. Patients with marked blood pressure elevations (generally greater than 200/120 mm Hg) and acute target-organ damage (e.g., encephalopathy, myocardial infraction, unstable angina, pulmonary edema, stroke) require hospitalization and parenteral drug therapy. Patients with markedly elevated blood pressure but without target organ damage usually do not require hospitalization but should be given immediate combination oral anti-hypertensive therapy. See question 7 for more details. In pregnant woman, preeclampsia may be the cause of hypertension. Waiting to treat in this setting can have devastating consequences to mother and fetus.

4. What are the conservative (i.e., nonpharmacologic) treatments for hypertension?
Dietary changes (i.e., low salt, low fat, low calorie), reduced smoking and alcohol intake, weight loss, and exercise may each have a positive effect on blood pressure and, in some cases, get the patient back into the normotensive range. For stage I hypertension, it is reasonable to give a 1- to 2-month trial of lifestyle modifications before starting medication. In patients with stage II hypertension or those with diabetes or renal disease, early pharmacologic treatment is often preferred.

5. List the first-line medications for treatment of hypertension.
Thiazide-type diuretics should be used as initial therapy for most patients with hypertension, either alone or in combination with one of the following classes: angiotensin-converting enzyme (ACE) inhibitors, angiotensin receptor blockers (ARBs), beta blockers, and calcium channel blockers. Which you should use often depends on the individual patient and his or her other medical problems. In some cases, medications from multiple classes may be needed to reach blood pressure goals.

Drug Class	Use in Patients with:	Avoid in Patients with:
Thiazides	Heart failure, diabetes, high risk for coronary artery disease or stroke, osteoporosis	Gout, electrolyte disturbances (e.g., hyponatremia), pregnancy
Beta blockers	Stable angina, acute coronary syndrome/unstable angina, acute or prior myocardial infarction, high risk for coronary artery disease, atrial tachycardia/fibrillation, thyrotoxicosis (short-term), essential tremor, migraines	Asthma, chronic obstructive pulmonary disease, heart block, sick sinus syndrome
ACE inhibitors	Heart failure, diabetes, acute coronary syndrome/unstable angina, acute or prior myocardial infarction, high risk for coronary artery disease or stroke, chronic kidney disease	Pregnancy, angioedema, renovascular hypertension (may cause renal failure)
ARBs	Heart failure, diabetes, chronic kidney disease	Pregnancy, renovascular hypertension (may cause renal failure)
Calcium channel blockers	Raynaud syndrome, atrial tachyarrhythmias	Heart block, sick sinus syndrome, congestive heart failure (all related to central-acting agents), pregnancy

Note: ACE inhibitors are first-line agents for congestive heart failure, because they reduce mortality rates. In diabetes, ACE inhibitors retard progression to nephropathy and neuropathy. All patients with stable congestive heart failure or diabetes should take an ACE inhibitor (if they can tolerate it) even in the absence of hypertension.

6. **What about women of reproductive age and pregnant women with hypertension?**
Labetalol, hydralazine, and alpha-methyldopa are safe. If preeclampsia is present, remember that magnesium sulfate lowers blood pressure.

7. **Define hypertensive urgency. How is it different from hypertensive emergency?**
Hypertensive **urgency** is defined as blood pressure greater than 200/120 mm Hg without symptoms. Hypertensive **emergency** is defined as blood pressure greater than 200/120 mm Hg with symptoms or evidence of end-organ damage. Examples include acute left ventricular failure, chest pain or angina, myocardial infarction, encephalopathy (watch for headaches, confusion, retinal hemorrhages, papilledema, mental status changes, vomiting, blurry vision, dizziness, and/or seizures), or acute renal failure (from necrotizing arteriolitis, Fig. 18-1). Both require immediate treatment, but hypertensive emergency is more worrisome. Hypertensive urgency typically is treated orally with furosemide, clonidine, or captopril. There are many treatment options for hypertensive emergency, but intravenous nitroprusside, labetalol, or nicardipine are the most common.

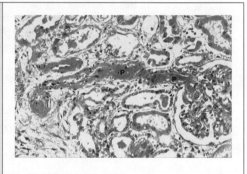

Figure 18-1. Fibrinoid necrosis secondary to malignant hypertension. This change is due to rapid intimal cell proliferation with leakage of plasma proteins into and beyond the arteriolar wall with resultant obliteration of the wall by intensely eosinophilic amorphous proteinaceous material (P) and, often, luminal occlusion. Damage to the vessel wall may also lead to thrombosis within the lumen. A glomerulus can be seen on the far right side of the image. (From Stevens A, et al.: Wheater's Basic Histopathology, 4th ed. New York, Churchill Livingstone, 2002, p 116, with permission.)

8. **What causes hypertension?**
Roughly 90% to 95% of cases are idiopathic, multifactorial, or essential hypertension. About 5% to 10% of cases are due to secondary (known) causes.

9. **What are the common causes of secondary hypertension in younger men and women?**
In younger men, a common cause of secondary hypertension is excessive alcohol intake (get the patient to quit!). In younger women, common and classic causes are birth control pills (stop them!) and renal artery stenosis from fibromuscular dysplasia (which may cause a bruit and should be treated with balloon angioplasty).

10. **List less common causes of secondary hypertension.**
Pheochromocytoma. Look for wild swings in blood pressure with diaphoresis and confusion. As a screening test, order 24-hour urine collection to assess catecholamine products (metanephrines, vanillylmandelic acid, homovanillic acid).
   Renal artery stenosis (RAS). Unlike young patients with fibromuscular dysplasia, elderly patients typically have RAS due to atherosclerosis. A renal artery bruit is classically present (although not sensitive); magnetic resonance or conventional angiography makes the definitive diagnosis (Fig. 18-2). Giving ACE inhibitors to patients with RAS may precipitate acute renal failure (sometimes the first diagnostic clue to its presence).

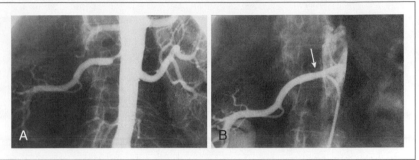

Figure 18-2. A, Baseline aortogram showing 70 percent diameter stenosis of the right renal artery. **B,** After stenting. Note the mild residual narrowing (*arrow*). (From Libby P, et al.: Braunwald's Heart Disease: A Textbook of Cardiovascular Medicine, 8th ed. Philadelphia, Saunders, 2008, Fig. 59-12.)

Polycystic kidney disease. Look for flank mass, positive family history (autosomal dominant pattern of inheritance), and elevations in creatinine and blood urea nitrogen.

Cushing syndrome. Look for stigmata of Cushing syndrome on exam. Order 24-urine collection to assess free cortisol or a dexamethasone suppression test

Conn syndrome. The cause is an aldosterone-secreting adrenal neoplasm. Look for high aldosterone levels, low renin levels, hypokalemia, metabolic alkalosis, and/or an adrenal mass on computed tomography.

Coarctation of the aorta. Look for hypertension in the upper extremities only, with unequal pulses, radiofemoral delay, and rib notching on chest radiograph; associated with Turner syndrome. MRI or angiography makes a definitive diagnosis.

Renal failure from any cause. In children, watch for poststreptococcal glomerulonephritis or hemolytic uremic syndrome.

11. **What does lowering blood pressure accomplish?**
    Hypertension is the number-one modifiable risk factor for strokes. Lowering blood pressure decreases heart disease, myocardial infarctions, atherosclerosis, renal failure, and dissecting aortic aneurysms.

12. **What is the most common cause of death among untreated patients with hypertension?**
    The same as for the general population—coronary artery disease.

13. **Which tests should be ordered for every patient with a diagnosis of hypertension? Why?**
    1. **Electrocardiogram:** to determine whether the heart has been affected (e.g., left ventricular hypertrophy).
    2. **Chemistry 7 panel** (i.e., basic metabolic panel): clues to possible secondary cause of hypertension (e.g., electrolyte disturbances in Conn syndrome) and evaluation for diabetes
    3. **Urinalysis:** clues to possible secondary cause of hypertension (e.g., red blood cell casts in poststreptococcal glomerulonephritis) and to kidney damage (proteinuria).
    4. **Hemoglobin and hematocrit:** to evaluate for anemia or polycythemia.
    5. **Lipid panel:** to evaluate for dyslipidemia as an additional risk factor for coronary artery disease.

1. **List the four classic types of hypersensitivity reactions.**
   ■ Anaphylactic (type I)
   ■ Cytotoxic (type II)
   ■ Immune complex-mediated (type III)
   ■ Cell-mediated/delayed (type IV)

2. **What causes type I hypersensitivity? Give the classic clinical examples.**
   Type I (anaphylactic) hypersensitivity is due to preformed IgE antibodies that cause release of vasoactive amines (e.g., histamine, leukotrienes) from mast cells and basophils. Examples are anaphylaxis, atopy, hay fever, urticaria, allergic rhinitis, and some forms of asthma. Anaphylaxis may be due to bee stings, food allergy (especially peanuts and shellfish), medications (especially penicillins and sulfa drugs), or rubber glove allergy.

3. **Describe the clinical findings with chronic type I hypersensitivity.**
   Look for eosinophilia, elevated IgE levels, positive family history, and seasonal exacerbations. Patients also may have allergic "shiners" (bilateral infraorbital edema), and a transverse nasal crease (due to frequent nose rubbing). Pale, bluish, edematous nasal turbinates with many eosinophils in clear, watery nasal secretions are also classic.

4. **What medication should be avoided in patients with nasal polyps?**
   Do not give aspirin, which may precipitate a severe asthma attack.

5. **How do you recognize and treat true anaphylaxis?**
   Look for the classic triggers mentioned above just before the patient becomes agitated and flushed and develops itching (urticaria), facial swelling (angioedema), and difficulty in breathing. Symptoms tend to develop rapidly and dramatically.
   Treat immediately by securing the airway (laryngeal edema may prevent intubation, in which case do a cricothyroidotomy, if needed) and give subcutaneous epinephrine. Antihistamines are only useful for cutaneous reactions and itching, not for more severe reactions. Use corticosteroids only if the initial treatment options are not available (not a first-line agent).

6. **What usually causes hereditary angioedema?**
   A deficiency of **C1 esterase inhibitor** (complement) is the usual cause of hereditary angioedema. Patients have diffuse swelling of lips, eyelids, and possibly the airway, unrelated to allergen exposure. The disease is autosomal dominant; look for a positive family history. C4 complement levels are low. Acute treatment is the same as for anaphylaxis. Androgens are used for long-term treatment because they increase liver production of C1 esterase inhibitor.

7. **What type of testing can identify an allergen if it is not obvious?**
   Skin or patch testing (Fig. 19-1).

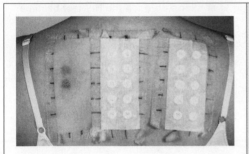

Figure 19-1. Patch testing. A battery of common and suspected allergens is applied to the back for 48 hours. The skin is then examined at 96 hours. Irritant reactions disappear, allergic ones do not. Two positives are present. (From du Vivier A: Atlas of Clinical Dermatology, 3rd ed. New York, Churchill Livingstone, 2002, p 65, with permission.)

8. **What causes type II hypersensitivity? List some classic clinical examples.**
   Type II (cytotoxic) hypersensitivity is due to preformed IgG and IgM antibodies that react with the antigen and cause secondary inflammation. Examples include the following:
   - Autoimmune hemolytic anemia (classically caused by methyldopa, penicillins, or sulfa drugs) or other cytopenias caused by antibodies (e.g., idiopathic thrombocytopenic purpura)
   - Transfusion reactions
   - Erythroblastosis fetalis (Rh incompatibility)
   - Goodpasture syndrome (watch for linear immunofluorescence on kidney biopsy)
   - Myasthenia gravis
   - Graves disease
   - Pernicious anemia
   - Pemphigus vulgaris
   - Hyperacute transplant rejection (as soon as the anastomosis is made at transplant surgery, the transplanted organ deteriorates in front of the surgeon's eyes)

9. **What lab test is usually positive with a type II hypersensitivity that causes anemia?**
   Coombs test (usually the direct Coombs test).

10. **What causes type III hypersensitivity? List some classic clinical examples.**
    Type III (immune complex-mediated) hypersensitivity is due to antigen–antibody complexes that usually are deposited in vessels and cause an inflammatory response. Examples include serum sickness, lupus erythematosus, rheumatoid arthritis, polyarteritis nodosa, cryoglobulinemia, and certain types of glomerulonephritis (e.g., from chronic hepatitis).

11. **What causes type IV hypersensitivity? How is it related to tuberculosis testing?**
    Type IV (cell-mediated/delayed) hypersensitivity is due to sensitized T lymphocytes that release inflammatory mediators. The tuberculosis skin test (purified protein derivative [PPD]) exploits this immune system reaction. Other examples include contact dermatitis (especially poison ivy, nickel earrings, cosmetics, and medications), chronic transplant rejection, and granulomas (e.g., sarcoidosis).

12. **What sexually transmitted infectious disease should be in the back of your mind when a patient presents with a sore throat and mononucleosis-like syndrome?**
    Human immunodeficiency virus (HIV) infection, because initial seroconversion may present as a mononucleosis-like syndrome (e.g., fever, malaise, pharyngitis, rash, lymphadenopathy).

13. **How is HIV diagnosed? How long after exposure does the HIV test become positive?**

Diagnosis is made with the enzyme-linked immunosorbent assay (ELISA), which, if positive, is confirmed with a Western blot test. All of these tests should be done before you tell the patient anything. It takes 6 to 12 weeks for antibodies to develop in the majority of patients. Antibodies are present by 6 months in 95% of patients. Therefore, if a patient wants testing because of recent risk-taking behavior, you should retest the patient in 6 months if the initial test is negative.

Rapid tests are available, but the predictive accuracy varies with the prevalence of HIV infection in the population. Positive tests require confirmatory testing with ELISA and Western blot. Negative test results are reliable unless the patient is in the window period of acute HIV infection.

14. **Are "control" tests needed when a PPD tuberculosis test is done in HIV-positive patients?**

Most authorities no longer recommend "control" (also known as anergy) testing when a PPD test is done in HIV-positive patients.

15. **How do you recognize *Pneumocystis carinii* pneumonia (PCP)?**

For the Step 2 exam, think of PCP first in any patient with HIV and pneumonia, even though community-acquired pneumonia is more common even in patients with AIDS. Look for severe hypoxia with normal radiographs or diffuse, bilateral interstitial infiltrates (Fig. 19-2). Patients usually have a dry, nonproductive cough. PCP may be detected with silver stains (Wright-Giemsa, Giemsa, or methenamine silver) applied to induced sputum; if not, you can use bronchoscopy with bronchoalveolar lavage and brush biopsy to make the diagnosis. High levels of lactate dehydrogenase are suspicious in the appropriate setting. PCP is now usually treated presumptively, with diagnostic testing reserved for those in whom the diagnosis is unclear or initial treatment fails.

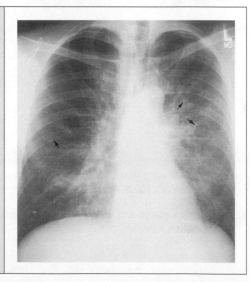

Figure 19-2. Posteroanterior chest radiograph of an HIV-seropositive patient with *Pneumocystis* pneumonia showing bilateral, predominantly perihilar, granular opacities and three pneumatoceles (*arrows*). Pneumatoceles may predispose patients to pneumothorax. (From Mason RJ, et al.: Murray and Nadel's Textbook of Respiratory Medicine, 4th ed. Philadelphia, Saunders, 2005, Fig. 75-5. Reproduced with permission from L. Huang.)

16. **What is the most common primary immunodeficiency? How do you recognize it?**

   IgA deficiency, which causes recurrent respiratory and gastrointestinal infections. IgA levels are always low, and levels of IgG subclass 2 may be low. Do not give immunoglobulins, which may cause anaphylaxis due to development of anti-IgA antibodies. Alternatively, if any patient develops anaphylaxis after immunoglobulin exposure, you should think of IgA deficiency.

17. **How do you recognize Bruton agammaglobulinemia?**

   Bruton agammaglobulinemia (X-linked agammaglobulinemia) is an X-linked recessive disorder with low or absent B cells that affects males. Infections begin after 6 months when maternal antibodies disappear. Look for recurrent lung or sinus infections with *Streptococcus* and *Haemophilus* species.

18. **What causes DiGeorge syndrome? How do you recognize it?**

   DiGeorge syndrome is caused by hypoplasia of the third and fourth pharyngeal pouches. Look for hypocalcemia and tetany (from hypocalcemia due to absent parathyroid glands) in the first 24 to 48 hours of life. The thymus also may be absent or hypoplastic, and congenital heart defects and typical facies often are present.

19. **What is the classic cause of severe combined immunodeficiency? How does it present?**

   Severe combined immunodeficiency may be autosomal recessive or X-linked. The classic cause is **adenosine deaminase deficiency** (autosomal recessive). Patients have B- and T-cell defects and severe infections in the first few months of life. Other symptoms include cutaneous anergy and absent or dysplastic thymus and lymph nodes.

20. **What triad indicates the diagnosis of Wiskott-Aldrich syndrome?**

   Wiskott-Aldrich deficiency is an X-linked recessive disorder that affects males. The classic triad consists of eczema, thrombocytopenia (look for bleeding), and recurrent infections (usually respiratory).

21. **How do you recognize Chediak-Higashi syndrome?**

   Chediak-Higashi syndrome is usually an autosomal recessive disorder characterized by giant granules in neutrophils, infections, and often oculocutaneous albinism. It is caused by a defect in microtubule polymerization.

22. **Describe the pathophysiology of chronic granulomatous disease.**

   Chronic granulomatous disease (CGD) is usually an X-linked recessive disorder that affects males. Because of a defect in the activity of the enzyme nicotinamide adenine dinucleotide phosphate (NADPH) oxidase, patients have recurrent infections with catalase-positive organisms (e.g., *Staphylococcus aureus, Pseudomonas* species). Diagnosis is clinched if the question mentions deficient nitroblue tetrazolium (NBT) dye reduction by granulocytes. This test measures the respiratory burst, which patients with chronic granulomatous disease lack. On the USMLE, if you see "CGD" then look for "NBT" in the answer.

23. Cover the right-hand column, and answer the questions about HIV management on the left.

Question	Answer
After HIV diagnosis, how often do you check the CD4 count?	Every 3–4 months. Every 6 months for patients who are adherent to therapy with sustained viral suppression and stable clinical status for more than 2–3 years.
When do you start antiretroviral therapy?	When the CD4 count is less than $350/mm^3$ or if there is a history of an AIDS-defining illness. Also should be initiated in pregnant women, in patients with HIV-associated nephropathy, and in patient with hepatitis B coinfection.
What are the AIDS-defining illnesses?	*Pneumocystic carinii* pneumonia Esophageal candidiasis Wasting Kaposi's sarcoma Disseminated *Mycobacterium avium* infection Tuberculosis Cytomegalovirus disease HIV-associated dementia Recurrent bacterial pneumonia Toxoplasmosis Immunoblastic lymphoma Chronic cryptosporidiosis Burkitt lymphoma Disseminated histoplasmosis Invasive cervical cancer Chronic Herpes simplex
When do you start PCP prophylaxis?	When the CD4 count is less than $200/mm^3$ or a history of oropharyngeal candidiasis
What is the drug of choice for PCP prophylaxis?	Trimethoprim-sulfamethoxazole (Bactrim)
What other agents are used in patients with allergy or intolerance to Bactrim?	Dapsone, aerosolized pentamidine, dapsone plus pyrimethamine plus leucovorin, and atovaquone
When should you start Mycobacterium avium complex (MAC) prophylaxis?	When the CD4 count is less than $50/mm^3$
What drugs are used for MAC prophylaxis?	Clarithromycin or azithromycin (rifabutin is an alterative)

(continued)

Question	Answer
True or false: Once the CD4 is less than 200/mm^3, the patient is automatically considered to have AIDS (even without opportunistic infections).	True.
True or false: Give the measles-mumps-rubella vaccine.	True (CD4 count must be greater than 200/mm^3)
True or false: Give the varicella vaccine.	True, if patient does not have evidence of immunity (CD4 count must be greater than 200/mm^3).
True or false: Do not give annual influenza vaccines.	False (give every year to all HIV-infected patients).
True or false: Pneumococcal vaccine should be given.	True. It should be given to all HIV-infected patients, and revaccination every 5 years should be considered.
True or false: Give hepatitis A vaccine.	True, if the patient has chronic liver disease or is at increased risk for hepatitis A infection.
True or false: Give hepatitis B vaccine.	True.
True or false: PPD testing should be done annually.	True, if the initial test is negative and the patient is high-risk.
True or false: Oral polio vaccine should be given to patients who are at risk of exposure through travel or work.	False (use inactive polio vaccine injection).
The risk of which cancer is increased on skin and in the mouth?	Kaposi sarcoma
The risk of which type of blood cell cancer is increased?	Non-Hodgkin lymphoma (usually primary B-cell lymphomas of CNS)
What do positive India ink preparations of the cerebrospinal fluid mean?	*Cryptococcus neoformans* meningitis
What do ring-enhancing lesions in the brain on CT or MR scans usually mean?	Toxoplasmosis, cysticercosis/*Taenia solium,* or lymphoma
True or false: HIV may cause thrombocytopenia.	True.
True or false: HIV can cause dementia.	True.
True or false: HIV protects against peripheral neuropathies.	False (HIV can cause them).
True or false: HIV-positive mothers may breast-feed their infants.	False (breast milk transmits HIV).
First-choice agent for cytomegalovirus retinitis.	Valganciclovir
Second-choice agents for cytomegalovirus retinitis.	Ganciclovir, foscarnet or cidofovir

(continued)

Question	Answer
True or false: Pregnant patients should receive anti-retroviral therapy.	True. Three-drug therapy is currently recommended, beginning at 28 weeks gestation.
True or false: Infants born to HIV-positive mothers should take zidovudine (ZDV).	True (for the first 6 weeks after delivery).
True or false: Cesarean section increases maternal HIV transmission.	False (it may decrease transmission to child).
Most likely cause of pneumonia in HIV-positive patient	*Streptococcus pneumoniae*
Most likely cause of opportunistic pneumonia in HIV-positive patient	*Pneumocystis carinii*
Stain used on sputum to detect PCP	Silver (Wright-Giemsa or Giemsa)
Two pathogens that cause chronic diarrhea only in AIDS.	*Cryptosporidium* and *Isospora* spp.
True or false: Herpes-zoster infection in young adults = possible HIV infection.	True (suggests immunodeficiency).
True or false: Thrush in young adults may mean HIV infection.	True (also associated with diabetes, leukemia, and steroids).
True or false: A positive HIV antibody test in a newborn is unreliable.	True (maternal antibodies in the neonate can give a false-positive result for the first 6 months).

24. **Complement deficiencies of C5 through C9 cause recurrent infections with which genus of bacteria?**
   Neisseria species.

25. **Define chronic mucocutaneous candidiasis.**
   Chronic mucocutaneous candidiasis is a cellular immunodeficiency specific for candidal infection. Patients have thrush and candidal infections of the scalp, skin, and nails as well as anergy to *Candida* sp. with skin testing. Often it is associated with hypothyroidism. The rest of the immune function is intact; no other types of infections are present.

26. **Give the classic description of hyper-IgE syndrome (Job-Buckley syndrome).**
   Patients with hyper-IgE syndrome have recurrent staphylococcal infections (especially of the skin) and have extremely high IgE levels. They also commonly have fair skin, red hair, and eczema.

CHAPTER 20

1. **Cover the middle and right-hand columns and specify which bugs are associated with each type of infection and what type of empiric antibiotic should be used while waiting for culture results.**

Condition	Main Organism(s)	Empirical Antibiotics
Urinary tract infection	*Escherichia coli*	Trimethoprim-sulfamethoxazole, nitrofurantoin, amoxicillin, quinolones
Bronchitis	Virus, *Haemophilus influenzae, Moraxella* spp.	Usually no benefit from antibiotics. May consider macrolides or doxycycline
Pneumonia (classic)	*Streptococcus pneumoniae, H. influenzae*	Third-generation cephalosporin, azithromycin
Pneumonia (atypical)	*Mycoplasma, Chlamydia* spp.	Macrolide antibiotic, doxycycline
Osteomyelitis	*Staphylococcus aureus, Salmonella* spp.	Oxacillin, cefazolin, vancomycin
Cellulitis	Streptococci, staphylococci	Cephalexin, dicloxacillin. Use clindamycin or trimethoprim-sulfamethoxazole if MRSA is suspected.
Meningitis (neonate)	Streptococci B, *E. coli, Listeria* spp.	Ampicillin + aminoglycoside, expanded spectrum third-generation cephalosporin (cefotaxime)
Meningitis (child/adult)	*S. pneumoniae, Neisseria meningitidis**	Cefotaxime or ceftriaxone + vancomycin
Endocarditis	Staphylococci, streptococci	Antistaphylococcal penicillin[†] (or vancomycin) + aminoglycoside
Sepsis	Gram-negative organisms, streptococci, staphylococci	Third-generation penicillin/ cephalosporin + aminoglycoside, or imipenem
Septic arthritis[‡]	*S. aureus*	Vancomycin
	Gram negative bacilli	Ceftazidime or ceftriaxone
	Gonococci	Ceftriaxone, ciprofloxacin, or spectinomycin

*H. influenzae is no longer as common a cause of meningitis in children because of widespread vaccination. In a child with no history of immunization, *H. influenzae* is the most likely cause of meningitis.
[†]Examples: dicloxacillin, methicillin.
[‡]Think of staphylococci if the patient is monogamous or not sexually active. Think of gonorrhea for younger adults who are sexually active.

2. **Cover the right-hand columns and specify the empirical antibiotic of choice for each organism.**

Organism*	Antibiotic	Other Choices
Streptococcus A or B	Penicillin, cefazolin	Erythromycin
S. pneumoniae	3rd-generation cephalosporin + vancomycin	Fluoroquinolone
Enterococcus	Penicillin or ampicillin + aminoglycoside	Vancomycin + aminoglycoside
Staphylococcus aureus	Anti-staphylococcus penicillin (e.g., methicillin)	Vancomycin (MRSA)
Gonococcus†	Ceftriaxone or cefixime	Spectinomycin
Meningococcus	Cefotaxime or ceftriaxone	Chloramphenicol or penicillin G if proven to be penicillin susceptible
Haemophilus	2nd or 3rd gen. cephalosporin	Ampicillin
Pseudomonas	Antipseudomonal penicillin (ticarcillin, piperacillin) +/- beta lactamase inhibitor (clavulanate, tazobactam)	Ceftazidime, cefepime, aztreonam, imipenem, ciprofloxacin
Bacteroides	Metronidazole	Clindamycin
Mycoplasma	Erythromycin, azithromycin	Doxycycline
Treponema pallidum	Penicillin	Doxycycline
Chlamydia	Doxycycline, azithromycin	Erythromycin, ofloxacin
Lyme disease (*Borrelia* spp)	Cefuroxime, doxycycline, amoxicillin	Erythromycin

*Always use culture sensitivities to guide therapy once available
†With genital infections, always treat for presumed *Chlamydia* co-infection with azithromycin or doxycycline

3. **Cover the right-hand column and specify what each Gram stain most likely represents.**

Gram Stain Result	Meaning
Blue/purple color	Gram-positive organism
Red color	Gram-negative organism
Gram-positive cocci in chains	Streptococci
Gram-positive cocci in clusters	Staphylococci
Gram-positive cocci in pairs (diplococci)	*Streptococcus pneumoniae*
Gram-negative coccobacilli (small rods)	*Haemophilus* sp.
Gram-negative diplococci	*Neisseria* sp. (sexually transmitted disease, septic arthritis, meningitis) or *Moraxella* sp. (lungs, sinusitis)

(continued)

Gram Stain Result	Meaning
Plump gram-negative rod with thick capsule (mucoid appearance)	*Klebsiella* sp.
Gram-positive rods that form spores	*Clostridium* sp., *Bacillus* sp.
Pseudohyphae	*Candida* sp.
Acid-fast organisms	*Mycobacterium* (usually *M. tuberculosis*), *Nocardia* sp.
Gram-positive with sulfur granules	*Actinomyces* sp. (pelvic inflammatory disease in intrauterine device users; rare cause of neck mass/cervical adenitis)
Silver-staining	*Pneumocystis jirovecii* and cat-scratch disease
Positive India ink preparation (thick capsule)	*Cryptococcus neoformans*
Spirochete	*Treponema* sp., *Leptospira* sp. (both seen only on dark-field microscopy), *Borrelia* sp. (seen on regular light microscope)

4. **What is the gold standard for diagnosis of pneumonia?**
Sputum culture. Try to get the culture before starting antibiotics, though many treat empirically without culture in routine cases. Get blood cultures, too, because bacteremia is common with pneumonia.

5. **What is the most common cause of pneumonia? How does it classically present?**
Streptococcus pneumoniae. Look for rapid onset of shaking chills after 1 to 2 days of upper respiratory infection symptoms (sore throat, runny nose, dry cough), followed by fever, pleurisy, and productive cough (yellowish-green or rust-colored from blood), especially in older adults. Chest radiograph shows lobar consolidation, and the white blood cell count is high with a large percentage of neutrophils. Treat with a macrolide (e.g., azithromycin, clarithromycin), doxycycline, third-generation cephalosporin with a macrolide or doxycycline, or a fluoroquinolone with atypical coverage (e.g., levofloxacin, moxifloxacin).

6. **What is the best prevention against *S. pneumoniae*?**
Vaccination. Give pneumococcal vaccine to all children as well as adult patients over 65 years old, splenectomized patients, patients with sickle-cell disease (who have autosplenectomy) or splenic dysfunction, immunocompromised patients (HIV, malignancy, organ transplant), and all patients with chronic disease (e.g., diabetes, cardiac, pulmonary, renal, or liver disease).

7. **How do you recognize and treat *Haemophilus influenzae* pneumonia?**
H. influenzae is now uncommon in children due to vaccination, but is still an important cause of pneumonia in the elderly and in those with underlying lung disease such as COPD. Often it resembles pneumococcal pneumonia clinically, but look for gram-negative coccobacilli on sputum Gram stain. Treat with amoxicillin or a third-generation cephalosporin.

8. **Describe the hallmarks of *Staphylococcus aureus* pneumonia.**
S. aureus tends to cause hospital-acquired (nosocomial) pneumonia and pneumonia in patients with cystic fibrosis (along with *Pseudomonas* sp.), intravenous drug abusers, and patients with chronic granulomatous disease (look for recurrent lung abscesses). Empyema and lung abscesses are relatively common with *S. aureus* pneumonia.

9. **In what clinical situations do you tend to see gram-negative pneumonias?**
Pseudomonas infection classically is associated with cystic fibrosis, *Klebsiella* infection with people who are alcoholics and people who are homeless (watch for classic description of currant jelly sputum), and enteric gram-negative organisms (e.g., *Escherichia coli*) with aspiration, neutropenia, and hospital-acquired pneumonia. These pneumonias often have a high mortality rate because of the type of patients affected and the severity of the pneumonia (abscesses are common). Treat empirically with an antipseudomonal penicillin (e.g., ticarcillin, piperacillin) with or without a beta lactamase inhibitor (e.g., clavulanate, tazobactam). Alternatives include ceftazidime or ciprofloxacin.

10. **How do you recognize *Mycoplasma* pneumonia?**
Mycoplasma infection is most common in adolescents and young adults (the classic patient is a college student or soldier who lives in a dormitory/barracks and has sick contacts). It is one of the atypical pneumonias because it is different from pneumonia due to *Streptococcus pneumoniae*. For example, it has a long prodrome with gradual worsening of malaise, headaches, dry, nonproductive cough, and sore throat; the fever tends to be low-grade. Chest radiograph shows a patchy, diffuse bronchopneumonia and classically looks terrible, although the patient often does not feel that bad. Look for positive **cold-agglutinin antibody titers,** which may cause hemolysis or anemia. Atypical pneumonia is treated empirically with a macrolide antibiotic (azithromycin) or broad-spectrum fluoroquinolone (e.g., levofloxacin or moxifloxacin).

11. **What about chlamydial pneumonia?**
Chlamydia sp. is second only to *Mycoplasma* sp. as the cause of atypical pneumonia in adolescents and young adults. It presents similarly but has negative cold-agglutinin antibody titers. Treat empirically with a macrolide antibiotic (azithromycin) or broad-spectrum fluoroquinolone (e.g., levofloxacin or moxifloxacin).

12. **In what setting do you see *Pneumocystis jirovecii* (PCP) and cytomegalovirus (CMV) pneumonia?**
In HIV-positive patients with CD4 counts less than $200/mm^3$ (AIDS) and other severely immunosuppressed patients (e.g., organ transplant recipients taking powerful immunosuppressants or patients on cancer chemotherapy). In AIDS, PCP is the most common opportunistic pneumonia and may require bronchoalveolar lavage for diagnosis. PCP can be seen with silver stains and typically causes bilateral interstitial lung infiltrates. Treat with trimethoprim-sulfamethoxazole; an alternative is pentamidine. CMV pneumonia is characterized by intracellular inclusion bodies. Treat with ganciclovir; foscarnet is an alternative.

13. **What is the best time to treat PCP?**
Before it happens! PCP is acquired when the CD4 count is below $200/mm^3$. At that point you should institute PCP prophylaxis in an HIV-positive patient with trimethoprim-sulfamethoxazole. Alternatives include atovaquone, dapsone, or pentamidine.

14. **Cover the two right-hand columns and specify the organism after looking at the scenario associated with it:**

Scenario	Organism(s)	Comments
Stuck with thorn or gardening	*Sporothrix schenckii*	Treat with oral potassium iodide or ketoconazole
Aplastic crisis in sickle cell disease	Parvovirus B19	

(continued)

Scenario	Organism(s)	Comments
Sepsis after splenectomy	*S. pneumoniae, H. influenzae, N. meningitis* (encapsulated bugs)	
Pneumonia in the Southwest (California, Arizona)	*Coccidioides immitis*	Treat with itraconazole or fluconazole, amphotericin B for severe disease
Pneumonia after cave exploring or exposure to bird droppings in Ohio and Mississippi River valleys	*Histoplasma capsulatum*	
Pneumonia after exposure to a parrot or exotic bird	*Chlamydia psittaci*	
Fungus ball/hemoptysis after tuberculosis or cavitary lung disease	*Aspergillus* sp.	Fig. 20-1. Treat with voriconazole.
Pneumonia in a patient with silicosis	Tuberculosis	
Diarrhea after hiking/drinking from a stream	*Giardia lamblia*	Stool cysts; treat with metronidazole.
Pregnant woman with cats	*Toxoplasma gondii*	Fig. 20-2. Treat with spiramycin.
B_{12} deficiency and abdominal symptoms	*Diphyllobothrium latum*	
Seizures with ring-enhancing brain lesion on CT	*Taenia solium* (cysticercosis) or toxoplasmosis	Treat neurocysticercosis with albendazole or praziquantel, usually with steroids. Consider anticonvulsants.
Squamous cell bladder cancer in Middle East or Africa	*Schistosoma haematobium*	
Worm infection in children	*Enterobius* sp.	Positive tape test, perianal itching. Treat with mebendazole or albendazole.
Fever, muscle pain, eosinophilia, and periorbital edema after eating raw meat	*Trichinella spiralis* (trichinosis)	
Gastroenteritis in young children	Rotavirus, Norwalk virus	

(continued)

Scenario	Organism(s)	Comments
Food poisoning after eating reheated rice	*Bacillus cereus*	Infection is usually self-limited.
Food poisoning after eating raw seafood	*Vibrio parahaemolyticus*	
Diarrhea after travel to Mexico	*E. coli* (Montezuma revenge)	Treat with ciprofloxacin.
Diarrhea after antibiotics	*Clostridium difficile*	Use metronidazole or vancomycin.
Baby paralyzed after eating honey	*Clostridium botulinum*	Toxin blocks acetylcholine release
Genital lesions in children in the absence of sexual abuse or activity	Molluscum contagiosum	
Cellulitis after cat/dog bites	*Pasteurella multocida*	Treat animal bite wounds with prophylactic amoxicillin-clavulanate.
Slaughterhouse worker with fever	Brucellosis	
Pneumonia after being in hotel or near air conditioner or water tower	*Legionella pneumophila*	Treat with azithromycin or levofloxacin.
Burn wound infection with blue/green color	*Pseudomonas* sp.	*S. aureus* is also a common burn infection, but it lacks blue-green color.

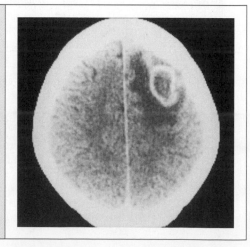

Figure 20-1. Ring-enhancing brain lesion. The differential is quite broad for such findings; thus the clinical history is important. In this case, which occurred as a complication of acute myelogenous leukemia and immune compromise, a biopsy yielded *Aspergillus* spp. (From Hoffbrand AV, Petti JE: Color Atlas of Clinical Hematology, 3rd ed. St. Louis, Mosby, 2000, p 142, with permission.)

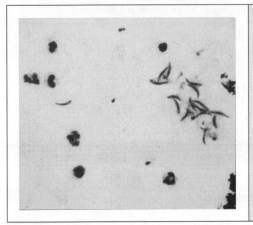

Figure 20-2. Acute toxoplasmosis. A thick peripheral blood film shows trophozoite forms of *Toxoplasma gondii* from a ruptured monocyte. (From Hoffbrand AV, Petti JE: Color Atlas of Clinical Hematology, 3rd ed. St. Louis, Mosby, 2000, p 317, with permission.)

15. How is syphilis diagnosed?

Screen for syphilis with a rapid plasma reagin (RPR) or Venereal Disease Research Laboratory (VDRL) test. Confirm a positive test with a fluorescent treponemal antibody absorbed (FTA-ABS) or microhemagglutination (MHA-TP) test because false positives occur with the RPR and VDRL tests, classically in patients with lupus erythematosus. Once syphilis is treated, the RPR and VDRL tests become negative, whereas the FTA-ABS and MHA-TP tests often remain positive for life. You also can scrape the base of a genital chancre or condyloma lata and look for spirochetes on dark-field microscopy.

16. Which group of patients should always be screened for syphilis?

Pregnant women. Early treatment can prevent birth defects.

17. How is syphilis treated?

With penicillin. Use doxycycline for penicillin-allergic patients.

18. Describe the three stages of syphilis.

Primary stage: look for painless chancre that resolves on its own within 8 weeks.

Secondary stage: roughly 6 weeks to 18 months after infection; look for condyloma lata, maculopapular rash (classically involves palms and soles of feet), and lymphadenopathy.

Tertiary stage: years after initial infection (between the secondary and tertiary stages is the latent phase, in which the disease is quiet and asymptomatic). Look for gummas (granulomas in many different organs), neurologic symptoms and signs (e.g., neurosyphilis, Argyll-Robertson pupil, dementia, paresis, tabes dorsalis, Charcot joints), and thoracic aortic aneurysms.

19. How do you recognize measles (rubeola) infection in a child?

Look for a reason for lack of immunization. Pathognomonic Koplik's spots (tiny white spots on buccal mucosa) are seen 3 days after high fever, cough, runny nose, and conjunctivitis with or without photophobia. On the next day, a maculopapular rash begins on the head and neck and spreads downward to cover the trunk (cephalocaudal progression). Treat supportively.

20. Describe the complications of measles.

Complications include giant-cell pneumonia, especially in very young and immunocompromised patients; otitis media; and encephalitis, either acute or late (**subacute sclerosing panencephalitis,** which usually occurs years later).

21. **Why is rubella infection (German measles) an important disease?**

    Rubella is important mainly because infection in pregnant mothers can cause severe birth defects in the fetus. Screen and immunize all women of reproductive age without evidence of rubella antibodies before pregnancy to avoid this complication. Remember, however, that the vaccine is contraindicated in pregnant women.

22. **How do you recognize a rubella infection in children? What are the complications?**

    Rubella is milder than measles. Signs and symptoms include low-grade fever, malaise, and tender swelling of the suboccipital and postauricular nodes; arthralgias are common. After a 2- to 3-day prodrome, a faint maculopapular rash appears on the face and neck and spreads to the trunk (cephalocaudal progression), just as in measles. Complications include encephalitis and otitis media.

23. **How do you recognize roseola infantum (exanthem subitum)? What causes it?**

    Roseola infantum is often easy to recognize because of the progression: high fever (may be higher than 40° C) with no apparent cause for 4 days, which may result in febrile seizures, followed by an abrupt return to normal temperature as a diffuse macular/maculopapular rash appears on the chest and abdomen. The disease is rare in children older than 3 years. It is caused by the human herpesvirus type 6 (a DNA herpes family virus).

24. **How do you recognize erythema infectiosum (fifth disease) in children? What causes it?**

    Look for the classic "slapped-cheek" rash (Fig. 20-3, confluent erythema over the cheeks looks like someone slapped the child across the face) accompanied by mild constitutional symptoms (e.g., low fever, malaise). One day later, a maculopapular rash appears on the arms, legs, and trunk. The disease is caused by parvovirus B19, the same virus that causes aplastic crisis in sickle cell disease.

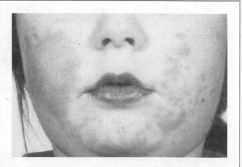

Figure 20-3. Erythema infectiosum. The blotchy erythema makes it look as though the cheeks have been slapped. (From du Vivier A: Atlas of Clinical Dermatology, 3rd ed. New York, Churchill Livingstone, 2002, p 287, with permission.)

25. **How do you recognize chickenpox? What causes it?**

    The description and progression of the rash should lead you to the diagnosis: discrete macules (usually on the trunk) turn into papules, which turn into vesicles that rupture and crust over. Such changes occur within 1 day. Because the lesions appear in successive crops, the rash will be in different stages of progression in different areas. The cause is the varicella virus.

26. **How can you make a definitive diagnosis of chickenpox? At what point is a patient with chickenpox no longer infectious?**

A Tzanck smear of tissue from the base of a vesicle shows multinucleated giant cells. A presumptive diagnosis can be made if the rash is classic. Infectivity ceases only when the last lesion crusts over.

27. **What are the complications of chickenpox?**

A major complication is infection of the lesions with streptococci or staphylococci, which causes erysipelas, cellulitis, and/or sepsis. The patient should be instructed to keep clean to avoid infection. Other complications include pneumonia (especially in very young children, adults, and immunocompromised patients), encephalitis, and **Reye syndrome.** Do not give aspirin to a child with a fever unless you have a diagnosis that requires its use. The varicella-zoster virus can reactivate years later to cause herpes zoster (also known as shingles, see Fig. 20-4), a rash that develops in a dermatomal distribution, often with preceding pain and paresthesias. A child who has not been immunized or exposed to chickenpox can catch the disease from someone with shingles.

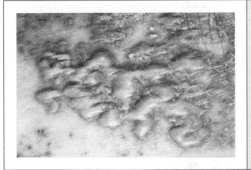

Figure 20-4. Herpes zoster. Grouped vesicopustules are noted to have a dermatomal distribution. (From du Vivier A: Atlas of Clinical Dermatology, 3rd ed. New York, Churchill Livingstone, 2002, p 7, with permission.)

28. **Describe the treatment and prophylaxis for chickenpox.**

In most cases, no treatment is needed except supportive care (e.g., acetaminophen, fluids, avoidance of infecting others). Acyclovir can be used in severe cases. Routine vaccination with the varicella vaccine is now recommended for all children in the United States. Varicella zoster immune globulin (VariZIG) is available for prophylaxis in patients with debilitating illness (e.g., leukemia, AIDS) if you see them within 4 days of exposure and for newborns of mothers with chickenpox. Intravenous immunoglobulin can be given if varicella zoster immune globulin is not available.

29. **What is scarlet fever? What causes it? How is it recognized and treated?**

Scarlet fever is a febrile illness with a rash caused by certain *Streptococcus* species. Look for a history of untreated streptococcal pharyngitis; only streptococcal species that produce erythrogenic toxin can cause scarlet fever. Pharyngitis is followed by a sandpaper-like rash on the abdomen and trunk with classic circumoral pallor and strawberry tongue. The rash tends to desquamate once the fever subsides. Oral penicillin V is the treatment of choice for streptococcal pharyngitis to prevent rheumatic fever. Alternative therapies include amoxicillin, cephalosporins, macrolides, or clindamycin.

30. **What are the diagnostic criteria for Kawasaki disease (mucocutaneous lymph node syndrome)?**

This rare disease is seen in patients younger than 5 years old on the Step 2 exam. The diagnostic criteria include fever for more than 5 days (mandatory for diagnosis); bilateral conjunctival injection; changes in the lips, tongue, or oral mucosa (e.g., strawberry tongue, fissuring, injection); changes in the extremities (e.g., skin desquamation, edema, erythema); polymorphous truncal rash, which usually begins one day after the fever starts; and cervical lymphadenopathy. Also look for arthralgia or arthritis.

31. What is the most feared complication of Kawasaki disease? How do you prevent it?

The most feared complications involve the heart (coronary artery aneurysms, congestive heart failure, arrhythmias, myocarditis, and even myocardial infarction). Include Kawasaki disease in the differential diagnosis of any child who has a myocardial infarction. If Kawasaki disease is suspected, give aspirin and intravenous immunoglobulins. Both have been proved to reduce cardiac lesions. Kawasaki disease is one of the few indications for aspirin in a child. Follow the child with echocardiography to detect heart involvement.

32. Describe the classic findings of Epstein-Barr virus (EBV) infection (infectious mononucleosis).

Look for fatigue, fever, pharyngitis, and cervical lymphadenopathy in a young adult. The signs and symptoms are similar to those of streptococcal pharyngitis, but malaise tends to be prolonged and pronounced in EBV infection. To differentiate from streptococcal pharyngitis, look for the following:

- Splenomegaly (patients may have splenic rupture and should avoid contact sports and heavy lifting)
- Hepatomegaly
- Atypical lymphocytes (bizarre forms that may resemble leukemia) with lymphocytosis, anemia, or thrombocytopenia
- Positive serology (heterophile antibodies [e.g., Monospot test] or specific EBV antibodies (viral capsid antigen, Epstein-Barr nuclear antigens).

33. What is an important differential diagnosis of EBV infection?

Acute HIV infection, which can cause a mononucleosis-type syndrome.

34. What is the association between EBV and cancer?

EBV is associated with nasopharyngeal cancer, African Burkitt lymphoma, and posttransplant lymphoproliferative disorder.

35. Describe the classic clinical vignette for Rocky Mountain spotted fever. What causes it? What is the treatment?

Look for history of a tick bite (especially in a patient on the East Coast) one week before the development of high fever/chills, severe headache, and prostration or severe malaise. A rash appears roughly 4 days later on the palms and wrists and soles and ankles and spreads rapidly to the trunk and face (unique pattern of spread). Patients often look quite ill (e.g., disseminated intravascular coagulation, delirium). The infection is caused by *Rickettsia rickettsii*. Treat with doxycycline; chloramphenicol is a second choice.

36. How do you recognize and treat the rash of impetigo? What causes it?

In patients with impetigo, which is caused by *Streptococcus* and *Staphylococcus* species, look for a history of a break in the skin (e.g., previous chickenpox, insect bite, scabies, cut). The rash starts as thin-walled vesicles that rupture and form yellowish crusts. The skin classically is described as "weeping." Typical lesions appear on the face and tend to be localized. The rash is infectious; look for a history of sick contacts. Treat with dicloxacillin, cephalexin, or clindamycin to cover both *Streptococcus* and *Staphylococcus* species. Topical mupirocin may also be used.

37. **Describe the two clinical types of endocarditis. What are the causative bugs?**
    1. **Acute** (fulminant) endocarditis, which typically affects normal heart valves and most commonly is caused by *Staphylococcus aureus*.
    2. **Subacute,** which has an insidious onset and typically affects previously damaged or mechanical valves. The most common cause is *Streptococcus viridans*, but other streptococcal and staphylococcal species also may cause endocarditis (e.g., *Staphylococcus epidermis, Streptococcus bovis,* and *Streptococcus faecalis* [also known enterococci]). Suspect colon cancer if *S. bovis* turns up on blood culture.

38. **How is endocarditis diagnosed and treated?**
    The diagnosis generally is made by blood cultures. Empiric treatment is begun with broad-spectrum intravenous antibiotics until the culture and sensitivity results are known. A third-generation penicillin or cephalosporin plus an aminoglycoside is a reasonable choice.

39. **What are the classic signs and symptoms of endocarditis?**
    Look for general signs of infection (e.g., fever, tachycardia, malaise) plus new-onset heart murmur, embolic phenomena (stroke and other infarcts), **Osler nodes** (painful nodules on tips of fingers), **Janeway lesions** (*nontender,* erythematous lesions on palms and soles), **Roth spots** (round retinal hemorrhages with white centers), and septic shock (more likely with acute than subacute disease).

40. **What elements of the history point to endocarditis?**
    Look for patients who are more likely to be affected by endocarditis:
    ■ Intravenous drug abusers, who usually have right-sided lesions, although left-sided lesions are much more common in the general population.
    ■ Patients with abnormal heart valves (e.g., prosthetic valves, rheumatic valvular disease, congenital heart defects such as ventricular septal defects or tetralogy of Fallot).
    ■ Postoperative patients (especially after gastrointestinal, genitourinary, or dental surgery).

41. **What are the recommendations for endocarditis prophylaxis?**
    The 2008 American Heart Association recommendations conclude that only an extremely small number of cases of infective endocarditis might be prevented by antibiotic prophylaxis for dental procedures. Cardiac conditions for which prophylaxis with dental procedures is recommended includes prosthetic cardiac valve, previous infectious endocarditis, congenital heart disease, and cardiac transplant recipients who develop valvulopathy. Antibiotic prophylaxis is no longer recommended for genitourinary or gastrointestinal procedures.
    If a prophylactic antibiotic is indicated, it should be administered in a single dose before the procedure. Amoxicillin is the preferred choice for oral therapy. Cephalexin, clindamycin, azithromycin, or clarithromycin may be used in patients with penicillin allergy. Ampicillin, cefazolin, ceftriaxone, or clindamycin may be used for patients unable to take oral medication.

42. **What is the classic age group for meningitis? Describe the physical findings.**
    Neonates are the classic age group for meningitis; 75% of all cases occur in children younger than 2 years. Deciding when to do a lumbar tap is difficult, because patients often do not have classic physical findings (Kernig sign and Brudzinski sign). Look for lethargy, hyper- or hypothermia, poor muscle tone, bulging fontanelle, vomiting, photophobia, altered consciousness, and signs of generalized sepsis (e.g., hypotension, jaundice, respiratory distress). Seizures also may be seen, but simple febrile seizures are common if the patient is between 5 months and 6 years old and has a fever greater than 102° F without other signs of meningitis.

43. **What should you do if you suspect meningitis?**
    In the absence of trauma, do a lumbar puncture immediately and begin broad-spectrum antibiotics and IV fluids. Do *not* wait for culture or other results to start antibiotics.

44. What is the most common neurologic sequela of meningitis?

Hearing loss. All pediatric and many adult patients need formal hearing evaluation after a bout of meningitis. Vision testing also is recommended. Other sequelae include mental retardation, motor deficits/paresis, epilepsy, and learning/behavioral disorders.

45. What are the common viral (aseptic) causes of meningitis in children?

Mumps and measles meningitis may be seen in children who are not immunized. The best treatment is prevention via immunization. Watch for neonatal herpes encephalitis (HSV-2) if the mother has genital lesions of herpes simplex virus at the time of delivery. Other children and adults can develop HSV-1 herpes encephalitis, which classically affects the **temporal lobes** on a head CT or MR scan. Give intravenous acyclovir.

46. Which types of bacterial meningitis require antibiotic prophylaxis in contacts?

N. meningitidis and *H. influenzae*. If a case of meningitis is due to *Neisseria,* give all contacts rifampin, ciprofloxacin, ceftriaxone, or azithromycin as prophylaxis; rifampin is used for *H. influenzae* meningitis prophylaxis.

47. What are the "big three" respiratory infections in patients younger than 5 years?

Croup, epiglottitis, and respiratory syncytial virus infection (bronchiolitis). These three diseases are high yield on the USMLE.

48. How do you recognize croup (acute laryngotracheitis)? Describe the cause and treatment.

Look for a child 1 to 2 years of age. Croup usually occurs in the fall or winter. Fifty to 75% of cases are due to infection with parainfluenza virus; the other causative agent is influenza virus. The disease begins with symptoms of viral upper respiratory infection (e.g., rhinorrhea, cough, fever). Roughly 1 to 2 days later patients develop a "barking" cough, hoarseness, and inspiratory stridor. The **"steeple sign"** (describes subglottic narrowing of the trachea) is classic on a frontal radiograph of the chest or neck. Treat supportively with a mist tent, humidified oxygen, and racemic epinephrine.

49. How do you recognize epiglottitis? Describe the cause and treatment.

Epiglottitis usually occurs in children 2 to 5 years old. The main cause is *Haemophilus influenzae* type b, thus widespread vaccination has significantly reduced the incidence of this condition. *Staphylococcus aureus, S. pyogenes*, and *S. pneumoniae* are other potential causes. Look for little or no prodrome, with rapid progression to high fever, toxic appearance, drooling, and respiratory distress with no coughing. The **"thumb sign"** (describes a swollen, enlarged epiglottis) is classic on lateral radiographs of the neck. Do not examine the throat or irritate the child in any way. You may precipitate airway obstruction. When a case of epiglottitis is diagnosed, the first step is to be prepared to establish an airway (intubation and, if needed, tracheostomy). Treat with a combination of oxacillin or cefazolin or clindamycin or vancomycin plus cefotaxime or ceftriaxone.

50. Describe the classic clinical vignette for bronchiolitis. What is the cause? How is it treated?

Bronchiolitis generally affects children aged 0 to 18 months and usually occurs in the fall or winter. More than 75% of cases are caused by respiratory syncytial virus (RSV); other causes are parainfluenza and influenza viruses. Patients first develop symptoms of viral upper respiratory infection, followed 1 to 2 days later by rapid respirations, intercostal retractions, and expiratory wheezing. The child may have crackles on auscultation of the chest. Diffuse hyperinflation of the lungs is classic on chest radiograph; look for flattened diaphragms. Treat supportively (e.g., oxygen, mist tent, bronchodilators, intravenous fluids). Use ribavirin in patients with severe symptoms or at high risk (e.g., patients with cyanosis or other chronic health problems).

51. **What "old-school" pediatric infection causes pseudomembranes and myocarditis? What about whooping cough?**
Diphtheria (*Corynebacterium diphtheriae*) and pertussis (*Bordetella pertussis*), respectively. Diphtheria is quite uncommon in the United States because of mandatory vaccination. Pertussis was uncommon, but the incidence has been increasing significantly over the last 20 years. If a child is unimmunized (e.g., child of immigrants), don't forget these two entities. Diphtheria causes grayish pseudomembranes (necrotic epithelium and inflammatory exudate) on the pharynx, tonsils, and uvula as well as myocarditis. Pertussis is associated with severe paroxysmal coughing and a high-pitched whooping inspiratory noise (traditionally called "whooping cough"), particularly in children and especially those under one year of age. Treat diphtheria with antitoxin and either penicillin or erythromycin. Treat pertussis with azithromycin or erythromycin.

52. **In what clinical scenario does rabies occur in the United States? Describe the classic physical findings.**
Rabies in the United States is due to bites from bats, skunks, raccoons, or foxes; rabies due to bites from dogs is rare due to vaccination. The incubation period is usually around 1 to 2 months. The classic findings are hydrophobia (fear of water due to painful swallowing) and central nervous system signs (e.g., paralysis).

53. **What should you do after a patient is bitten by an animal?**
1. Treat the local wound. Cleanse thoroughly with soap. Do *not* cauterize or suture the wound. Amoxicillin-clavulanate is often given for cellulitis prophylaxis.
2. Observe the animal. If possible, capture and observe the dog or cat to see if it develops rabies. If a wild animal is caught, it should be killed and the brain tissue examined for rabies.
3. If the wild animal escapes or has rabies, give rabies immunoglobulin and vaccinate the patient. In cases of a dog or cat bite, do *not* give prophylaxis or vaccine unless the animal acted strangely or bit the patient without provocation and rabies is prevalent in the area (rare). Do not give prophylaxis or vaccine for rabbit or small rodent bites (e.g., rats, mice, squirrels, chipmunks).

54. **What are the two main infections caused by *Streptococcus pyogenes* (group A streptococci)? What are the common sequelae?**
S. pyogenes causes pharyngitis and skin infections. Sequelae include rheumatic fever, scarlet fever, and poststreptococcal glomerulonephritis.

55. **How does streptococcal pharyngitis present? How do you diagnosis and treat it?**
Look for sore throat with fever, tonsillar exudate, enlarged tender cervical nodes, and leukocytosis. A positive streptococcal throat culture confirms the diagnosis. Elevated titers of antistreptolysin O (ASO) and anti-DNase antibody can be used for a retrospective diagnosis in patients with rheumatic fever or poststreptococcal glomerulonephritis. Treat streptococcal pharyngitis with penicillin, amoxicillin, cephalosporin, macrolide, or clindamycin to avoid rheumatic fever and scarlet fever.

56. **What are the major and minor Jones criteria for rheumatic fever? Why is rheumatic fever less common today?**
The five major Jones criteria include migratory polyarthritis, carditis, chorea, erythema marginatum, and subcutaneous nodules. The minor Jones criteria include elevations in

erythrocyte sedimentation rate, C-reactive protein, white blood cell count, and ASO titer; prolonged PR interval on EKG; and arthralgia. The diagnosis of rheumatic fever requires a history of streptococcal pharyngitis plus at least one major criterion. Treatment of streptococcal pharyngitis with antibiotics markedly reduces the incidence of rheumatic fever; thus, it is less common today. Give all patients affected by rheumatic fever endocarditis prophylaxis before surgical procedures.

57. **How do you recognize poststreptococcal glomerulonephritis? How is it treated?**
Poststreptococcal glomerulonephritis occurs most commonly after a streptococcal skin infection, but it also may occur after pharyngitis. Patients are usually children and generally present with a history of infection with a nephritogenic strain of *Streptococcus* species 1 to 3 weeks earlier and abrupt onset of hematuria, proteinuria (mild, not in nephrotic range), red blood cell casts, hypertension, edema (especially periorbital), and elevated blood urea nitrogen/creatinine. Treat supportively. Control blood pressure, and use diuretics for severe edema. Treatment of streptococcal infections does not reduce the incidence of poststreptococcal glomerulonephritis.

58. **Distinguish between impetigo and erysipelas.**
Both are superficial skin infections due to streptococci or *S. aureus* and often occur after a break in the skin (e.g., trauma, scabies, insect bite). **Impetigo** classically changes first from maculopapules to vesicopustules and bullae and then to honey-colored, crusted lesions. Staphylococci are a more frequent cause than streptococci. Definitely think of staphylococci if a furuncle or carbuncle is present; think of streptococci if glomerulonephritis develops. Impetigo is contagious; watch for sick contacts. **Erysipelas** is a superficial cellulitis that appears red, shiny, and swollen; it is tender and may be associated with vesicles and bullae, fever, and lymphadenopathy. Treat both empirically with dicloxacillin, cephalexin, or clindamycin, though erysipelas may require parenteral therapy with a cephalosporin if systemic symptoms such as fever and chills are present.

59. **What organisms typically cause cellulitis? What special circumstances should make you think of atypical causes?**
Streptococci and staphylococci cause most cases. Think of *Pseudomonas* species with burns or severe trauma; of *Pasteurella multocida* after dog or cat bites (treat with ampicillin); of *Vibrio vulnificus* in fishermen or other patients exposed to salt water (treat with tetracycline). Diabetic patients with foot ulcers tend to have polymicrobial infections and need powerful, broad-spectrum antibiotic coverage.

60. **Describe the physical findings of cellulitis. Define necrotizing fasciitis. How is it treated?**
In patients with cellulitis, the involved overlying skin is red, hot, and frequently tender. It looks like erysipelas but involves deeper subcutaneous tissues. Treat with anti-staphylococcal antibiotics to cover both streptococcus and staphylococcus. Necrotizing fasciitis is defined as the progression of cellulitis to necrosis and gangrene. Watch for crepitus and signs of systemic toxicity (e.g., tachycardia, fever, and hypotension). Often multiple organisms are involved (aerobes and anaerobes). Treat with intravenous fluids, incision and drainage/surgical debridement, and broad-spectrum antibiotics (e.g., ampicillin plus either clindamycin or metronidazole).

61. **What is the most common cause of endometritis (puerperal fever)? How do you recognize and treat it?**
Watch for endometritis, an infection of the endometrial lining, as a cause of postpartum fever. The hallmark is uterine tenderness, and the most common cause is *Streptococcus* species. Treat with clindamycin plus gentamicin after getting local cultures.

62. **What infection in neonates is caused by *Streptococcus agalactiae* (group B streptococci)?**
Streptococcus agalactiae is the most common cause of neonatal meningitis or sepsis. The organism is often part of normal vaginal flora and may be acquired from the birth canal. Group B streptococci are penicillin-sensitive. Expectant mothers are cultured for group B strep, and if it is present around the time of delivery, then prophylactic penicillin or ampicillin is given to the mother to prevent meningitis in the newborn.

63. **Other than pneumonia, what infections does *Streptococcus pneumoniae* commonly cause?**
Otitis media, meningitis, sinusitis, and spontaneous bacterial peritonitis.

64. **What are the main infections caused by *S. aureus*?**
The list is long. *S. aureus* is a common cause of the following infections:
- Skin and soft-tissue abscesses (especially in the breast after breast-feeding or in the skin after a furuncle)
- Endocarditis (especially in drug users)
- Osteomyelitis (the most common cause unless sickle cell disease is present)
- Septic arthritis
- Food poisoning (via a preformed toxin)
- Toxic shock syndrome (via a preformed toxin)
- Scalded skin syndrome (via a preformed toxin; affects younger children who often present with impetigo, then desquamate; Fig. 20-5)
- Impetigo
- Cellulitis
- Wound infections
- Pneumonia (often forms lung abscess or empyema)
- Furuncles and carbuncles

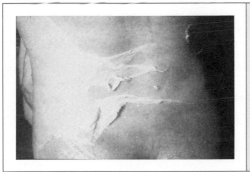

Figure 20-5. Staphylococcal scalded skin syndrome. The skin is typically raw and desquamates in sheets. (From du Vivier A: Atlas of Clinical Dermatology, 3rd ed. New York, Churchill Livingstone, 2002, p 252, with permission.)

65. **Who are the classic spreaders of nosocomial staphylococcal infections?**
Health care workers who are chronic nasal carriers can cause nosocomial infections. Carriers should be treated with antibiotics.

66. **What is the treatment of choice for staphylococcal infections on the USMLE?**
An antistaphylococcal penicillin (e.g., methicillin, dicloxacillin). Use vancomycin, clindamycin, doxycycline, or trimethoprim-sulfamethoxazole if the staphylococcal species is known to be methicillin-resistant or if methicillin-resistant *S. aureus* (MRSA) is suspected. MRSA is a rapidly growing problem. Most abscesses (regardless of the causative organism) must be

treated first with surgical incision and drainage because antibiotics cannot penetrate through the walls of an abscess cavity.

67. **Cover up the right-hand column in the table below and describe the preferred treatment for tuberculosis based on the clinical scenario.**

Clinical Setting/Findings	Treatment
Exposed adult with negative PPD skin test	None
Exposed child younger than 5 years old with negative PPD	Isoniazid (INH) for 3 mo., then repeat PPD
Prophylaxis for PPD conversion (negative to positive), no active disease	INH for 9 mo.
Active pulmonary disease/positive culture	INH/rifampin/pyrazinamide/ethambutol for 2 mo., then INH/rifampin for 4 mo. in most patients

PPD = purified protein derivative.

Other important tuberculosis treatment issues:
- Multidrug resistant strains are an increasing problem and require four drug therapy in most circumstances.
- If the patient is noncompliant, directly observed therapy (someone watches the patient take medications every day) is recommended.
- Consider supplementation with vitamin B_6 (pyridoxine) for patients on isoniazid (INH), or watch for signs of deficiency, such as neuropathy, confusion, angular chilitis, or a seborrheic dermatitis-like rash.
- Watch for liver dysfunction in patients on therapy.

CHAPTER 21

LABORATORY MEDICINE

1. **What may cause a false lab report of hyperkalemia?**
   Hemolysis of the blood sample. Repeat the test if a high value doesn't make sense (e.g., high level with no EKG changes or symptoms).

2. **What can cause a "false" hyponatremia?**
   Hyponatremia may be caused by hyperglycemia, hyperproteinemia, or hyperlipidemia. The hyponatremia resolves with correction of the glucose, lipid, or protein levels.

3. **What may result from rapid correction of hyponatremia?**
   Brainstem damage (**central pontine myelinolysis**). For this reason you should generally not give hypertonic saline to correct hyponatremia except in severe or symptomatic cases, and then it should be given in limited quantities.

4. **What effect do serum acidosis and serum alkalosis have on potassium and calcium levels?**
   Alkalosis may cause hypokalemia and symptoms of hypocalcemia (perioral numbness, tetany) due to cellular shift, whereas acidosis may cause hyperkalemia by the same mechanism. Correction of acid-base status will correct the potassium and calcium derangements.

5. **Other than pancreatic disease, what else can cause elevated levels of amylase and lipase?**
   Damage of the salivary glands or bowel, renal failure, and ruptured tubal pregnancy may cause amylase and lipase elevations. Elevation of both amylase and lipase in the same patient, however, is usually due to pancreatitis. The boards may try to trick you with an isolated elevation of amylase.

6. **Which diseases can cause elevated levels of alkaline phosphatase? What lab test is used to distinguish among these diseases?**
   Alkaline phosphatase can be elevated in biliary disease, bone disease, or pregnancy (the placenta produces alkaline phosphatase). If the elevation is due to biliary disease, gamma-glutamyltranspeptidase (GGT) and/or 5'-nucleotidase (5'-NT) also should be elevated; both values, however, are normal in bone disease and pregnancy.

7. **True or false: Hypothyroidism can cause elevated cholesterol.**
   True. Thyroid hormone replacement corrects the elevated cholesterol.

8. **Injury to what organ (other than the heart) causes elevated levels of creatine kinase (CK)?**
   Muscle. Watch for trauma, rhabdomyolysis, HMG-CoA reductase inhibitors (which can cause muscle damage), and burns.

9. **What is the relationship of low calcium and potassium levels to low levels of magnesium?**
Hypokalemia and/or hypocalcemia may be due to hypomagnesemia. In addition, if hypomagnesemia is present, it is often impossible to correct the hypokalemia or hypocalcemia until you correct the hypomagnesemia. If a patient has hypokalemia that does not correct with potassium supplements, check the magnesium level.

10. **Which two electrolytes are classically depleted in the setting of diabetic ketoacidosis or diabetic hyperosmolar, hyperglycemic state?**
Potassium and phosphorus.

11. **What does a blood urea nitrogen (BUN)-to-creatinine ratio greater than 15 or 20 generally imply?**
Dehydration.

12. **What disease classically causes a false-positive result on the rapid plasma reagin (RPR) or Venereal Disease Research Laboratory (VDRL) syphilis test?**
Systemic lupus erythematosus (SLE). A false-positive result on the RPR or VDRL test is actually one of the diagnostic criteria for SLE.

13. **Define isosthenuria. What condition does it suggest?**
Isosthenuria is the inability to concentrate or dilute the urine. The specific gravity of urine and serum is the same—classically 1.010. Isosthenuria is often associated with sickle cell trait or disease.

14. **What does an elevated erythrocyte sedimentation rate mean in pregnancy?**
Nothing. This is a normal finding in pregnancy (i.e. not a good test to order in a pregnant patient).

15. **True or false: A high-normal level of BUN or creatinine during pregnancy often indicates renal disease.**
True. BUN and creatinine are decreased significantly in pregnancy after the first trimester in women with normal renal function.

CHAPTER 22

NEPHROLOGY

1. **What are the symptoms and signs of acute renal failure?**
   Symptoms: fatigue, nausea and vomiting, anorexia, shortness of breath, mental status changes.
   Signs: increased levels of blood urea nitrogen (BUN) and creatinine, metabolic acidosis, hyperkalemia, tachypnea (due to acidosis and hypervolemia), and hypervolemia (bilateral rales on lung exam, elevated jugular venous pressure, dilutional hyponatremia).

2. **What are the three broad categories of renal failure?**
   Prerenal, renal/intrarenal, and postrenal.

3. **Define prerenal failure? What are the causes? How do you recognize it?**
   In prerenal failure the kidney is not adequately perfused. The most common cause is hypovolemia (dehydration, hemorrhage). Look for a BUN-to-creatinine ratio greater than 20 and signs of hypovolemia (e.g., tachycardia, weak pulse, depressed fontanelle). Give intravenous fluids and/or blood. Other common prerenal causes are sepsis (treat the sepsis and give intravenous fluids), heart failure (give digitalis and diuretics), liver failure (hepatorenal syndrome; treat supportively), and renal artery stenosis.

4. **Define postrenal failure. What causes it?**
   In postrenal failure, urine is blocked from being excreted at some point beyond the kidneys (ureters, prostate, urethra). The most common cause is benign prostatic hypertrophy (BPH). Patients are men over age 50 with BPH symptoms (e.g., hesitancy, dribbling); ultrasound demonstrates bilateral hydronephrosis. Treat with catheterization (suprapubic, if necessary) to relieve the obstruction and prevent further renal damage. Then consider surgery (transurethral resection of the prostate). Other causes are nephrolithiasis (but remember that stones generally have to be bilateral to cause renal failure), retroperitoneal fibrosis (watch for a history of methysergide use), and pelvic malignancies.

5. **What is the most common cause of intrarenal failure?**
   Intrarenal failure, which results from a problem within the kidney itself, is most commonly due to **acute tubular necrosis** from various causes.

6. **What do you need to know about intravenous contrast and renal failure?**
   Intravenous contrast can precipitate renal failure, usually in diabetics and patients with preexisting renal disease. Avoid contrast in such patients if possible. If you must give intravenous contrast, give lots of intravenous hydration (i.e., IV fluids) before and after the contrast is given to decrease the chance of renal shutdown. Also consider the use of oral acetylcysteine on the day before and the day of contrast administration.

7. **True or false: Muscle breakdown can cause renal failure.**
   True. Myoglobinuria or rhabdomyolysis due to strenuous exercise (e.g., marathon runners), alcohol, burns, muscle trauma, heat stroke, and neuroleptic malignant syndrome may cause renal failure. The cellular debris that results from muscle breakdown plugs the renal

filtration system. Look for very high levels of creatine phosphokinase (CPK). Treat with hydration and diuretics.

8. **What medications commonly cause renal insufficiency or failure?**
Chronic use of nonsteroidal anti-inflammatory drugs (may cause acute tubular necrosis or papillary necrosis), cyclosporine, aminoglycosides, and methicillin.

9. **Define Goodpasture syndrome. How does it present?**
Goodpasture syndrome is due to the presence of measurable antiglomerular basement membrane antibodies, which cause a linear immunofluorescence pattern on renal biopsy. These antibodies react with and damage both kidneys and lungs. Look for a young man with hemoptysis, dyspnea, and renal failure. Treat with steroids and cyclophosphamide.

10. **Define Wegener granulomatosis. How does it present?**
Wegener granulomatosis is a vasculitis that also affects the lungs and kidneys. Look for nasal involvement (bloody nose, nasal perforation) or hemoptysis and pleurisy as presenting symptoms, along with renal disease. Patients test positive for titers of **antineutrophil cytoplasmic antibody (ANCA)**. Treat with cyclophosphamide and glucocorticoids. Methotrexate is an alternative.

11. **What is the prototypical cause of glomerulonephritis? How does it present?**
Poststreptococcal glomerulonephritis is the classic example on board exams. It usually affects children with a history of upper respiratory infection or strep throat 1 to 3 weeks earlier. Patients present with edema, hypervolemia, hypertension, hematuria, and oliguria. *Red blood cell casts* on urinalysis clinch the diagnosis. Treat supportively. Also watch for lupus erythematosus as a cause of glomerulonephritis. Renal failure is a major cause of morbidity and mortality in patients with lupus.

12. **What are the indications for dialysis in patients with renal failure?**
Whenever renal failure is present, first try to determine the cause and fix it, if possible, to correct the renal failure. Indications for acute dialysis include uremic encephalopathy, pericarditis, severe metabolic acidosis (roughly, pH < 7.25), heart failure, and hyperkalemia severe enough to cause arrhythmia.

13. **Define nephrotic syndrome. What causes it? How is it diagnosed?**
Nephrotic syndrome is defined by proteinuria (> 3.5 g/day), hypoalbuminemia, edema (the classic pattern is morning periorbital edema), and hyperlipidemia with lipiduria. In children it is usually due to minimal change disease (podocytes with missing "feet" on electron microscopy), which often follows an infection. Measure 24-hour urine protein to clinch the diagnosis, and treat with steroids. Causes in adults include diabetes, hepatitis B, amyloidosis, lupus erythematosus, and drugs (e.g., gold, penicillamine, captopril).

14. **Define nephritic syndrome. What is the classic cause? How is it treated?**
Nephritic syndrome generally is defined as oliguria, azotemia (rising BUN/creatinine), hypertension, and hematuria. The patient may have some degree of proteinuria, but not in the nephrotic range. The classic cause is poststreptococcal glomerulonephritis. Treatment is supportive, including control of hypertension and maintenance of urine output with intravenous fluids and diuretics.

15. **What causes chronic renal failure (CRF)?**
Any of the causes of acute renal failure can cause chronic renal failure if the insult is severe or prolonged. Most cases of CRF are due to diabetes mellitus (number-one cause) or hypertension (number-two cause). A popular Step 2 cause is polycystic kidney disease.

Watch for multiple cysts in the kidney, look for a positive family history (usually autosomal dominant; autosomal recessive form presents in children), hypertension, hematuria, palpable renal masses, berry aneurysms in the circle of Willis, and cysts in liver (Fig. 22-1).

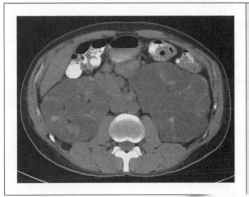

Figure 22-1. This noncontrast CT image demonstrates autosomal dominant polycystic kidney disease. The kidneys are markedly enlarged bilaterally with multiple low density cysts throughout both kidneys. The little remaining renal parenchyma is noted by the sparse higher density material squeezed by the cysts. (From Brenner B: Brenner and Rector's The Kidney, 8th ed. Philadelphia, Saunders, 2008, Fig. 27-30.)

16. **What metabolic derangements are seen in CRF?**
   ■ Azotemia (high levels of BUN and creatinine)
   ■ Metabolic acidosis
   ■ Hyperkalemia
   ■ Fluid retention (may cause hypertension, edema, congestive heart failure, and pulmonary edema)
   ■ Hypocalcemia and hyperphosphatemia (impaired vitamin D production; bone loss leads to renal osteodystrophy)
   ■ Anemia (due to lack of erythropoietin; give synthetic erythropoietin to correct)
   ■ Anorexia, nausea, vomiting (from build-up of toxins)
   ■ Central nervous system disturbances (mental status changes and even convulsions or coma from toxin build-up)
   ■ Bleeding (due to disordered platelet function)
   ■ Uremic pericarditis (friction rub may be heard)
   ■ Skin pigmentation and pruritus (skin turns yellowish-brown and itches because of metabolic byproducts)
   ■ Increased susceptibility to infection (due to decreased cellular immunity)

17. **How is CRF treated?**
   Treat CRF with regular hemodialysis (usually 3 times/week), water-soluble vitamins (which are removed during dialysis), phosphate restriction and binders (calcium carbonate, calcium acetate, or sevelamer), erythropoietin, and hypertension control. The only cure is renal transplant.

18. **What are the signs and symptoms of urinary tract infection (UTI)? What are the most likely organisms?**
   Symptoms and signs include urgency, dysuria, suprapubic and/or low back pain, and low grade fever. UTIs usually are caused by *Escherichia coli* (75% to 85% of cases) but also may be caused by *Staphylococcus saprophyticus* or *Proteus, Pseudomonas, Klebsiella, Enterobacter,* and/or *Enterococcus* species (or other enteric organisms). Patients who acquire UTIs in the hospital or from a chronic, indwelling Foley catheter are more likely to have organisms other than *E. coli.*

19. **What factors increase the likelihood of UTIs?**

Female gender and conditions that promote urinary stasis (BPH, pregnancy, stones, neurogenic bladder, vesicoureteral reflux) or bacterial colonization (indwelling catheter, fecal incontinence, surgical instrumentation) predispose to UTI.

20. **How do you diagnose and treat UTIs?**

The gold standard for diagnosis is a positive urine culture with at least 100,000 colony-forming units (measure of bacterial load) of specific bacteria. At the least, get a midstream sample; the best method is a catheterized sample or suprapubic tap. Urinalysis shows white blood cells, bacteria (on Gram stain of the urine), positive leukocyte esterase, and/or positive nitrite.

Empiric treatment usually is based on symptoms and urinalysis while awaiting culture results. Commonly used antibiotics include trimethoprim-sulfamethoxazole, amoxicillin, nitrofurantoin, ciprofloxacin, or a first-generation cephalosporin for about 5 days.

21. **Why are UTIs in children of special concern?**

In children, a UTI is cause for concern because it may be the presenting symptom of a genitourinary malformation. The most common examples are vesicoureteral reflux and posterior urethral valves. Urine culture should be obtained. Order an ultrasound and either a voiding cystourethrogram (VCUG) or radionuclide cystogram (RNC) to evaluate the urinary tract in any child 2 months to 2 years with a first UTI. Recommendations for imaging in older children are less clear-cut.

22. **True or false: You should treat asymptomatic bacteriuria in most patients.**

False. The exception is the pregnant patient, in whom asymptomatic bacteriuria is treated because of the high risk of progression to pyelonephritis. Use antibiotics that are safe in pregnancy, such as penicillins.

23. **How does pyelonephritis usually occur? What are the signs and symptoms? How is it treated?**

Pyelonephritis most often is due to an ascending UTI caused by *E. coli* (> 80% of cases). Patients present with high fever, shaking chills, costovertebral angle tenderness, flank pain, and/or UTI symptoms. Order urinalysis and urine and blood cultures to establish the diagnosis, but treat this life-threatening infection on an inpatient basis with intravenous antibiotics while awaiting results. A typical regimen consists of an oral fluoroquinolone or intravenous ceftriaxone or fluoroquinolone in uncomplicated pyelonephritis. Always choose an antibiotic regimen with good *E. coli* coverage.

24. **How do you differentiate among the common pediatric hematologic disorders that affect the kidney?**

	HUS	HSP	TTP	ITP
Most common age	Children	Children	Young adults	Children or adults
Previous infection	Diarrhea (*E. coli*)	URI	None	Viral (especially in children)
Red blood cell count	Low	Normal	Low	Normal
Platelet count	Low	Normal	Low	Low
Peripheral smear	Hemolysis	Normal	Hemolysis	Normal

(continued)

	HUS	HSP	TTP	ITP
Kidney effects	ARF, hematuria	Hematuria	ARF, proteinuria	None
Treatment	Supportive*	Supportive*	Plasmapheresis, NSAIDs; no platelets[‡]	Steroids,[†] Splenectomy if drugs fail
Key differential points	Age, diarrhea	Rash, abdominal pain, arthritis, melena (Fig. 22-2)	CNS changes, age	Antiplatelet antibodies

HUS = hemolytic uremic syndrome, HSP = Henoch-Schönlein purpura, TTP = thrombotic thrombocytopenic purpura, ITP = idiopathic thrombocytopenia, URI = upper respiratory infection, ARF = acute renal failure, NSAIDs = nonsteroidal anti-inflammatory drugs, CNS= central nervous system.
*In HUS and HSP, patients may need dialysis and transfusions.
[†]Give steroids only if the patient is bleeding or platelet counts are very low ($< 20,000-30,000/\mu L$).
[‡]Do not give platelet transfusions to patients with TTP; clots may form.

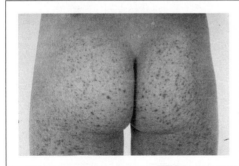

Figure 22-2. Henoch-Schönlein purpura. Purpuric lesions of the buttocks and lower extremities are characteristic of this IgA-mediated, vasculitic disorder, which also commonly affects the joints, GI tract and/or kidneys. (From du Vivier A: Atlas of Clinical Dermatology, 3rd ed. New York, Churchill Livingstone, 2002, p 382, with permission.)

25. **Which is more likely to be seen on a plain abdominal radiograph: kidney stones or gallbladder stones?**
Kidney stones (85%), which more commonly calcify (Fig. 22-3), are more likely to be seen than gallstones (15%).

26. **What are the signs and symptoms of renal stones? How are they diagnosed and treated?**
Kidney stones (nephrolithiasis) generally present with severe, intermittent, unilateral flank and/or groin pain when the stone dislodges and gets stuck in the ureter (ureterolithiasis). Most stones can be seen on abdominal radiographs and are composed of calcium. Renal ultrasound or CT scan can be used to detect a stone if clinical suspicion is high but plain abdominal radiographs are negative. Symptomatic urolithiasis should be treated with lots of hydration and pain control (to see if the stone will pass). If the stone does not pass, it needs to be removed surgically (preferably endoscopically) or by lithotripsy.

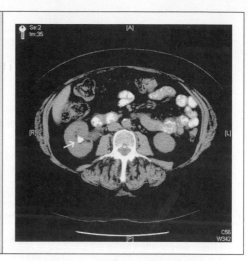

Figure 22-3. CT image of a urinary calculus in the right kidney. All stones (with the exception of some medication calculi) appear as dense, white objects within the urinary collecting system. (From Wein A, et al.: Campbell-Walsh Urology, 9th ed. Philadelphia, Saunders, 2007, Fig. 43-2.)

27. **What causes kidney stones?**

Nephrolithiasis is often idiopathic, but on the Step 2 exam watch for one of the following underlying disorders that predispose to the development of kidney stones:

Hypercalcemia: due to hyperparathyroidism or malignancy (calcium stones).

Infection: from ammonia-producing bugs (Proteus sp., staphylococci). Look for **staghorn calculi** (large stones composed of magnesium, ammonia, and phosphate [struvite] that fill the renal calyceal system; Fig. 22-4).

Hyperuricemia: uric acid stones due to gout or leukemia treatment (allopurinol and intravenous hydration are given before leukemia chemotherapy to prevent this complication).

Cystinuria/aminoaciduria: should be suspected if the stone is made of cystine or you are presented with a repetitive stone-forming patient.

Note: Send any recovered stones to the lab to determine the type.

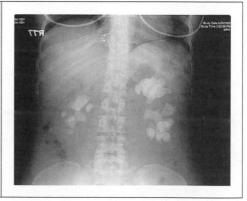

Figure 22-4. Plain film of a patient with bilateral staghorn calculi composed entirely of struvite. This patient had a 15 year history of recurrent urinary tract infections. (From Wein A, et al.: Campbell-Walsh Urology, 9th ed. Philadelphia, Saunders, 2007, Fig. 43-9.)

CHAPTER 23

NEUROLOGY

1. **In what common situation is a lumbar puncture contraindicated?**
   In the setting of acute head trauma, signs of intracranial hypertension (e.g., papilledema), or suspicion for subarachnoid hemorrhage. You should do a lumbar tap only after you have a negative computed tomography (CT) or magnetic resonance (MR) scan of the head in these settings. Otherwise, you may cause uncal herniation and death.

2. **Cover all but the left-hand column and describe the classic findings of cerebrospinal fluid (CSF) analysis in the following conditions:**

Condition	CELLS (mL)*	Glucose (mg/dL)	Protein (mg/dL)	Pressure (mmHg)
Normal CSF	0–3 (L)	50–100	20–45	100–200
Bacterial meningitis	> 1000 (PMN)	< 50	Around 100	> 200
Viral/aseptic meningitis	> 100 (L)	Normal	Normal/slightly increased	Normal/slightly increased
Pseudotumor cerebri	Normal	Normal	Normal	> 200
Guillain-Barré syndrome	0–100 (L)	Normal	> 100	Normal
Cerebral hemorrhage†	Bloody (RBC)	Normal	> 45	> 200
Multiple sclerosis‡	Normal/slightly increased (L)	Normal	Normal/slightly increased	Normal

*Main cell type is in parenthesis after number (L = lymphocytes, PMN = neutrophils, RBC = red blood cells).
†Think of subarachnoid hemorrhage, but this pattern also may occur after an intracerebral bleed.
‡On electrophoresis of CSF look for oligoclonal bands due to increased IgG production and an increased level of myelin basic protein in the CSF during active demyelination.
Note: Tuberculous and fungal meningitis have low glucose (< 50) with increased cells (> 100), which are predominantly lymphocytes. In patients with fungal meningitis, a positive India ink preparation equals *Cryptococcus neoformans*.

3. **Give a classic case description of multiple sclerosis.**
   Multiple sclerosis classically presents with an insidious onset of neurologic symptoms in white women aged 20 to 40 years with exacerbations and remissions. Common presentations

include paresthesias and numbness, weakness and clumsiness, visual disturbances (decreased vision and pain due to optic neuritis, diplopia due to cranial nerve involvement), gait disturbances, incontinence and urgency, and vertigo. Also look for emotional lability or other mental status changes. Internuclear ophthalmoplegia and scanning speech are classic; the patient may have a positive Babinski sign.

4. **What is the most sensitive test for diagnosis of multiple sclerosis? How is it treated?**
MRI is the most sensitive diagnostic tool and shows demyelination plaques. Also look for increased IgG/oligoclonal bands and possibly myelin basic protein in the CSF. Treatment is not highly effective but includes interferon, glatiramer, mitoxantrone, natalizumab, cyclophosphamide, and methotrexate. Acute exacerbations are treated with glucocorticoids.

5. **Define Guillain-Barré syndrome.**
Guillain-Barré syndrome is a postinfectious polyneuropathy. Look for a history of mild infection (especially upper respiratory infection) or immunization roughly 1 week before onset of symmetric, distal weakness or paralysis with mild paresthesias that starts in the feet and legs with loss of deep tendon reflexes in affected areas. The hallmark of the disease is that motor function is often affected with intact or only minimally impaired sensation. As the ascending paralysis or weakness progresses, respiratory paralysis may occur. Watch carefully; usually spirometry is done to follow inspiratory ability. Intubation may be required. Diagnosis is by clinical presentation. CSF is usually normal except for markedly increased protein. Nerve conduction velocities are slowed. The disease usually resolves spontaneously. Plasmapheresis (for adults) and intravenous immune globulin (for children) reduce the severity and length of disease. Do *not* use steroids; they no longer have a role in the treatment of Guillain-Barré syndrome.

6. **What causes nerve conduction velocity to be slowed?**
Demyelination. Watch for Guillain-Barré syndrome and multiple sclerosis as causes.

7. **What causes an electromyography (EMG) study to show fasciculations or fibrillations at rest?**
A lower motor neuron lesion (i.e., a peripheral nerve problem).

8. **What causes an EMG study with no muscle activity at rest and decreased amplitude of muscle contraction upon stimulation?**
Intrinsic muscle disease. You now know enough about EMG for the USMLE.

9. **What is the most common cause of syncope? What other conditions should you consider?**
Vasovagal syncope is the most common cause and classically is seen after stress or fear. The other three categories to worry about:
1. Cardiac problems (arrhythmias; always check an EKG)
2. Vascular disease (consider transient ischemic attacks or carotid stenosis, which can be ruled out with carotid artery ultrasound/duplex scanning)
3. Neurologic disorders (especially seizures; consider an electroencephalogram or CT/MR scan if history suggests seizures or intracranial lesion)

10. **Cover the right-hand column and localize the neurologic lesion for each of the following symptoms and signs:**

Symptom/Sign	Area
Decreased or no reflexes, fasciculations, atrophy	Lower motor neuron disease (or possibly muscle problem)
Hyperreflexia, clonus, increased muscle tone	Upper motor neuron lesion (cord or brain)
Apathy, inattention, disinhibition, labile affect	Frontal lobes
Broca (motor) aphasia	Dominant frontal lobe*
Wernicke (sensory) aphasia	Dominant temporal lobe*
Memory impairment, hyperaggression, hypersexuality	Temporal lobes
Inability to read, write, name, or do math	Dominant parietal lobe*
Ignoring one side of body, trouble with dressing	Nondominant parietal lobe*
Visual hallucinations/illusions	Occipital lobes
Cranial nerves 3 and 4	Midbrain
Cranial nerves 5, 6, 7 and 8	Pons
Cranial nerves 9, 10, 11, and 12	Medulla
Ataxia, dysarthria, nystagmus, intention, tremor, dysmetria, scanning speech	Cerebellum

*The left side is dominant in more than 95% of population (99% of right-handed people and 60% to 70% of left-handed people).

11. **For delirious or unconscious patients in the emergency department with no history of trauma, for what three common causes should you think about giving empiric treatment?**
    1. Hypoglycemia (give glucose)
    2. Opioid overdose (give naloxone)
    3. Thiamine deficiency (give thiamine before giving glucose in a suspected alcoholic)
    Other common causes are alcohol, illicit drugs, prescription drugs, diabetic ketoacidosis, stroke, and epilepsy or postictal state.

12. **What are the classic differential points between delirium and dementia?**

	Delirium	Dementia
Onset	Acute and dramatic	Chronic and insidious
Common causes	Illness, toxin, withdrawal	Alzheimer disease, multi-infarct dementia, HIV/AIDS
Reversible	Usually	Usually not
Attention	Poor	Usually unaffected
Arousal level	Fluctuates	Normal

13. **What symptoms and signs do delirium and dementia have in common?**
Both may have hallucinations, illusions, delusions, memory impairment (usually global in delirium, whereas remote memory is spared in early dementia), orientation difficulties (unawareness of time, place, person), and "sundowning" (worse at night).

delirium- ↓consciousness

14. **Define pseudodementia.**
Depression can cause some clinical symptoms and signs of dementia, classically in the elderly. This type of "dementia" is reversible with treatment. Step 2 questions will give you other signs and symptoms of depression (e.g., sadness, loss of loved one, weight or appetite loss, suicidal ideation, poor sleep, feelings of worthlessness).

15. **What treatable causes of dementia must always be ruled out?**
Treatable causes of dementia include vitamin B$_{12}$ deficiency, hyperhomocysteinemia, endocrine disorders (especially thyroid and parathyroid), uremia, hypercalcemia, syphilis, Lyme disease, brain tumors, and normal-pressure hydrocephalus. Treatment of Parkinson disease may reverse dementia if it is present.

16. **Define Wernicke encephalopathy and Korsakoff syndrome. What causes them?**
Thiamine deficiency, classically in alcoholics, causes the acute delirium of **Wernicke encephalopathy,** which results in ataxia, ophthalmoplegia, nystagmus, and confusion. If untreated, this acute encephalopathy may progress to **Korsakoff syndrome,** which is characterized by memory loss with confabulation, because patients cannot remember, they invent things. Korsakoff syndrome usually is irreversible. Always give thiamine before glucose in an alcoholic to prevent precipitating Wernicke encephalopathy.

17. **Differentiate among tension, cluster, and migraine headaches. How is each treated?**
Tension headaches are the most common; look for a long history of headaches and stress, plus a feeling of tightness or stiffness, usually frontal or occipital and bilateral. Treat with stress reduction and acetaminophen/nonsteroidal anti-inflammatory drugs (NSAIDs).
Cluster headaches are unilateral, severe, and tender; they occur in clusters (e.g., three in 1 week, then none for 2 months) and are usually accompanied by autonomic symptoms such as ptosis, lacrimation, rhinorrhea, and nasal congestion. Supplemental oxygen and subcutaneous sumatriptan are first-line therapy for acute attacks.
Migraine headaches classically are associated with an aura (a peculiar sensation, such as a noise or a flash of light, that lets the patient know that an attack is about to start). Often signs and symptoms include photophobia, nausea/vomiting, and a positive family history. Occasionally neurologic symptoms are seen during attacks. Migraines usually begin between the ages of 10 and 30 years. Medications used for the acute treatment of migraines includes NSAIDs, triptans, ergotamine, and antiemetics. Prophylaxis can be achieved with beta-blockers, tricyclic antidepressants, topiramate, valproic acid, and calcium channel blockers.

18. **How do you recognize a headache secondary to brain tumor or intracranial mass?**
By the presence of associated neurologic symptoms and signs of intracranial hypertension (papilledema; nausea/vomiting, which may be projectile; and mental status changes or ataxia). The classic headache occurs every day and is worse in the morning. Watch for a headache that wakes the patient from sleep. Headaches from an intracranial mass get worse with a Valsalva maneuver, exertion, or sex. Get a CT or MR scan of the head.

19. **Define pseudotumor cerebri. How is it diagnosed and treated?**
Pseudotumor cerebri is a fairly benign condition that can mimic a tumor because both cause intracranial hypertension with papilledema and daily headaches that classically are worse in

the morning and may be accompanied by nausea and vomiting. The difference, however, is that pseudotumor cerebri usually is found in young, obese females who are unlikely to have a brain tumor. Negative CT and MR scans rule out a tumor or mass. The main worrisome sequela is vision loss. Treatment is supportive; weight loss usually helps and repeated lumbar punctures or a CSF shunt may be needed. Large doses of vitamin A, tetracyclines, and withdrawal from corticosteroids are possible causes of pseudotumor cerebri.

20. **How do you recognize a headache due to meningitis?**
The adult patient has a fever, **Brudzinski sign** or **Kernig sign,** and positive CSF findings if a lumbar tap is done. Photophobia is also common.

21. **What causes the "worst headache" of a patient's life?**
This is a classic description for a subarachnoid hemorrhage. The most common causes are congenital berry aneurysm rupture or trauma. Look for blood around the brain or within sulci on a CT/MR scan or grossly bloody CSF on lumbar puncture. Treatment is supportive. Aneurysms require surgical treatment to prevent rebleeding and death.

22. **What are the common extracranial causes of headache?**
- Eye pain (optic neuritis, eyestrain from refractive errors, iritis, glaucoma)
- Middle ear pain (otitis media, mastoiditis)
- Sinus pain (sinusitis)
- Oral cavity pain (toothache)
- Herpes zoster infection with cranial nerve involvement
- Nonspecific headache (malaise from any illness, studying for the Step 2 exam)

23. **What does a lesion of the first cranial nerve (CN I) cause? What exotic syndrome should you watch for clinically?**
CN I lesions cause anosmia (inability to smell). Watch for **Kallmann syndrome,** which is anosmia plus hypogonadism due to gonadotropin-releasing hormone deficiency.

24. **True or false: Brain lesions can be localized based on the visual field defect.**
True. Remember this stuff from basic science? Review it again for at least one easy point (Fig. 23-1). If you really hate this stuff, at least remember bitemporal hemianopsia due to an optic chiasm lesion, usually caused by a pituitary tumor.

Visual Field Defect	Location of Lesion
Right anopsia (monocular blindness)	Right optic nerve
Bitemporal hemianopsia	Optic chiasm (classically due to pituitary tumor)
Left homonymous hemianopsia	Right optic tract
Left upper quadrant anopsia	Right optic radiations in the right temporal lobe
Left lower quadrant anopsia	Right optic radiations in the right parietal lobe
Left homonymous hemianopsia with macular sparing	Right occipital lobe (from posterior cerebral artery occlusion)

25. **How do you distinguish between a benign and serious cause of CN III deficit?**
With benign causes (i.e., hypertension and diabetes) of a CN III palsy, the pupil is normal in size and reactive; no treatment is needed. With serious causes (i.e., aneurysm, tumor,

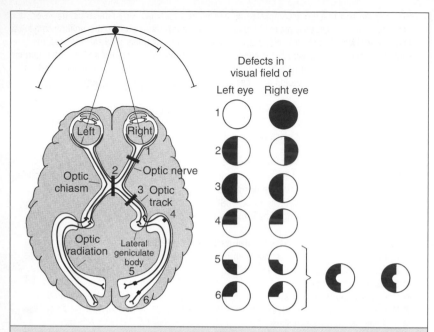

Figure 23-1. Visual field defects produced by lesions at various levels of the visual pathway. 1, Right optic nerve; 2, optic chiasm; 3, optic tract; 4, Meyer's loop; 5, cuneus; 6, lingual gyrus; *bracket,* occipital lobe (with macular sparing). (From Berne R: Physiology, 5th ed. Philadelphia, Mosby, 2003, Fig. 8-10.)

or uncal herniation), the pupil is dilated and nonreactive ("blown"). Urgent diagnosis and treatment are required. Additional neurologic symptoms also indicate a serious cause.

The first step in serious cases is to get a CT/MR scan of the head. Careful observation is preferred in benign cases, but if the patient does not improve within a few months or does not have hypertension or diabetes, you should order a CT/MR scan of the head just in case.

26. What does CN V (trigeminal nerve) innervate? What classic peripheral nerve disorder affects its function?
CN V innervates the muscles of mastication and facial sensation, including the afferent limb of the corneal reflex. Watch for **trigeminal neuralgia** (tic douloureux), which classically is described as unilateral shooting pains in the face in older adults and often triggered by activity (e.g., brushing the teeth). This condition is best treated with antiepilepsy medications (e.g., carbamazepine). If the patient is younger and female or the symptoms are bilateral, consider multiple sclerosis and rule out other causes, such as tumor or stroke.

27. What structures does CN VII innervate? What is the difference between an upper and lower motor neuron lesion of the facial nerve?
CN VII (facial nerve) innervates the muscles of facial expression, taste in the anterior two-thirds of the tongue, skin of the external ear, lacrimal and salivary glands (except the parotid gland), and stapedius muscle. With an upper motor neuron lesion of CN VII, the forehead is spared on the affected side, and the cause is usually a stroke or tumor. With a lower motor neuron lesion, the forehead is involved on the affected side, and the cause is usually Bell palsy or tumor.

28. **What problems other than facial droop affect patients with a CN VII lesion?**
Patients may be unable to close their eyes. Give artificial tears to prevent corneal ulceration. Also watch for **hyperacusis** (quiet noises sound extremely loud) in Bell palsy due to stapedius muscle paralysis.

29. **What rare tumor is a classic cause of lower motor neuron lesions of CN VII and CN VIII?**
Cerebellopontine angle tumors (e.g., acoustic neuroma, classically seen in patients with neurofibromatosis).

30. **Describe the function of CN VIII. What symptoms do lesions cause?**
CN VIII (the vestibulocochlear nerve) is needed for hearing and balance. Lesions can cause deafness, tinnitus, and/or vertigo. In children, think of meningitis as a cause. In adults, symptoms may be due to a toxin or medication (e.g., aspirin, aminoglycosides, loop diuretics, cisplatin), infection (labyrinthitis), tumor, or stroke.

31. **What does CN IX innervate? What physical findings are associated with a lesion?**
CN IX (the glossopharyngeal nerve) innervates the pharyngeal muscles and mucous membranes (afferent limb of gag reflex), parotid gland, taste in the posterior third of the tongue, skin of the external ear, and the carotid body/sinus. With lesions (due to stroke or tumor) look for loss of gag reflex and loss of taste in the posterior third of the tongue.

32. **Describe the function of CN X. Specify the physical findings and causes of lesions.**
CN X innervates muscles of the palate, pharynx, and larynx (efferent limb of gag reflex); taste buds in the base of the tongue; abdominal viscera; and skin of the external ear. Look for hoarseness, dysphagia, and loss of gag or cough reflex. Commonly lesions are due to stroke, but do not forget aortic aneurysms or tumors (especially apical/Pancoast lung tumors) as a cause of recurrent laryngeal nerve palsy and hoarseness.

33. **What muscles does CN XI innervate? How do you know on which side the lesion is located?**
CN XI (the spinal accessory nerve) innervates the sternocleidomastoid and trapezius muscles. Patients with CN XI lesions have trouble in turning their head to the side opposite the lesion and have ipsilateral shoulder droop.

34. **What does a lesion of CN XII cause?**
CN XII (the hypoglossal nerve) innervates the muscles of the tongue. A protruded tongue deviates to the same side as the lesion.

35. **Which vitamin deficiencies may present with neurologic signs or symptoms?**
Vitamin B_{12}: dementia, peripheral neuropathy, loss of vibration sense in lower extremities, loss of position sense, ataxia, spasticity, hyperactive reflexes, and positive Babinski sign.
Thiamine: peripheral neuropathy, confusion, ophthalmoplegia, nystagmus, ataxia, confusion, delirium, dementia.
Vitamin E: loss of proprioception/vibratory sensation, areflexia, ataxia, and gaze palsy.
Vitamin A: vision loss.
Vitamin B_6: peripheral sensory neuropathy (watch for isoniazid as a cause, and give prophylactic B_6 to patients taking isoniazid, if given the choice).

36. **What are the six general types of seizures that you should be able to recognize?**
    1. Simple partial
    2. Complex partial
    3. Absence (petit mal)
    4. Tonic-clonic
    5. Febrile
    6. Secondary

37. **Describe a simple partial seizure. How is it treated?**
    Simple partial (local or focal) seizures may be motor (e.g., Jacksonian march), sensory (e.g., hallucinations), or psychic (cognitive or affective symptoms). The key point is that consciousness is *not* impaired. The first-line agents for treatment are carbamazepine, lamotrigine, oxcarbazepine, and levetiracetam.

38. **Describe complex partial seizures. How are they treated?**
    Complex partial (psychomotor) seizures are any simple partial seizure followed by impairment of consciousness. Patients perform purposeless movements and may become aggressive if restraint is attempted (however, people who get in fights or kill other people are not having a seizure). The first-line agents for treatment are valproate, lamotrigine, and levetiracetam.

39. **Give the classic description of an absence seizure.**
    Absence (petit mal) seizures do not begin after the age of 20 years. They are brief (10 to 30 seconds in duration), generalized seizures in which the main manifestation is loss of consciousness, often with eye or muscle fluttering. The classic description is a child in a classroom who stares into space in the middle of a sentence, then 20 seconds later resumes the sentence where he left off. The child is *not* daydreaming; he or she is having a seizure. There is no postictal state (an important differential point). The first-line treatment agents are ethosuximide and valproate.

40. **How do you recognize a tonic-clonic seizure?**
    Tonic-clonic (grand mal) seizures are the classic seizures that we knew about before we went to medical school. They may be associated with an aura. Tonic muscle contraction is followed by clonic contractions, usually lasting 2 to 5 minutes. Associated symptoms may include incontinence and tongue lacerations. The postictal state is characterized by drowsiness, confusion, headache, and muscle soreness. The first-line agents for treatment are valproate, lamotrigine, or levetiracetam.

41. **Define febrile seizure.**
    Children between the ages of 6 months and 5 years may have a seizure caused by fever. Always assume another cause outside this age range. The seizure is usually of the tonic-clonic, generalized type. No specific seizure treatment is required, but you should treat the underlying cause of the fever, if possible, and give acetaminophen to reduce fever. Such children do *not* have epilepsy, and the chances of their developing it are just barely higher than in the general population. Make sure that the child does not have meningitis, tumor, or another serious cause of the seizure. The Step 2 question will give clues in the case description if you should pursue work-up for a serious condition.

42. **What are the common causes of secondary seizures? How are they treated?**
    - Mass effect (tumor [Fig. 23-2], hemorrhage)
    - Metabolic disorder (hypoglycemia, hypoxia, phenylketonuria, hyponatremia)
    - Toxins (lead, cocaine, carbon monoxide poisoning)
    - Drug withdrawal (alcohol, barbiturates, benzodiazepines, withdrawing anticonvulsants too rapidly)

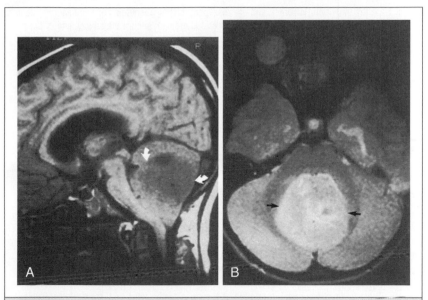

Figure 23-2. MRI scan of medulloblastoma. **A,** Sagittal T1-weighted image shows a hypointense mass involving the vermis (*arrows*). **B,** Axial T2-weighted image shows a hyperintense mass (*arrows*) with areas of hypointensity representing acute hemorrhagic infarction within the medulloblastoma. (From Kuhn JP, Slovis TL, Haller JO: Caffey's Pediatric Diagnostic Imaging, 10th ed. Philadelphia, Mosby, 2004, p 574.)

- Cerebral edema (severe or malignant hypertension; also watch for pheochromocytoma and eclampsia)
- Central nervous system infections (meningitis, encephalitis, toxoplasmosis [Fig. 23-3], cysticercosis)
- Trauma
- Stroke

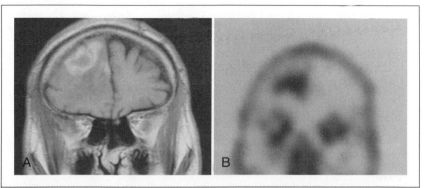

Figure 23-3. A, MR (post-contrast T1-weighted image) demonstrating a focal mass-like lesion with ring enhancement within the right frontoparietal area in a 30-year-old HIV-positive patient who presented with mental status changes. The primary differential diagnosis is between lymphoma and toxoplasmosis. **B,** Thallium SPECT scan in the same patient shows abnormal increased uptake representing a primary CNS lymphoma. (From Goetz C: Textbook of Clinical Neurology, 3rd ed. Philadelphia, Saunders, 2007, Fig. 23-34.)

Treat the underlying disorder, and use diazepam and/or phenytoin (or fosphenytoin) acutely to control seizures. For all seizures (primary or secondary), secure the airway, and, if possible, roll the patient onto his or her side to prevent aspiration.

43. Define status epilepticus. How is it treated?
Status epilepticus is defined as a seizure that lasts for a sufficient length of time (usually 30 minutes or longer) or is repeated frequently enough that the individual does not regain consciousness between seizures. Status epilepticus may occur spontaneously or result from withdrawing anticonvulsants too rapidly. Treat with intravenous lorazepam. Give fosphenytoin if the seizures persist. As with all seizures, remember your ABCs (**a**irway, **b**reathing, **c**irculation). Protect the airway. Intubate if necessary, and roll the patient on his or her side to prevent aspiration.

44. True or false: Hypertension can cause seizures.
True. Always remember hypertension as a cause of seizures or convulsions, headache, and/or confusion, stupor, and mental status changes.

45. What do you need to remember when giving anticonvulsants to women?
All anticonvulsants are teratogenic, and women of reproductive age need counseling about the risks of pregnancy. Do a pregnancy test before starting an anticonvulsant and offer birth control. Valproic acid is a major contributor to the risk. Polypharmacy increases the risk. There is limited human information of the risks to the fetus with the newer antiepileptic medications.

46. What causes strokes? How common are they?
Cerebrovascular disease (stroke) is the most common cause of neurologic disability in the United States—and the third leading cause of death. Ischemia due to atherosclerosis (atherothrombotic ischemia) is by far the most common type of stroke (more than 85% of cases). Hypertension is another cause of stroke and typically causes hemorrhagic stroke, most commonly in the basal ganglia, thalamus or cerebellum. Having said this, be aware of more exotic causes of stroke, such as atrial fibrillation with resultant clot formation and emboli to the brain, septic emboli from endocarditis, and sickle cell disease.

47. How is an acute stroke treated?
Treatment for an acute stroke in evolution is supportive (e.g., airway, oxygen, intravenous fluids). The first step is to get a CT scan of the head without contrast to evaluate for bleeding or mass (Fig. 23-4). If no blood is seen on CT scan, aspirin is usually the medication of choice. Heparin is not recommended for the treatment of acute ischemic stroke and should be avoided on the USMLE. Chapter 33 ("Vascular Surgery") discusses the role of carotid endarterectomy, which is not done emergently. Thrombolysis with t-PA (tissue-plasminogen activator) can be attempted if patients present within 3 hours and meet strict criteria for its use (although benefit has been shown up to 4.5 hours after symptom onset).

48. Define transient ischemic attack (TIA). How is it managed?
TIA is a focal neurologic deficit that lasts minutes to hours (generally up to 24 hours, though this classic definition is being reconsidered), then resolves spontaneously. It is often a precursor to stroke and is due to ischemia. The classic presentation is ipsilateral blindness (amaurosis fugax) and/or unilateral hemiplegia, hemiparesis, weakness, or clumsiness that lasts less than 5 minutes.

Order a carotid duplex scan to look for carotid stenosis. The correct choice for long-term therapy is aspirin and antiplatelet medications. Choose carotid endarterectomy over aspirin if the degree of carotid stenosis is 70% to 99%.

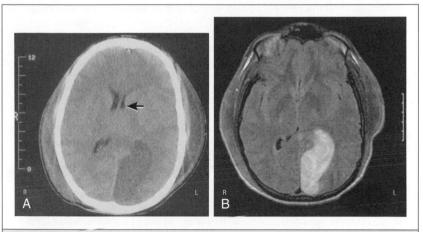

Figure 23-4. Stroke on computed tomography (CT) and magnetic resonance imaging (MRI) scans. The CT scan (**A**) done three days after a stroke shows a low-density area posteriorly on the left with mass effect and clear midline shift (*arrow*). The MRI scan (**B**) done on the same day shows the infarcted area much more clearly. (From Mettler F: Essentials of Radiology, 2nd ed. Philadelphia, Saunders, 2004, Fig. 2-17.)

49. **Describe the signs and symptoms of Huntington disease. How is it acquired? What is the classic CT finding?**

Huntington disease is an autosomal dominant condition that usually presents between the ages of 35 and 50 years. Look for choreiform movements (irregular, spasmodic, involuntary movements of the limbs or facial muscles) and progressive intellectual deterioration, dementia, or psychiatric disturbances. **Atrophy of the caudate nuclei** may be seen on CT or MR scan. Treatment is supportive; antipsychotics may help.

50. **Define Parkinson disease. How do you recognize it on the Step 2 exam?**

Parkinson disease has a classic tetrad of (1) slowness or poverty of movement, (2) muscular ("lead pipe" and "cog-wheel") rigidity, (3) "pill-rolling" tremor at rest (which disappears with movement and sleep), and (4) postural instability (manifested by the classic shuffling gait and festination). Patients also may have dementia and depression. The mean age of onset is around 60 years.

51. **Describe the pathophysiology of Parkinson disease. How is it treated pharmacologically?**

The cause is thought to be a loss of dopaminergic neurons, especially in the **substantia nigra**, which project to the basal ganglia. The result is decreased dopamine in the basal ganglia. Drug therapy, which aims to increase dopamine, includes dopamine precursors (levodopa with carbidopa), dopamine agonists (bromocriptine, apomorphine, pergolide, pramipexole, and ropinirole), monoamine oxidase-B inhibitors (selegiline), COMT inhibitors (entacapone and tolcapone), anticholinergics (trihexyphenidyl and benztropine), and amantadine.

52. **What is the classic iatrogenic cause of parkinsonian signs and symptoms?**

Antipsychotics may cause parkinsonian symptoms in schizophrenics. This is a favorite Step 2 question. Treat this side-effect of antipsychotic medication with anticholinergics (benztropine, trihexyphenidyl) or antihistamines (diphenhydramine).

53. **What brain lesions cause a resting tremor and an intention tremor? What about hemiballismus?**

A resting tremor, if due to a brain lesion, is generally a sign of basal ganglia disease, as is chorea. An intention tremor is usually due to cerebellar disease. Hemiballismus (random, violent, unilateral flailing of the limbs) is classically due to a lesion in the **subthalamic nucleus.**

54. **What conditions other than Parkinson disease cause a resting tremor?**

A resting tremor may be due to hyperthyroidism, anxiety, drug withdrawal or intoxication, or benign (essential) hereditary tremor. Benign hereditary tremor is usually autosomal dominant; look for a positive family history, and use beta blockers to reduce the tremor. Also watch for Wilson disease (hepatolenticular degeneration), which can cause chorea-like movements; asterixis (slow, involuntary flapping of outstretched hands) may be seen in patients with liver failure.

55. **What diseases should come to mind in children with cerebellar findings?**

- Brain tumor (cerebellar astrocytoma, medulloblastomas)
- Hydrocephalus (enlarging head in an infant under the age of 6 months, Arnold-Chiari or Dandy-Walker malformations)
- Friedreich ataxia (starts between ages 5 and 15 years; autosomal recessive; look for areflexia, loss of vibration/position sense, and cardiomyopathy)
- Ataxia-telangiectasia (progressive cerebellar ataxia, oculocutaneous telangiectasias, and immune deficiency)

56. **What diseases should come to mind in adults with cerebellar findings?**

Alcoholism, tumor, ischemia or hemorrhage, and multiple sclerosis.

57. **How do you recognize amyotrophic lateral sclerosis (ALS) on the Step 2 exam?**

ALS (Lou Gehrig disease) is the only condition that you are likely to be asked about that causes both upper and lower motor neuron lesion signs and symptoms. This idiopathic neurodegenerative disease is more common in men, and the mean age at onset is 55. The key is to notice a combination of upper motor neuron lesion signs (spasticity, hyperreflexia, positive Babinski sign) and lower motor neuron lesion signs (fasciculations, atrophy, flaccidity) present at the same time. Treatment is supportive. Fifty percent of patients die within 3 years of disease onset.

58. **What are the two classic causes of a "floppy" (flaccid) baby? How do you differentiate the two?**

Genetic disorders, the most common of which is Werdnig-Hoffmann disease (WHD), and infant botulism. History easily differentiates the two. WHD is an autosomal recessive degeneration of anterior horn cells in the spinal cord and brainstem (lower motor neuron disease). Most infants are hypotonic at birth, and all are affected by 6 months. Look for a positive family history and a long, slowly progressive disease course. Treatment is supportive only.

Infant botulism is caused by a *Clostridium botulinum* toxin. Look for sudden onset and a history of ingesting honey or other home-canned foods. Diagnosis is made by finding *C. botulinum* toxin or organisms in the feces. Treatment involves inpatient monitoring and support with a close watch of respiratory status. The child may need intubation for respiratory muscle paralysis. Spontaneous recovery usually occurs within 1 week, and supportive care is all that is needed.

59. **List the causative categories of peripheral neuropathy and give examples of each.**

1. Metabolic/endocrine: diabetes mellitus (autonomic and sensory neuropathy), uremia, hypothyroidism.
2. Nutritional: deficiencies of vitamin B_{12}, vitamin B_6 (look for history of isoniazid), thiamine ("dry" beriberi), and vitamin E.

3. Toxins/medications: lead (the classic symptom is wrist drop or foot drop; look for coexisting central nervous system or abdominal symptoms) or other heavy metals, isoniazid, vincristine, ethambutol (optic neuritis), aminoglycosides (especially CN VIII).

4. Immunization and autoimmune disorders: Guillain-Barré syndrome, lupus erythematosus, polyarteritis nodosa, scleroderma, sarcoidosis, amyloidosis.

5. Trauma: carpal tunnel syndrome (entrapment of the median nerve at the wrist; usually due to repetitive physical activity but may be a presentation of acromegaly or hypothyroidism; look for positive Tinel and Phalen signs), pressure paralysis (radial nerve palsy in alcoholics), fractures.

6. Infectious: Lyme disease, diphtheria, HIV, leprosy.

60. **What test can be used to prove the presence of a peripheral neuropathy, regardless of etiology?**
Nerve conduction velocity is slowed with a peripheral neuropathy.

61. **Describe the pathophysiology of myasthenia gravis (MG). Who is affected? What are the classic physical findings?**
MG is an autoimmune disease that destroys acetylcholine receptors. Most patients have antibodies to acetylcholine receptors in their serum. The disease usually presents in women between the ages of 20 and 40 years. Look for ptosis, diplopia, and general muscle fatigability, especially toward the end of the day.

62. **How is MG diagnosed? What tumor is associated with it?**
Diagnosis is made with the Tensilon test. After injection of edrophonium (Tensilon), a short-acting anticholinesterase inhibitor, muscle weakness improves. Nerve stimulation studies can also be used. Watch for associated **thymomas** (a tumor of the thymus). Most patients with MG improve after removal of the thymus, which is considered part of standard treatment. Chronic medical treatment consists of long-acting anticholinesterase inhibitors (pyridostigmine), immunotherapy (glucocorticoids, mycophenolate, azathioprine, and cyclosporine), and thymectomy.

63. **What three conditions may cause an MG-like clinical picture?**
1. **Eaton-Lambert syndrome** is a paraneoplastic syndrome (classically seen with small cell lung cancer) associated with muscle weakness. The extraocular muscles are spared, whereas MG almost always is characterized by prominent involvement of extraocular muscles. Eaton-Lambert syndrome has a different mechanism of action (impaired release of acetylcholine from nerves) and a differential response to repetitive nerve stimulation. The weakness in MG worsens with repetitive use or stimulation, whereas the weakness in Eaton-Lambert syndrome improves.
2. **Organophosphate poisoning** also causes MG-like muscle weakness. Poisoning usually is due to agricultural exposure. Look for symptoms of parasympathetic excess (e.g., miosis, excessive bronchial secretions, urinary urgency, and diarrhea). Edrophonium causes worsening of the muscular weakness. Treat with atropine and pralidoxime.
3. **Aminoglycosides in high doses** may cause MG-like muscular weakness and/or prolong the effects of muscular blockade after anesthesia.

64. **What is the most common type of muscular dystrophy? How is it inherited? What are the classic findings?**
The most common type is Duchenne muscular dystrophy, an X-linked recessive disorder of dystrophin that usually presents in boys between the ages of age 3 and 7. Look for muscle weakness, markedly elevated levels of creatine phosphokinase, pseudohypertrophy of the calves (due to fatty and fibrous infiltration of the degenerating muscle), and often

a lower-than-normal IQ. Gower sign is also classic: the patient "walks" his hands and feet toward each other to rise from a prone position. Muscle biopsy establishes the diagnosis. Treatment is supportive. Most patients die by age 20.

65. **List the five less common types of muscular dystrophies.**
    1. Becker muscular dystrophy: also an X-linked recessive dystrophin disorder but milder.
    2. Fascioscapulohumeral dystrophy: an autosomal dominant disorder that affects the areas in the name (face, shoulder girdle). Symptoms begin between the age of 7 and 20 years. Life expectancy is normal.
    3. Limb-girdle dystrophy: affects pelvic and shoulder muscles; begins in adulthood.
    4. Mitochondrial myopathies: of interest because they are inherited mitochondrial defects (passed only from mother to offspring; cannot be transmitted by men). The key phrase is "ragged red fibers" on biopsy specimen. Ophthalmoplegia is usually present.
    5. Myotonic dystrophy: an autosomal dominant disorder that presents between the ages of 20 and 30 years. Myotonia (inability to relax muscles) classically presents as an **inability to relax the grip or release a handshake.** Look for coexisting mental retardation, baldness, and testicular or ovarian atrophy. Treatment is supportive, including genetic counseling. The diagnosis is clinical.

66. **What class of inherited metabolic disorders affect muscle and may resemble muscular dystrophy?**
    The rare glycogen storage diseases (autosomal recessive inheritance) can cause muscular weakness, especially **McArdle disease,** a deficiency in glycogen phosphorylase that is relatively mild and presents with weakness and cramping after exercise due to lactic acid build-up.

CHAPTER 24

NEUROSURGERY

1. **List the four major types of intracranial hemorrhage.**
   1. Subdural hematoma
   2. Epidural hematoma
   3. Subarachnoid hemorrhage
   4. Intracerebral hemorrhage

2. **What causes a subdural hematoma? How do you recognize and treat it?**
   Subdural hematomas are due to bleeding from veins that bridge the cortex and dural sinuses. On computed tomography (CT) scan the hematoma is crescent-shaped (Fig. 24-1). Subdural hematomas are common in alcoholics and victims of head trauma. They may present immediately after trauma or as long as 1 to 2 months later. If the patient has a history of head trauma, always consider the diagnosis of subdural hematoma. If large, expanding, or accompanied by neurologic deficits, treat with surgical evacuation.

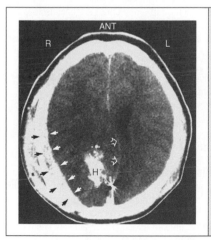

Figure 24-1. Subdural hematomas. A noncontrast computed tomography (CT) scan of an acute subdural hematoma shows a crescentic area of increased density (*arrows*) in the right posterior parietal region between the brain and the skull. An area of intraparenchymal hemorrhage (H) also is seen; in addition, mass effect causes a midline shift to the left (*open arrows*). (From Mettler F: Essentials of Radiology, 2nd ed. Philadelphia, Saunders, 2004, Fig. 2-13A.)

3. **What causes an epidural hematoma? How do you recognize and treat it?**
   Epidural hematomas are due to bleeding from meningeal arteries (classically, the middle meningeal artery). On CT scan, the hematoma is lenticular in shape (Fig. 24-2). At least 85% of epidural hematomas are associated with a skull fracture (classically, a temporal bone fracture), and many patients have an ipsilateral "blown" pupil (dilated, fixed, nonreactive pupil on the side of the hematoma). The classic history includes head trauma with loss of consciousness, followed by a lucid interval of minutes to hours, then neurologic deterioration. Treatment usually includes surgical evacuation.

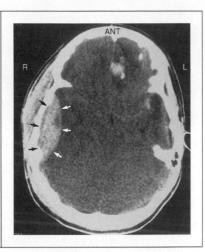

Figure 24-2. Epidural hematoma. In this patient, who was in a motor vehicle accident, a lenticular area of increased density is seen on a noncontrasted axial computed tomography (CT) scan in the right parietal region. Areas of hemorrhage also are seen in the left frontal lobe. (From Mettler F: Essentials of Radiology, 2nd ed. Philadelphia, Saunders, 2004, Fig. 2-14.)

4. Define subarachnoid hemorrhage. What causes it? How is it treated?

A subarachnoid hemorrhage describes bleeding between the arachnoid and pia mater. The most common cause is trauma, followed by ruptured berry aneurysms. Blood can be seen in the cerebral ventricles and surrounding the brain or brainstem on CT scan. The classic patient describes the "worst headache of my life," although many die or are unconscious before they reach the hospital. Patients who are awake have signs of meningitis (positive Kernig sign and Brudzinski sign). Remember the association between polycystic kidney disease and berry aneurysms. CT is the test of choice. A lumbar tap shows grossly bloody cerebrospinal fluid (CSF).

Treat with support of vital functions, anticonvulsants, and observation. Once the patient is stable, do a cerebral or MR angiogram to look for aneurysms or arteriovenous malformations, which may be treatable with surgical clipping or catheter-directed angiographic procedures.

5. What causes an intracerebral hemorrhage? How do you recognize and treat it?

Intracerebral hemorrhage describes bleeding into the brain parenchyma. The most common cause is hypertension, but it also may be due to other forms of stroke, trauma, arteriovenous malformations, coagulopathies, or tumors. Two-thirds of intracerebral hemorrhages occur in the basal ganglia (especially with hypertension). The patient may present with coma or, if awake, contralateral hemiplegia and hemisensory deficits. Blood (which appears white on CT scan) can be seen in the brain parenchyma and may extend into the ventricles. Surgery is reserved for large, accessible hemorrhages, although usually it is not helpful.

6. After a history of head trauma, what does a dilated, unreactive pupil on one side mean until proved otherwise?

In the setting of head trauma, a dilated, unreactive pupil on one side most likely represents impingement of the ipsilateral third cranial nerve and impending uncal herniation due to increased intracranial pressure. Of the different intracranial hemorrhages, this scenario is seen most commonly with epidural hemorrhages. Do *not* do a lumbar puncture in any patient with a "blown" pupil, because you may precipitate uncal herniation and death. Instead, order a CT or magnetic resonance (MR) scan of the head.

7. **List the four classic signs of a basilar skull fracture.**
   1. Periorbital ecchymosis ("raccoon eyes")
   2. Postauricular ecchymosis (Battle sign)
   3. Hemotympanum (blood behind the eardrum)
   4. CSF otorrhea or rhinorrhea (leakage of CSF, which is clear in appearance, from the ears or nose)

8. **What is the imaging test of choice for skull fractures of the calvarium? How are they managed?**
   Skull fractures of the calvarium (roof of the skull) are best seen on CT scan (preferred over plain x-rays). Surgical indications include contamination (surgical cleaning and debridement), depression with impingement on brain parenchyma, or open fracture with CSF leak. Otherwise, such fractures can be observed and generally heal on their own.

9. **True or false: Severe, permanent neurologic deficits may occur after head trauma, even with a negative CT or MR scan of the head.**
   True. Head trauma can cause cerebral contusion or shear injury of the brain parenchyma, both of which may not show up on a CT or MR scan but may cause temporary or permanent neurologic deficits.

10. **What finding suggests increased intracranial pressure?**
    Increased intracranial pressure (intracranial hypertension) is highly suggested in the setting of bilaterally dilated and fixed pupils. Normal intracranial pressure is between 5 and 15 mmHg. Less specific symptoms include headache, papilledema, nausea and vomiting, and mental status changes. Look also for the classic Cushing triad, which consists of increasing blood pressure, bradycardia, and respiratory irregularity.

11. **How should increased intracranial pressure be managed?**
    The first step is to intubate the patient in reverse Trendelenburg position (head up). Once intubated, the patient should be hyperventilated for rapid lowering of intracranial pressure through decreased intracranial blood volume (due to cerebral vasoconstriction). For longer-term treatment, **mannitol** diuresis can be tried to lessen cerebral edema. Furosemide is also used but less effective. Ventriculostomy should be performed if hydrocephalus is identified. Barbiturate coma and decompressive craniotomy (burr holes) are last-ditch measures. Anticonvulsant therapy should be started if seizures are suspected; prophylactic anticonvulsants are controversial but may be warranted in some cases.

    Remember that cerebral perfusion pressure equals blood pressure minus intracranial pressure. In other words, do *not* treat hypertension initially in a patient with increased intracranial pressure because hypertension is the body's way of trying to increase cerebral perfusion. Lowering blood pressure in this setting may worsen symptoms or even cause a stroke.

12. **True or false: Lumbar puncture is the first test that should be performed in a patient with increased intracranial pressure.**
    False. *Never* do a lumbar tap in any patient with signs of increased intracranial pressure until a CT scan is done first. If the CT is totally negative, you can proceed to a tap, if needed. If you do a lumbar puncture first, you may precipitate uncal herniation and death.

13. **How do patients with spinal cord trauma present? How are they managed?**
    Patients with spinal cord trauma often present with "spinal shock" (loss of reflexes and motor function, hypotension). Order standard trauma radiographs (cervical spine, chest, pelvis) as well as additional spine radiographs or CT scans based on physical exam. Also give corticosteroids (proven to improve outcome). Surgery is done for incomplete neurologic

injury (some residual function maintained) with external compression (e.g., subluxation, bone chip). MRI can visualize cord injury non-invasively.

14. **What causes spinal cord compression? How do patients present?**
Spinal cord compression usually is defined as acute or subacute. Most cases of acute cord compression result from trauma. Look for the appropriate history. Subacute compression is often due to metastatic cancer but also may result from a primary neoplasm, subdural or epidural abscess (classically seen in diabetics and due to *Staphylococcus aureus*), or hematoma (especially after a lumbar tap or epidural/spinal anesthesia in a patient with a bleeding disorder or a patient taking anticoagulation).
Patients present with local spinal pain (especially with bone metastases) and neurologic deficits below the lesion (e.g., hyperreflexia, positive Babinski sign, weakness, sensory loss).

15. **How should patients with subacute spinal cord compression be diagnosed and treated?**
The first step in the emergency department is to give high-dose corticosteroids and order an MRI scan (preferred over CT; see Fig. 24-3). If the cause is cancer or tumor, give local radiation if the metastases are from a known primary tumor that is radiosensitive. Surgical decompression can be used if the tumor is not radiosensitive. For a hematoma or subdural/epidural abscess, surgery is indicated for decompression and drainage. Prognosis is related most closely to pretreatment function; the longer you wait to treat, the worse the prognosis.

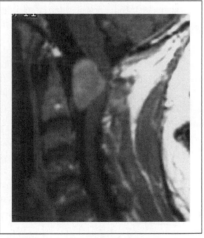

Figure 24-3. Post-contrast MR image of C1-C2 meningioma demonstrates that this discrete tumor mass (bright ovoid area) arose outside the spinal cord and is compressing and displacing the cord posteriorly. (From Katz DS, Math KR, Groskin SA, [eds]: Radiology Secrets. Philadelphia, Hanley & Belfus, 1998, p 376, with permission.)

16. **Define syringomyelia. What causes it? How does it usually present?**
Syringomyelia is a central pathologic cavitation of the spinal cord, usually in the cervical or upper thoracic region. Most cases are idiopathic, but syringomyelia also may follow trauma or be related to congenital cranial base malformations (e.g., Arnold-Chiari malformation). The classic presentation, due to involvement of the lateral spinothalamic tracts, is bilateral loss of pain and temperature sensation below the lesion in the distribution of a "cape." The cavitation in the cord gradually widens to involve other tracts, causing motor and sensory deficits. MR scan is the diagnostic imaging study of choice. The primary treatment available is surgical creation of a shunt.

17. Define spina bifida. How can it be prevented?

Spina bifida is a congenital abnormality in which lack of fusion of the spinal column, specifically the posterior vertebral arches, allows protrusion of spinal membranes, with or without spinal cord. Spina bifida occulta, the mildest form of the disease (bone deficiency without dural membrane or cord protrusion), is often asymptomatic and should be suspected in patients with a triangular patch of hair over the lumbar spine. More serious defects are usually obvious and occur most often in the lumbosacral region. A **meningocele** is protrusion of the meninges outside the spinal canal, whereas a **myelomeningocele** is protrusion of meninges plus central nervous system tissue outside the spinal canal. Patients with a myelomeningocele almost always have an associated Arnold-Chiari malformation. Giving folate to potential mothers reduces the incidence of spina bifida and other neural tube defects.

18. Define hydrocephalus. How is it recognized in children?

Hydrocephalus is excessive accumulation of CSF in the cerebral ventricles. In children, look for increasing head circumference, increased intracranial pressure, bulging fontanelle, scalp vein engorgement, and paralysis of upward gaze. The most common causes include congenital malformations, tumors, and inflammation (e.g., hemorrhage, meningitis). Treat the underlying cause, if possible; otherwise a surgical shunt is created to decompress the ventricles.

19. In what setting does dural venous sinus thrombosis occur? How is it diagnosed and treated?

The risk factors are similar to those for deep venous thrombosis in other areas, including hypercoagulable state, trauma, dehydration, pregnancy, oral contraceptive use, infections (e.g., extension of sinusitis or mastoiditis intracranially), nephrotic syndrome and local tumor invasion. The diagnostic test of choice is MRI (Fig. 24-4). Though hemorrhagic infarcts are common with dural venous thrombosis, treatment with anticoagulation improves outcomes.

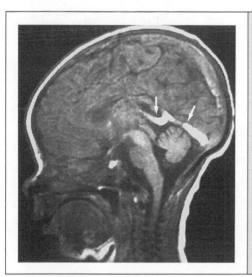

Figure 24-4. Venous thrombosis is seen as a high signal area on MR (sagittal image). The great vein of Galen and straight sinus are involved *(white arrows)*. (From Katz DS, Math KR, Groskin SA [eds]: Radiology Secrets. Philadelphia, Hanley & Belfus, 1998, p 364, with permission.)

CHAPTER 25

OBSTETRICS

1. **A patient who is taking birth control pills presents with amenorrhea. What is the likely cause?**
   Pregnancy. No form of contraception is 100% effective (including tubal ligation), especially when patient compliance is required.

2. **List the symptoms and signs of pregnancy.**
   - Amenorrhea
   - Morning sickness
   - Weight gain
   - Hegar sign (softening and compressibility of the lower uterine segment)
   - Chadwick sign (dark discoloration of the vulva and vaginal walls)
   - Linea nigra
   - Melasma (also known as chloasma or the "mask of pregnancy")
   - Auscultation of fetal heart tones
   - Gestational sac or fetus seen on ultrasound
   - Uterine contractions
   - Palpation/ballottement of fetus

3. **Which vitamin should all pregnant women take? Why?**
   Give all pregnant patients folate to prevent neural tube defects. Ideally, all woman of reproductive age should take folate, because it is most effective in the first trimester, when most women do not know that they are pregnant. Iron supplements are given frequently to pregnant women to help prevent anemia.

4. **Define macrosomia. What is the likely cause?**
   Macrosomia is defined as a newborn that weighs more than 4 kg (roughly 9 pounds). The cause is maternal diabetes mellitus until proven otherwise.

5. **What routine tests should be obtained for all pregnant patients?**
   - **Pap smear:** if the patient is due. Pregnancy does not change the frequency of screening.
   - **Urinalysis:** at the first visit and every visit thereafter (to screen for proteinuria, preeclampsia, and bacteriuria; not a good screen for diabetes).
   - **Urine culture:** obtained at 12 to 16 weeks to screen for asymptomatic bacteriuria.
   - **Hemoglobin and hematocrit:** at the first visit to see if the patient is anemic (because pregnancy may aggravate anemia). Should be repeated in the third trimester.
   - **Blood type, rhesus (Rh) type, and antibody screen:** at first visit (for identification of possible isoimmunization).
   - **Syphilis test:** at first visit (mandated in most states) and subsequent visits (for high-risk patients).
   - **Rubella antibody screen:** if the patient if found to be nonimmune, counsel her to get postpartum immunization.
   - **Glucose screen for gestational diabetes:** at first visit in patients with risk factors for diabetes mellitus (obesity, positive family history, or age over 30 years old); otherwise,

screen at 24 to 28 weeks. Use fasting serum glucose and serum glucose levels 1 or 2 hours after an oral glucose load.

- **Serum alpha-fetoprotein:** performed at 15 to 20 weeks, primarily to detect open spina bifida and anencephaly.
- **Hepatitis B antigen testing:** to prevent perinatal transmission.
- **Varicella:** all pregnant women should be tested for immunity to varicella.
- **Thyroid function:** maternal hypothyroidism may affect fetal neurologic development. Maternal hyperthyroidism can lead to fetal and maternal complications.
- **HIV test:** the American College of Obstetrics and Gynecology (ACOG) advocates an "opt-out" approach to screening rather than an "opt-in" approach to increase screening.
- **Chlamydia screening:** the Centers for Disease Control advocates testing all pregnant women while the ACOG recommends screening women at higher risk (e.g., age greater than 25 years, new sexual partner or more than one sexual partner, history of STD, drug use).
- **Down syndrome screening:** should be offered to all pregnant patients. There are multiple ways to screen. See questions 21 to 23.
- **Group B beta-hemolytic streptococcus (GBS):** screen at 35 to 37 weeks with a swab of the lower vagina and rectum.
- **Others:** tuberculosis skin test for women at higher risk. Testing for gonorrhea for women at higher risk of infection. Testing for toxoplasmosis is controversial. If asked, you should do chlamydia and gonorrhea cultures for any pregnant teenager. Testing for sexually transmitted diseases should be repeated in the third trimester for women who continue to be at risk or for women who acquire a risk factor during pregnancy.

6. **On every prenatal visit, listen to fetal heart tones and evaluate uterine size. When can these factors first be noticed? What constitutes a size/date discrepancy?**
Fetal heart tones can be heard with Doppler ultrasound at 10 to 12 weeks and with a normal stethoscope at 16 to 20 weeks. At 12 weeks of gestation, the uterus enters the abdomen and is palpable at the symphysis pubis; at roughly 20 weeks, it reaches the umbilicus.
Uterine size is evaluated by measuring the distance from the symphysis pubis to the top of the fundus in centimeters. At roughly 20 to 35 weeks, the measurement in centimeters should equal the number of weeks of gestation. A discrepancy greater than 2 to 3 cm is called a **size/date discrepancy.** Ultrasound should be done for further evaluation (e.g., intrauterine growth retardation, multiple gestations).

7. **When is ultrasound most accurate at estimating the fetal age?**
At 16 to 20 weeks the biparietal diameter (measured on ultrasound) gives the most accurate estimate of fetal age.

8. **What is a hydatiform mole? What are the clues to its presence?**
A hydatiform mole is one form of gestational trophoblastic neoplasia, in which the products of conception basically become a tumor. Look for the following clues:
- Preeclampsia before the third trimester
- An hCG level that does not return to zero after delivery (or abortion/miscarriage) or one that rises rapidly during pregnancy
- First- or second-trimester bleeding with possible expulsion of "grapes" from the vagina (grossly, the tumor looks like a "bunch of grapes") and excessive nausea/hyperemesis.
- Uterine size/date discrepancy
- "Snow-storm" pattern on ultrasound

9. **Distinguish between complete and partial moles. How are hydatiform moles treated?**
   Complete moles have a karyotype of 46 XX (with all chromosomes from the father) and no fetal tissue. **Incomplete moles** usually have a karyotype of 69 XXY with fetal tissue in the tumor.
   Treat hydatiform moles with uterine dilation and curettage. Then follow with serial measurements of hCG levels until they fall to zero. If the hCG level does not fall to zero or rises, the patient has either an invasive mole or a choriocarcinoma (increasingly aggressive forms of gestational trophoblastic neoplasia) and needs chemotherapy (usually methotrexate or dactinomycin, both of which are extremely effective).

10. **How is intrauterine growth retardation (IUGR) defined? What causes it?**
    IUGR is defined as fetal size below the tenth percentile for age. Causes are best understood in broad terms as maternal (e.g., smoking, alcohol or drugs, lupus erythematosus), fetal (e.g., TORCH infections, congenital anomalies), or placental (e.g., hypertension, preeclampsia). For a discussion of TORCH infections, see question 33.

11. **When should ultrasound be used to evaluate the fetus?**
    The indications for ultrasound are now quite liberal. Order ultrasound for all patients who have a size/date discrepancy greater than 2 to 3 cm or risk factors for pregnancy-related problems (e.g., hypertension, diabetes, renal disease, lupus erythematosus, smoking, alcohol or drug use, and history of previous pregnancy-related problems). Ultrasound also is used when fetal death, distress, or abortion or miscarriage is suspected (e.g., a baby that stops kicking, vaginal bleeding, or slow fetal heartbeat on auscultation).

12. **How is fetal well-being evaluated?**
    A **nonstress** test is the easiest initial screen. It is performed with the mother at rest. A fetal heart rate tracing is obtained for 20 minutes. A normal strip has at least 2 accelerations of heart rate, each at least 15 beats per minute above baseline and lasting at least 15 seconds.
    A **biophysical profile** is slightly more involved and includes a nonstress test as well as a measure of amniotic fluid (to determine whether oligo- or polyhydramnios is present; Fig. 25-1), a measure of fetal breathing movements, and a measure of general fetal movements.

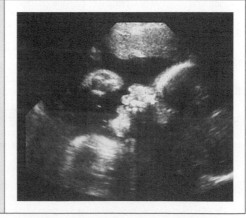

Figure 25-1. Fetal profile with a normal amount of amniotic fluid around the fetal face. (From Katz DS, Math KR, Groskin SA [eds]: Radiology Secrets. Philadelphia, Hanley & Belfus, 1998, p 233, with permission.)

If the fetus scores poorly on the biophysical profile, the next test is the **contraction stress test,** which looks for uteroplacental dysfunction. Oxytocin is given, and a fetal heart strip is monitored. If late decelerations are seen on the fetal heart strip with each contraction, the test is positive. In most cases of a positive contraction stress test, a cesarean section is performed.

13. **True or false: A biophysical profile often is used in high-risk pregnancies in the absence of obvious problems.**
    True. A biophysical profile may be done once or twice a week from the start of the third trimester until delivery to monitor for potential problems.

14. **True or false: Aspirin should be avoided during pregnancy.**
    True. Use acetaminophen instead. One important exception is patients with antiphospholipid syndrome, in whom aspirin may improve pregnancy outcome (subcutaneous unfractionated heparin or low molecular weight heparin also can be used to treat antiphospholipid syndrome in pregnancy).

15. **Define postterm pregnancy. Why is it a major concern? How is it treated?**
    Postterm pregnancy is defined as more than 42 weeks of gestation. Both prematurity and postmaturity increase perinatal morbidity and mortality rates. With postmaturity, **dystocia** (or difficult delivery) becomes more common because of the increased size of the infant.
    In general, if the gestational age is known to be accurate and the cervix is favorable, labor is induced (with oxytocin, for example). If the cervix is not favorable or the dates are uncertain, twice-weekly biophysical profiles are done. At 41 weeks, most obstetricians advise induction of labor.

16. **What two rare disorders are associated with prolonged gestation?**
    Anencephaly and placental sulfatase deficiency.

17. **What are the normal changes and complaints in pregnancy?**
    Normal changes in pregnancy include nausea or vomiting (morning sickness), amenorrhea, heavy (possibly even painful) feeling of the breasts, increased pigmentation of the nipples and areolae, Montgomery tubercles, backache, linea nigra, melasma (chloasma), striae gravidarum, and mild ankle edema. Heartburn and increased frequency of urination are also common problems.

18. **What test is used to screen for neural tube defects? At what time during pregnancy is it measured? Explain the significance of a low or high alpha-fetoprotein (AFP) level in maternal serum.**
    Maternal AFP is most accurate when measured between 15 and 20 weeks of gestation. A low AFP may represent **Down syndrome,** fetal demise, or inaccurate dates. A high AFP may represent **neural tube defects** (e.g., anencephaly, spina bifida), **ventral wall defects** (e.g., omphalocele, gastroschisis), multiple gestation, or inaccurate dates.

19. **What should be done if the AFP is elevated?**
    Repeat the test. As many as 30% of elevated maternal serum AFP test results may be elevated but are normal upon repeat testing. The initial elevation is not associated with an increased risk of neural tube defects.

20. **What further testing should a patient undergo if the AFP remains elevated?**
    If the AFP remains elevated the patient is advised first to undergo ultrasound to determine whether a neural tube defect or other anomaly is present. The ultrasound is also used to confirm gestational age, number of fetuses, and fetal viability. Further evaluation with

amniocentesis may be required if the ultrasound findings are uncertain or there is a concern for nonvisualized neural tube defects (via elevated AFP level in amniotic fluid or detection of acetylcholinesterase in amniotic fluid). There is a small risk of miscarriage after amniocentesis.

21. **What prenatal tests are available to screen for Down syndrome?**
   The first trimester combined test, integrated tests, and the quadruple test. The American College of Obstetricians and Gynecologists recommends that all women be offered screening before 20 weeks of gestation.

22. **What is the first trimester combined test? When is it performed?**
   The first trimester combined test is performed at 11 to 13 weeks of gestation. The test involves determination of nuchal translucency (NT) by ultrasound, combined with serum pregnancy-associated plasma protein-A (PAPP-A) and serum human chorionic gonadotropin (hCG). Chorionic villus sampling (CVS) is used for women who have this first trimester screening and test positive.

23. **Describe the integrated tests.**
   The full integrated test includes an ultrasound measurement of nuchal translucency at 10 to 13 weeks of gestation, PAPP-A at 10 to 13 weeks of gestation, and alpha fetoprotein (AFP), unconjugated estradiol (uE3), hCG, and inhibin A at 15 to 18 weeks of gestation. Results of the full integrated test are not available until the second trimester.
   The serum integrated test is the same as the full integrated test but without the ultrasound evaluation of nuchal translucency. This test is used in areas where expertise in the ultrasound measurement of nuchal translucency is not available. Results of the serum integrated test are not available until the second trimester.
   Step-wise sequential testing has been developed to provide a risk estimate during the first trimester. The first trimester portion of the integrated screen is performed. If the tests indicate a very high risk of having an affected fetus, CVS is offered. Those women whose results do not place them at very high risk of having an affected fetus go on to have the second trimester portion of the screening.
   Contingent testing is being evaluated in clinical trials, and concerns exist about the performance of this screening modality.

24. **What is the quadruple test? For whom is it typically used? When is it performed?**
   The quadruple test includes the serum markers AFP, uE3, hCG, and inhibin A. The quadruple test is the best available test for women who present for prenatal care in the second trimester, but can be used for women who receive earlier prenatal care. It is performed at 15 to 18 weeks of gestation.

25. **What is the next step if a woman has a positive screening test for Down syndrome?**
   Offer fetal karyotype determination. This is done by chorionic villus sampling in the first trimester and by amniocentesis in the second trimester.

26. **Why is chorionic villus sampling done instead of amniocentesis in some cases?**
   Chorionic villus sampling can be done at 9 to 12 weeks of gestation (earlier than amniocentesis) and generally is reserved for women with previously affected offspring or known genetic disease. It offers the advantage of a first-trimester abortion if the fetus is affected. Chorionic villus sampling is associated with a slightly higher miscarriage rate than amniocentesis.

27. **True or false: Chorionic villus sampling can detect neural tube defects but not genetic disorders.**
    False. Chorionic villus sampling can detect genetic or chromosomal disorders but not neural tube defects.

28. **Cover the right-hand column and specify the effects of the following classic teratogens on an exposed fetus.**

Agent	Defect(s) Caused
Thalidomide	Phocomelia (absence of long bones and flipper-like appearance of hands)
Antineoplastics	Many
Tetracycline	Yellow or brown teeth
Aminoglycosides	Deafness
Valproic acid	Spina bifida, hypospadias
Progesterone	Masculinization of female fetus
Cigarettes	Intrauterine growth retardation, low birth weight, prematurity
Oral contraceptive pills	VACTERL syndrome*
Lithium	Cardiac (Ebstein's) anomalies
Radiation	Intrauterine growth retardation, central nervous system defects, eye defects, malignancy (e.g., leukemia)
Alcohol	Fetal alcohol syndrome
Phenytoin	Craniofacial, limb, and cerebrovascular defect, mental retardation
Warfarin	Craniofacial defects, intrauterine growth retardation, central nervous system malformation, stillbirth
Carbamazepine	Fingernail hypoplasia, craniofacial defects
Isotretinoin[†]	Central nervous system, craniofacial, ear, and cardiovascular defects
Iodine	Goiter, cretinism
Cocaine	Cerebral infarcts, mental retardation
Diazepam	Cleft lip and/or palate
Diethylstilbestrol	Clear cell vaginal cancer, adenosis, cervical incompetence

*VACTERL = **V**ertebral anomalies, imperforate **A**nus, **C**ardiac anomalies, **T**racheo**E**sophageal fistula, **R**enal anomalies, **L**imb anomalies.
[†]Vitamin A in general is considered teratogenic when recommended intake levels are exceeded.

29. **List the teratogenic effects of maternal diabetes mellitus. What is the best way to reduce these complications?**
    - Cardiovascular malformations
    - Cleft lip and/or palate
    - Caudal regression (lower half of the body is incompletely formed)
    - Neural tube defects

- Left colon hypoplasia/immaturity
- Macrosomia (most common and classic)
- Microsomia (can occur if the mother has long-standing diabetes)
  Tight control of glucose during pregnancy dramatically reduces these complications.

30. **What other problems does maternal diabetes cause in pregnancy?**
In the mother, diabetes can result in polyhydramnios and preeclampsia (as well as the complications of diabetes). Problems in infants born to a diabetic mother (other than birth defects) include an increased risk of respiratory distress syndrome and postdelivery hypoglycemia (from fetal islet-cell hypertrophy due to maternal and thus fetal hyperglycemia). After birth, the infant is cut off from the mother's glucose and the hyperglycemia resolves, but the infant's islet cells still overproduce insulin and cause hypoglycemia. Treat with intravenous glucose.

31. **True or false: Oral hypoglycemic agents should not be used during pregnancy.**
True. Use insulin to treat diabetes if diet and exercise cannot control glucose levels. Oral hypoglycemics, unlike insulin, may cross the placenta and cause fetal hypoglycemia.

32. **What commonly used drugs are generally considered safe in pregnancy?**
A short list of drugs that are generally safe in pregnancy includes acetaminophen, penicillins, cephalosporins, erythromycin, nitrofurantoin, histamine-2 receptor blockers, antacids, heparin, hydralazine, methyldopa, labetalol, insulin, and docusate.

33. **What are the TORCH syndromes? What do they cause?**
TORCH is an acronym for several maternal infections that can cross the placenta and can cause intrauterine fetal infections that may result in birth defects. Most TORCH infections can cause mental retardation, microcephaly, hydrocephalus, hepatosplenomegaly, jaundice, anemia, low birth weight, and IUGR.
   T = **T**oxoplasma gondii: look for exposure to cats. Specific defects include intracranial calcifications and chorioretinitis.
   O = **O**ther: varicella-zoster causes limb hypoplasia and scarring of the skin. Syphilis causes rhinitis, saber shins, Hutchinson's teeth, interstitial keratitis, and skin lesions.
   R = **R**ubella: worst in the first trimester (some recommend abortion if the mother has rubella in the first trimester). Always check antibody status on the first visit in patients with a poor immunization history. Look for cardiovascular defects, deafness, cataracts, and microphthalmia.
   C = **C**ytomegalovirus: most common infection of the TORCH group. Look for deafness, cerebral calcifications, and microphthalmia.
   H = **H**erpes: look for vesicular skin lesions (with positive Tzanck smears) and history of maternal herpes lesions.

34. **True or false: With most in utero infections that can cause birth defects, obvious clues are present in the mother and/or fetus at birth.**
False. Although the USMLE probably will give clues, the mother may be asymptomatic (i.e., she may have a subclinical infection), and the infant may be asymptomatic at birth, developing only later such symptoms as learning disability, mental retardation, or autism.

35. **What do you need to know about HIV testing and transmission in mother and child?**
In untreated HIV-positive patients, HIV is transmitted to the fetus in roughly 25% of cases. When zidovudine is given to the mother prenatally and to the infant for 6 weeks after birth, HIV transmission is reduced to roughly 2%. A noninfected infant may still have a positive HIV antibody test at birth, because maternal antibodies can cross the placenta.

Within 6-18 months, however, the test reverts to negative. This is why infants of infected mothers are tested using a direct HIV DNA PCR (polymerase chain reaction) test at birth, at 4-6 weeks of age, and 2 months after the second test. Babies who have these three negative tests should have an HIV antibody test at 12 and 18 months of age. Cesarean section may reduce HIV transmission to the child.

36. **What should you do if a pregnant woman has genital herpes?**
A decision is generally made when the mother goes into labor (not beforehand). If, at the time of true labor, the mother has active, visible genital herpes lesions, do a cesarean section to prevent transmission to the fetus. If, at the time of true labor, the mother has no visible genital herpes lesions, the child can be delivered vaginally.

37. **What should you do for the child if the mother has chronic hepatitis B or chickenpox?**
If the mother has chronic hepatitis B, give the infant the first hepatitis B vaccine shot and hepatitis B immunoglobulin at birth. If the mother contracts chickenpox in the last 5 days of pregnancy or the first 2 days after delivery, give the infant varicella-zoster immunoglobulin.

38. **How do you treat gonorrheal and chlamydial genital infections during pregnancy?**
The treatment for gonorrhea remains unchanged, because ceftriaxone is safe during pregnancy. For chlamydial infection, give azithromycin, amoxicillin, or erythromycin base instead of doxycycline or erythromycin estolate.

39. **How is tuberculosis treated in pregnancy?**
In a similar way as in a nonpregnant patient. Use isoniazid, rifampin, and ethambutol if the risk of a drug-resistant organism is low. Pyrazinamide should be used with caution because of a lack of data on the risk of teratogenicity. However, pyrazinamide should be added if a drug-resistant organism is suspected. Streptomycin, which is a rarely used second-line agent, should be avoided. Give vitamin B_6 to pregnant patients treated with isoniazid to avoid a deficiency.

40. **What are the signs of placental separation during delivery?**
The signs of placental separation include a fresh show of blood from the vagina, lengthening of the umbilical cord, and a rising fundus that becomes firm and globular.

41. **True or false: After cesarean section, a patient may have a vaginal delivery in the future.**
It depends. After a classic (vertical) uterine incision, patients must have cesarean sections for all future deliveries because of the increased rate of uterine rupture with vaginal delivery. After a lower (horizontal) uterine incision (the incision of choice), a patient may deliver future pregnancies vaginally with only a slightly increased (i.e., acceptable) risk of uterine rupture.

42. **Define lochia. When is it a problem?**
For the first several days after delivery, some vaginal discharge (known as lochia) is normal. It is red for the first few days and gradually turns white or yellowish-white by day 10. If the lochia is foul smelling, suspect endometritis.

43. **What treatment may be given to a woman who does not want to breast-feed?**
Because the breasts can be become engorged with milk and thus quite painful, you may prescribe tight-fitting bras, ice packs, and analgesia to reduce symptoms. Medications for the suppression of lactation (e.g., bromocriptine and estrogens or oral contraceptive pills) are generally no longer recommended due to risks of thromboembolism and stroke.

44. List the common contraindications for breast-feeding.
- Hepatitis
- Use of alcohol or illicit drugs
- HIV infection
- Scheduled substances

45. What is the preferred method of anesthesia in obstetric patients? Why?
Epidural anesthesia is the preferred method in obstetric patients. General anesthesia involves a higher risk of aspiration and its resulting pneumonia, because the gastroesophageal sphincter is relaxed in pregnancy and patients usually have not refrained from eating before going into labor. There also is concern about the effect of general anesthetic agents on the fetus. Spinal anesthesia can interfere with the mother's ability to push and is associated with a higher incidence of hypotension than epidural anesthesia.

46. True or false: Asymptomatic bacteriuria, detected on routine urinalysis, should be treated during pregnancy.
True. Up to 20% of patients develop cystitis or pyelonephritis if untreated. This rate is much higher than in nonpregnant patients, who should not be treated for asymptomatic bacteriuria. In pregnancy, the gravid uterus can compress the ureters, and increased progesterone can decrease the tone of the ureters, increasing urinary stasis and the risk of urinary tract infection.

47. What do you need to know about vaginal group B streptococcal colonization and pregnancy?
Pregnant women should be tested for vaginal group B streptococci. Women who are carriers should be treated during labor and delivery with penicillin G or ampicillin. Earlier treatment (e.g., second trimester) is ineffective, because group B streptococci frequently return—and usually they are dangerous only during labor and delivery. The reason for treating asymptomatic carriers is to prevent neonatal sepsis and endometritis, both of which are commonly caused by group B streptococci.

48. When does mastitis occur? How do you recognize and treat it?
Mastitis (inflammation of the breast) usually develops in the first 2 months postpartum. Breasts are red, indurated, and painful, and nipple cracks or fissuring may be seen. *Staphylococcus aureus* is the usual cause. Treat with analgesics (e.g., acetaminophen, ibuprofen), warm and/or cold compresses, and continued breast feeding with the affected breast(s) even though it is painful (use breast pump to empty breast if needed) to prevent further milk duct blockage and abscess formation. Antistaphylococcal antibiotic (e.g., cephalexin, dicloxacillin) is usually given for more than mild symptoms. If a fluctuant mass develops or there is no response to antibiotics within a few days, an abscess is likely present and must be drained.

49. What are the diagnostic signs and symptoms of preeclampsia? When does it occur?
Preeclampsia causes **hypertension,** defined as a greater than 30-point increase in systolic or a greater than 15-point increase in diastolic blood pressure over baseline. Other signs and symptoms include **proteinuria** (2+ or more protein on urinalysis), oliguria, edema of the hands or face, headache, visual disturbances, or the HELLP syndrome (hemolysis, elevated liver enzymes, low platelets, and right upper quadrant or epigastric pain). Preeclampsia usually occurs in the third trimester.

50. What are the main risk factors for preeclampsia? How is it treated?
The risk factors (in decreasing order of importance) include chronic renal disease, chronic hypertension, family history of preeclampsia, multiple gestations, nulliparity, extremes of

reproductive age (the classic patient is a young woman with her first child), diabetes, and black race. The definitive treatment is delivery. This is the treatment of choice if the patient is at term. In a preterm patient with mild disease, the hypertension can be treated with hydralazine, labetalol or methyldopa. Advise bed rest and observe. If the patient has severe disease (defined as oliguria, mental status changes, headache, blurred vision, pulmonary edema, cyanosis, HELLP syndrome, blood pressure greater than 160/110 mmHg, or progression to eclampsia [seizures]), deliver the infant once the mother is stabilized. Otherwise, both mother and infant may die.

51. **True or false: The combination of hypertension and proteinuria during pregnancy means preeclampsia until proved otherwise.**
True.

52. **When is edema normal during pregnancy? When is it not?**
Mild ankle edema is normal in pregnancy, but moderate-to-severe edema of the ankles or hands is likely to be preeclampsia.

53. **What should you consider if preeclampsia develops before the third trimester?**
The possibility of gestational trophoblastic disease (i.e., hydatiform mole or choriocarcinoma).

54. **Distinguish between preeclampsia and eclampsia. How can eclampsia be prevented?**
Preeclampsia plus seizures equals eclampsia. Eclampsia can be prevented by regular prenatal care so that you catch the disease in the preeclamptic stage and treat appropriately.

55. **What should you use to treat seizures in eclampsia? What are the toxic effects?**
Use **magnesium sulfate** for eclamptic seizures; it also lowers blood pressure. Toxic effects include hyporeflexia (first sign of toxicity), respiratory depression, central nervous system depression, coma, and death. If toxicity occurs, the first step is to stop the magnesium infusion.

56. **True or false: When eclampsia occurs, you must deliver the infant immediately, regardless of maternal status.**
False. Do *not* try to deliver the infant until the mother is stable (e.g., do not perform a cesarean section while the mother is having seizures).

57. **Why are preeclampsia and eclampsia so important?**
Preeclampsia and eclampsia cause uteroplacental insufficiency, IUGR, fetal demise, and increased maternal morbidity and mortality rates.

58. **True or false: Preeclampsia and eclampsia are risk factors for development of hypertension in the future.**
False.

59. **What are the major causes of maternal mortality associated with child birth?**
In decreasing order: pulmonary embolism, pregnancy-induced hypertension (preeclampsia/eclampsia), and hemorrhage.

60. **How do you recognize an amniotic fluid pulmonary embolism?**
Look for a recently postpartum mother who develops sudden shortness of breath, tachypnea, chest pain, hypotension, and disseminated intravascular coagulation. Treatment is supportive.

61. Define oligohydramnios. What causes it? Why is it worrisome?
Oligohydramnios means a deficiency of amniotic fluid (less than 500 mL or an amniotic fluid index less than 5). Causes include IUGR, premature rupture of the membranes, postmaturity, and renal agenesis (Potter disease). Oligohydramnios may cause fetal problems, including pulmonary hypoplasia, cutaneous or skeletal abnormalities due to compression, and hypoxia due to cord compression.

62. Define polyhydramnios. What causes it? Why is it worrisome?
Polyhydramnios means an excess of amniotic fluid (greater than 2 L or an amniotic fluid index greater than 25). Causes include maternal diabetes, multiple gestation, neural tube defects (anencephaly, spina bifida), gastrointestinal anomalies (omphalocele, esophageal atresia), and hydrops fetalis. Polyhydramnios can cause maternal problems, including postpartum uterine atony (with resultant postpartum hemorrhage) and maternal dyspnea (an overdistended uterus compromises pulmonary function).

63. When does a standard home pregnancy test become positive?
Roughly 2 weeks after conception (about the time when the woman realizes that her period is late).

64. Define the characteristics and duration of the normal stages of labor.

Stage	Characteristics	Nulligravida	Multigravida
First stage	Onset of true labor to full cervical dilation	< 20 hrs	< 14 hrs
Latent phase	From 0 to 3–4 cm dilation (slow, irregular)	Highly variable	Highly variable
Active phase	From 3–4 cm to full dilation (rapid, regular)	> 1 cm/hr dilation	> 1.2 cm/hr dilation
Second stage	From full dilation to birth of baby	30 min–3 hr	5–30 min
Third stage	Delivery of baby to delivery of placenta	0–30 min	0–30 min
Fourth stage	Placental delivery to maternal stabilization	Up to 48 hr	Up to 48 hr

65. Distinguish between a protraction disorder and an arrest disorder. What should you do when either occurs?
A **protraction disorder** (dystocia) occurs once true labor has begun if the mother takes longer than the previous chart indicates, but labor nonetheless is progressing slowly. An **arrest disorder** (failure to progress) occurs once true labor has begun if no change in dilation is seen over 2 hours or no change in descent is seen over 1 hour.

In either situation, first rule out an abnormal lie and cephalopelvic disproportion. If neither is present, the mother can be treated with labor augmentation (e.g., oxytocin, prostaglandin). If these steps fail, manage expectantly and do a cesarean section at the first sign of trouble.

66. What is the most common cause of protraction or arrest disorder?
Cephalopelvic disproportion, defined as a disparity between the size of the infant's head and the mother's pelvis. Labor augmentation is contraindicated in this setting.

67. **Distinguish between true labor and false labor.**
In true labor, normal contractions occur at least every 3 minutes, are fairly regular, and are associated with cervical changes (effacement and dilation). In false labor (Braxton-Hicks contractions), contractions are irregular and no cervical changes occur.

68. **What problems may be encountered when oxytocin is used to augment labor?**
On Step 2, watch for uterine hyperstimulation (painful, overly frequent, and poorly coordinated uterine contractions), uterine rupture, fetal heart rate decelerations, and water intoxication/ hyponatremia (due to the antidiuretic hormone effect of oxytocin). Treat all of these complications first by discontinuing the oxytocin infusion; the half-life is less than 10 minutes.

69. **What problems are associated with the use of intravaginal prostaglandin and amniotomy?**
Prostaglandin E2 (dinoprostone) or misoprostol may be used locally to induce the cervix (a process sometimes called "ripening") and is highly effective in combination with (or before) oxytocin. It also may cause uterine hyperstimulation. **Amniotomy** (creating a manual opening in the amniotic membrane) also hastens labor but exposes the fetus and uterine cavity to possible infection if labor does not occur promptly.

70. **What are the contraindications to labor induction or augmentation?**
The list is almost the same as the list of contraindications to vaginal delivery: placenta or vasa previa, umbilical cord prolapse, prior classic cesarean section, transverse fetal lie, active genital herpes, cephalopelvic disproportion, and cervical cancer.

71. **Define abortion.**
Abortion is defined as the termination (intentional or not) of a pregnancy at less than 20 weeks of gestation or when the fetus weighs less than 500 grams. Miscarriage describes a spontaneous abortion.

72. **What are the different terms for an unintentional abortion?**
Threatened abortion: uterine bleeding without cervical dilation and no expulsion of tissue. Treat with bed rest and pelvic rest.
    Inevitable abortion: uterine bleeding with cervical dilation and crampy abdominal pain and no tissue expulsion.
    Incomplete abortion: passage of some products of conception through the cervix.
    Complete abortion: expulsion of all products of conception from the uterus. Treat with serial testing of hCG level to make sure that it goes down to zero.
    Missed abortion: fetal death with no expulsion of tissue (in some cases not for several weeks). Treat with dilation and curettage if less than 14 weeks of gestation, attempted delivery if more than 14 weeks of gestation.
    All of the above terms imply less than 20 weeks of gestation. Treat all abortions with intravenous fluids (and blood transfusions if necessary) and consider dilation and curettage (once the fetus is confirmed as dead or expelled). Give the mother RhoGAM if she has an Rh-negative blood type.

73. **Define induced and recurrent abortions. What do recurrent abortions suggest?**
Induced abortion is an intentional termination of pregnancy at less than 20 weeks of gestation; it may be elective (requested by patient) or therapeutic (done to maintain the health of the mother).
    Recurrent abortion is defined as two or three successive, unplanned abortions. History and physical exam may suggest the cause:
■ Infection (*Listeria, Mycoplasma,* or *Toxoplasma* species, syphilis)

- Inherited thrombophilia (Factor V Leiden, G20210A gene mutation, antithrombin deficiency, deficiency of protein C or protein S)
- Environmental factors (alcohol, tobacco, drugs)
- Diabetes
- Hypothyroidism
- Systemic lupus erythematosus (especially with positive antiphospholipid/lupus anticoagulant antibodies, sometimes an isolated syndrome without coexisting lupus)
- Cervical incompetence (watch for a history of exposure to diethylstilbestrol [DES] in the patient's mother during pregnancy and/or a patient with recurrent painless second-trimester abortions; treat future pregnancies with cervical cerclage)
- Congenital female tract abnormalities (correct if possible to restore fertility)
- Fibroids (remove them)
- Chromosomal abnormalities (e.g., maternal or paternal translocations)

74. **True or false: hCG roughly doubles every 2 days in the first trimester.**
True. An hCG level that stays the same or increases only slowly with serial testing indicates a fetus in trouble (e.g., threatened abortion, ectopic pregnancy) or fetal demise. A rapidly increasing hCG level or one that does not decrease after delivery may indicate hydatiform mole or choriocarcinoma.

75. **When can ultrasound detect an intrauterine gestational sac? Why do you need to know this information?**
At roughly 5 weeks after the last menstrual period (or when hCG is greater than 2000 mIU), evidence of intrauterine pregnancy can be detected by transvaginal sonography. A definite fetus and fetal heartbeat can be detected by transvaginal ultrasound at 5 to 6 weeks of gestation.
Use this information when trying to determine the possibility of an ectopic pregnancy. For example, if the patient's last menstrual period was 4 weeks ago and a pregnancy test is positive, you cannot rule out an ectopic pregnancy with ultrasound. If, however, the patient's last menstrual period was 10 weeks ago with a positive pregnancy test and an ultrasound of the uterus does not show a gestational sac, be suspicious of an ectopic pregnancy.

76. **What are the risk factors for developing an ectopic pregnancy?**
The major risk factor for ectopic pregnancy is a previous history of pelvic inflammatory disease (PID) (10-fold increase in ectopic pregnancy rate). Other risk factors include a previous ectopic pregnancy, history of tubal sterilization or tuboplasty, pregnancy that occurs with an intrauterine device in place, and a history of DES exposure, which can cause tubal abnormalities in women who were exposed in utero.

77. **What are the classic symptoms and signs of a ruptured ectopic pregnancy?**
A recent history of amenorrhea with current vaginal bleeding and abdominal pain. Patients also have a positive hCG pregnancy test. If you palpate an adnexal mass, it may be an ectopic pregnancy or a corpus luteum cyst.

78. **What should you do if you suspect an ectopic pregnancy?**
Order an ultrasound to look for a gestational sac or fetus. When the diagnosis is in doubt and the patient is doing poorly (e.g., hypovolemia, shock, severe abdominal pain, rebound tenderness), do a laparoscopy for definitive diagnosis and treatment, if necessary. Culdocentesis is rarely done in a stable patient to check for blood in the pouch of Douglas (with a ruptured ectopic pregnancy) because it has a high false-negative rate.

79. **How is symptomatic ectopic pregnancy managed?**
With surgery. A tubal pregnancy, if stable and less than 3 cm in diameter, can be treated with salpingostomy and removal of the products of conception. The tube is left open to heal on its own; this strategy retains normal tubal function and fertility. If the patient is unstable or the ectopic pregnancy has ruptured or is greater than 3 cm in diameter, a salpingectomy is required. In Rh-negative patients, give RhoGAM after treatment. Methotrexate (causes fetal demise) is an alternative treatment for small (less than 3 cm), unruptured tubal pregnancies.

80. **What are the problems with [preexisting] maternal hypertension in pregnancy?**
Preexisting hypertension (present before conception) increases the risk for IUGR and preeclampsia.

81. **What does a basic fetal heart monitoring strip contain?**
The fetal heart rate and the uterine contraction pattern over time.

82. **In fetal heart monitoring, what is the difference between early decelerations, late decelerations, and variable decelerations?**
In **early decelerations** (Fig. 25-2), the peaks match up (nadir of fetal heart deceleration and peak of uterine contraction). This pattern signifies **head compression** (probably a vagal response) and is normal.

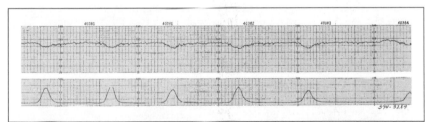

Figure 25-2. Early decelerations are caused by compression of the fetal head. They are shallow, symmetric, uniform decelerations that begin early in the contraction, have their nadir coincident with the peak of the contraction, and return to the baseline by the time the contraction is over. (From Gabbe S, et al.: Obstetrics: Normal and Problem Pregnancies, 5th ed. Philadelphia, Churchill Livingstone, 2007, Fig. 15-13.)

Variable decelerations (Fig. 25-3) are so-called because fetal heart rate deceleration varies in relation to uterine contractions. This is the most commonly encountered type of deceleration pattern and signifies **cord compression.** If it is seen, place the mother in the lateral decubitus position, administer oxygen by face mask, and stop any oxytocin infusion. If the fetal bradycardia is severe (less than 80 to 90 beats/min) or fails to resolve, check the fetal oxygen saturation or scalp pH.
Late decelerations (Fig. 25-4) occur when fetal heart rate deceleration comes after uterine contraction. This pattern signifies **uteroplacental insufficiency** and is the most worrisome. If it is seen, first place the mother in the lateral decubitus position; then give oxygen by face mask and stop oxytocin, if applicable. Next, give a tocolytic ($beta_2$ agonist such as ritodrine or magnesium sulfate) if the mother is not in active labor and intravenous fluids (if the mother is hypotensive). If the late decelerations persist, measure the fetal oxygen saturation or scalp pH. Consider preparing for operative delivery.

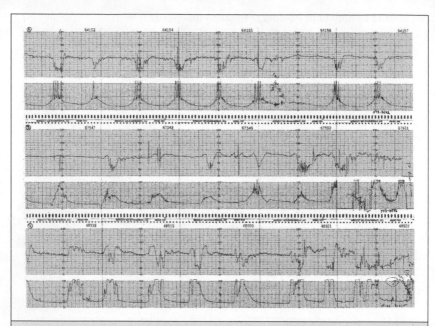

Figure 25-3. These are typical variable decelerations. Variable decelerations are often recognized by the accelerations that precede and follow the decelerations. (From Gabbe S, et al.: Obstetrics: Normal and Problem Pregnancies, 5th ed. Philadelphia, Churchill Livingstone, 2007, Fig. 15-18.)

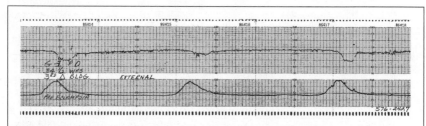

Figure 25-4. Late decelerations are seen in a case complicated by third-trimester bleeding. Note the presence of persistent late decelerations with only three contractions in 20 minutes as well as the apparent loss of variability of the fetal heart rate. The rise in baseline tone of the uterine activity channel cannot be evaluated with the external system. (From Gabbe S, et al.: Obstetrics: Normal and Problem Pregnancies, 5th ed. Philadelphia, Churchill Livingstone, 2007, Fig. 15-14.)

83. **What other patterns of fetal distress may be seen on a fetal heart tracing? What is a normal fetal heart rate?**
    Loss of short-term (beat-to-beat) variability, loss of long-term variability (or normal baseline changes in heart rate over 1 minute), and prolonged fetal tachycardia (greater than 160 beats/min). The normal fetal heart rate is 120 to 160 beats/min.

84. **What if the question gives you a value for fetal oxygen saturation or scalp pH?**
    Any fetal scalp pH less than 7.2 or abnormally decreased oxygen saturation is an indication for immediate cesarean delivery. If the pH is greater than 7.2 or oxygenation is normal, you can generally continue to observe the mother and fetus.

85. **What should you do if shoulder dystocia or impaction occurs during vaginal delivery?**
The first step is to try the McRoberts maneuver. Have the mother sharply flex her thighs against her abdomen, which may free the impacted shoulder. Other maneuvers include applying suprapubic pressure, Woods screw maneuver (rotates the fetus so the anterior shoulder emerges from behind the maternal symphysis), delivery of the posterior arm, and fracture of the clavicle (risky). If these maneuvers fail, options are limited. A cesarean section is usually the procedure of choice (after pushing the infant's head back into the birth canal).

86. **What causes third-trimester bleeding?**
■ Placenta previa
■ Abruptio placentae
■ Uterine rupture
■ Fetal bleeding
■ Cervical or vaginal infections (e.g., herpes simplex virus, gonorrhea, chlamydial or candidal infection)
■ Cervical or vaginal trauma (usually from sexual intercourse)
■ Bleeding disorders (rare before delivery; more common after delivery)
■ Cervical cancer (which may occur in pregnant patients)
■ "Bloody show"

87. **True or false: The initial work-up of third-trimester bleeding, like most conditions, requires a history and thorough physical exam, including a good pelvic exam.**
False. You should do a history and partial physical exam, but *always* do an ultrasound before you do a pelvic exam.

88. **Why should you do ultrasound before you do a pelvic exam for third-trimester bleeding?**
In case placenta previa is present. Disturbing the placenta may make the bleeding worse and turn a worrisome case into an emergency.

89. **Define placenta previa. How does it present? How is it diagnosed and treated?**
True placenta previa occurs when the placenta implants in an area where it covers the cervical opening (os). Predisposing factors include multiparity, increasing maternal age, multiple gestation, and a history of prior placenta previa. Because of this condition you *always* do an ultrasound before a pelvic exam for third-trimester bleeding. The bleeding is painless and may be profuse. Ultrasound is 95% to 100% accurate in diagnosis. Mandatory cesarean section is required for delivery, but patients may be admitted to the hospital for bed and pelvic rest and tocolysis if they are preterm and stable and if the bleeding has stopped.

90. **Define abruptio placentae. How does it present? How is it treated?**
Abruptio placentae is premature detachment of a normally situated placenta. Predisposing factors include hypertension (with or without preeclampsia), trauma, polyhydramnios with rapid decompression after membrane rupture, cocaine or tobacco use, and preterm premature rupture of membranes. Patients can have this condition without visible vaginal bleeding; the blood may be contained behind the placenta. Usual symptoms include pain, uterine tenderness, increased uterine tone with a hyperactive contraction pattern, and fetal distress. Abruptio placentae also may cause disseminated intravascular coagulation if fetal products enter the maternal circulation. Ultrasound detects only a small percentage of cases. Treat with intravenous fluids (and blood if needed) and rapid delivery (vaginal preferred).

91. **What factors predispose to uterine rupture? How does it present? How is it treated?**

    Predisposing factors include previous uterine surgery (especially prior caesarian section with vertical incision), trauma, oxytocin, grand multiparity (several previous deliveries), excessive uterine distention (e.g., multiple gestation, polyhydramnios), abnormal fetal lie, cephalopelvic disproportion, and shoulder dystocia. Uterine rupture is very painful, has a sudden and dramatic onset, and often is accompanied by maternal hypotension or shock. Other classic signs are the ability to feel fetal body parts on abdominal exam and a change in the abdominal contour. Maternal distress usually is more pronounced than fetal distress (unlike abruptio placentae, in which fetal distress is greater). Treat with immediate laparotomy and delivery. Hysterectomy usually is required after delivery.

92. **What causes fetal bleeding to present as third-trimester vaginal bleeding?**

    Visible fetal bleeding usually is due to vasa previa or velamentous insertion of the cord, which occurs when umbilical vessels present in advance of the fetal head, usually traversing the membranes and crossing the cervical os. The biggest predisposing risk factor is multiple gestation (the higher the number of fetuses, the higher the risk). Bleeding is painless, and the mother is completely stable, whereas the fetus shows worsening distress (tachycardia initially, then bradycardia as the fetus decompensates). An Apt test performed on vaginal blood is positive for fetal blood (this test differentiates fetal from maternal blood). Treat with immediate cesarean section.

93. **Explain the term "bloody show." How is it diagnosed?**

    With cervical effacement, a blood-tinged mucous plug may be released from the cervical canal and heralds the onset of labor. This normal occurrence is a diagnosis of exclusion in the evaluation of third-trimester bleeding.

94. **Describe the initial management of third-trimester bleeding.**

    For all cases of third-trimester bleeding, start intravenous fluids, give blood if needed, start the patient on oxygen, and start fetal and maternal monitoring. Then order a complete blood count, coagulation profiles, ultrasound, and drug screen (if drug use is suspected, as cocaine causes placental abruption). Give RhoGAM if the mother is Rh-negative. A Kleihauer-Betke test can quantify fetal blood in maternal circulation and can be used to calculate the dose of RhoGAM.

95. **Define preterm labor. How is it treated?**

    Preterm labor is defined as labor between 20 and 37 weeks of gestation. Put the mother in the lateral decubitus position, order bed and pelvic rest, and give oral or intravenous fluids and oxygen. In some cases these maneuvers stop the contractions. If they fail, you can give a tocolytic (beta$_2$ agonist or magnesium sulfate) if no contraindications (heart disease, hypertension, diabetes, hemorrhage, ruptured membranes, cervix dilated more than 4 cm) are present. The mother can be managed as an outpatient with an oral tocolytic once she is stable.

96. **What are tocolytics? When is it not appropriate to give them?**

    Tocolytics stop uterine contractions. Common examples are beta$_2$ agonists (terbutaline, ritodrine) and magnesium sulfate. Do not give tocolytics to the mother in the presence of preeclampsia, severe hemorrhage, chorioamnionitis, IUGR, fetal demise, or fetal anomalies incompatible with survival.

97. **What is the role of steroids in preterm labor?**

    Often steroids are given with tocolytics (at 24 to 34 weeks of gestation) to hasten fetal lung maturity and thus decrease the risk of respiratory distress syndrome in the neonatal period.

98. **Define quickening. When does it occur?**
Quickening is the term used to describe when the mother first detects fetal movements, usually at 18 to 20 weeks of gestation in a primigravida and 16 to 18 weeks of gestation in a multigravida.

99. **Give the order of fetal positions during normal labor and delivery.**
1. Descent
2. Flexion
3. Internal rotation
4. Extension
5. External rotation
6. Expulsion

100. **What subtype of maternal antibody can cross the placenta?**
IgG is the only type of maternal antibody that crosses the placenta. This may be an important diagnostic point: an elevated neonatal IgM concentration is never normal, whereas an elevated neonatal IgG often represents maternal antibodies.

101. **Explain Rh incompatibility. In what situations does it occur?**
Rh (or rhesus factor) blood-type incompatibility is of concern because it can lead to hemolytic disease of the newborn. Rh incompatibility occurs when the mother is Rh-negative and her infant is Rh-positive. The boards assume an understanding of inheritance of the Rh factor. If both the mother and the father are Rh-negative, there is nothing to worry about because their infant will be Rh negative. If the father is Rh-positive, the infant has a 50/50 chance of being Rh-positive.

102. **How do you detect and manage potential hemolytic disease of the newborn?**
If indicated by maternal and potential fetal blood type, check maternal titers of Rh antibody every month, starting in the seventh month of gestation. Give RhoGAM automatically at 28 weeks and within 72 hours after delivery as well as after any procedures that may cause transplacental hemorrhage (see question 107).

103. **True or false: The first child is usually the most severely affected by Rh incompatibility.**
False. Previous maternal sensitization is required for disease to occur. In other words, if a nulliparous Rh-negative mother has never received blood products, her first Rh-positive infant will not be affected by hemolytic disease—except in the rare case of sensitization during the first pregnancy from undetected fetomaternal bleeding, which commonly occurs later in the pregnancy and in most instances can be prevented by RhoGAM administration at 28 weeks. The second Rh-positive infant, however, will be affected—unless you, the astute board taker, administer RhoGAM at 28 weeks and within 72 hours after delivery during the first pregnancy. Any history of blood transfusion, abortion, ectopic pregnancy, stillbirth, or delivery can cause sensitization.

104. **How much RhoGAM should you give if the maternal Rh antibody titer is extremely high?**
In this setting RhoGAM is worthless, because sensitization has already occurred. RhoGAM administration is a good example of primary prevention. Close fetal monitoring for hemolytic disease is required.

105. **How do you recognize, monitor, and treat hemolytic disease of the newborn?**
Hemolytic disease of the newborn in its most severe form causes fetal hydrops (edema, ascites, pleural and/or pericardial effusions) and death. Amniotic fluid spectrophotometry

and ultrasound can help gauge the severity of fetal hemolysis. Treatment of hemolytic disease involves (1) delivery, if the fetus is mature (check lung maturity with a lecithin-to-sphingomyelin ratio); (2) intrauterine transfusion; and (3) phenobarbital, which helps the fetal liver break down bilirubin by inducing enzymes.

106. True or false: ABO blood group incompatibility can cause hemolytic disease of the newborn.

True. ABO blood group incompatibility can cause hemolytic disease of the newborn when the mother is type O and the infant is type A, B, or AB. This condition does not require previous sensitization, because IgG antibodies (which can cross the placenta) occur naturally in mothers with blood type O—but not in mothers with other blood types. The hemolytic disease is usually less severe than with Rh incompatibility, but treatment is the same. In rare instances, other minor blood antigens also may cause a reaction.

107. When should RhoGAM be given?

To reiterate, give RhoGAM only when the mother is Rh-negative and the father is Rh-positive or his blood type is unknown. During routine prenatal care, check for Rh antibodies at the first visit. If the test is positive, do not give RhoGAM—you are too late. Otherwise, give RhoGAM routinely at 28 weeks and immediately after delivery. Also give RhoGAM after an abortion, stillbirth, ectopic pregnancy, amniocentesis, chorionic villus sampling, and any other invasive procedure that may cause transplacental bleeding during pregnancy.

108. Define premature rupture of membranes (PROM). How is it diagnosed?

PROM is rupture of the amniotic sac before the onset of labor. Diagnosis of rupture of membranes (whether premature or not) is based on history, sterile speculum exam, and/or a positive nitrazine test. The sterile speculum exam shows pooling of amniotic fluid and a ferning pattern when the fluid is placed on a microscopic slide and allowed to dry. Nitrazine paper turns blue in the presence of amniotic fluid. Ultrasound should be done in cases of PROM to assess amniotic fluid volume as well as gestational age and any anomalies that may be present.

109. What usually follows membrane rupture? What should you do if it does not occur?

Spontaneous labor usually follows membrane rupture; for this reason, an amniotomy may be done in an attempt to induce labor if membranes do not rupture spontaneously. If labor does not occur within 6 to 8 hours of membrane rupture, and the mother is term, and if the cervix is favorable, labor should be induced.

Labor is induced because the main risk of PROM is infection, which may occur in the mother (chorioamnionitis) and/or the infant (neonatal sepsis, pneumonia, meningitis). The usual culprits are group B streptococci, *Escherichia coli,* or *Listeria* sp.

110. Define preterm premature rupture of membranes (PPROM). How is it managed?

PPROM is defined as premature rupture of membranes before 36 to 37 weeks of gestation. The risk of infection increases with the duration of ruptured membranes. Do a culture and Gram stain of the amniotic fluid. If it is negative, treatment simply involves pelvic and bed rest with frequent follow-up. If the culture is positive for group B streptococci, treat the mother with penicillin G or ampicillin, even if she is asymptomatic.

111. How does chorioamnionitis present and how is it treated?

Patients with chorioamnionitis present with fever and a tender, irritable uterus, usually after delivery. Antepartum chorioamnionitis may occur in patients with PROM. Do a culture and

Gram stain of the cervix and amniotic fluid, and treat with antibiotics such as ampicillin plus gentamicin while awaiting culture results.

112. Define postpartum hemorrhage. What are the common causes?
Postpartum hemorrhage is defined as a blood loss greater than 500 mL during vaginal delivery or greater than 1 L during cesarean section. The most common cause is **uterine atony** (75% to 80% of cases). Other causes include lacerations, retained placental tissue, coagulation disorders, low placental implantation, and uterine inversion. Retained placental tissue results from placenta accreta (penetration of the placenta through the endometrium into the myometrium), increta (deeper penetration of the placenta into the myometrium), or percreta (penetration of the placenta through the myometrium to the uterine serosa); the placenta grows more deeply into the uterine wall than it should. The major risk factor for this condition is previous uterine surgery or cesarean section, and the usual treatment is hysterectomy.

113. What causes uterine atony? How is it treated?
Uterine atony is caused by overdistention of the uterus (due to multiple gestation, polyhydramnios, or macrosomia), prolonged labor, oxytocin usage, grand multiparity (a history of five or more deliveries), and precipitous labor (too fast or less than 3 hours). Treat with a dilute oxytocin infusion, and use bimanual compression to massage the uterus while the infusion is running. If this approach fails, use ergonovine (contraindicated with maternal hypertension), prostaglandin f_2-alpha, or misoprostol. If these strategies also fail, the patient may need a hysterectomy; ligation of the uterine vessels can be attempted if the patient wants to retain fertility.

114. What is the treatment for retained products of conception?
With retained products of conception (which is probably the most common cause of a *delayed* postpartum hemorrhage), remove the placenta manually to stop the bleeding. Next try curettage in the operating room under anesthesia. If placenta accreta, increta, or percreta is present, hysterectomy is usually necessary to stop the bleeding.

115. What causes uterine inversion? How is it treated?
When the uterus inverts, it usually can be seen outside the vagina. It is usually iatrogenic, a result of *pulling too hard on the cord*. If it occurs, put the uterus back in place manually; you may need to use anesthesia because of pain. Give intravenous fluids and oxytocin.

116. Define postpartum fever. What are the common causes?
Postpartum fever is defined as a temperature greater than 100.4° F (38° C) for at least 2 consecutive days and is classically due to endometritis. However, do not forget easy causes of postpartum fever, such as a urinary tract infection or atelectasis/pneumonia. Pulmonary problems are especially common after a cesarean section. Other causes include pelvic abscess and pelvic thrombophlebitis.

117. What should you do if a patient has postpartum fever?
Look for clues in the history and physical exam. For example, in a patient with a history of PROM and a tender uterus on exam, endometritis is almost certainly the cause of the fever. Next, get cultures of the endometrium, vagina, blood, and urine. Start empiric antibiotics if indicated. Clindamycin plus gentamicin is a good choice; add "big-gun" antibiotics if the patient is crashing.

118. What should you do if postpartum fever does not improve with antibiotics?
If a postpartum fever does not resolve with broad-spectrum antibiotics, there are two main possibilities: progression to pelvic abscess or pelvic thrombophlebitis. CT scan will show a

pelvic abscess, which needs to be drained, and sometimes demonstrates thrombophlebitis. Pelvic thrombophlebitis presents with persistent spiking fevers, lack of response to antibiotics, and no abscess on CT. Give heparin or low molecular weight heparin for a cure (and diagnosis in retrospect).

119. **What should you consider if a postpartum patient goes into shock without evident bleeding?**
    ■ Amniotic fluid embolism
    ■ Uterine inversion
    ■ Concealed hemorrhage (e.g., uterine rupture with bleeding into the peritoneal cavity)

120. **What normal lab changes of pregnancy may be encountered on the Step 2 exam?**
    ■ The erythrocyte sedimentation test becomes markedly elevated; hence, this test is essentially worthless in pregnancy.
    ■ Total thyroxine (T_4) and thyroid-binding globulin increase, but free T_4 remains normal.
    ■ Hemoglobin increases, but plasma volume increases even more; thus the net result is a decrease in hemoglobin and hematocrit.
    ■ Blood urea nitrogen (BUN) and creatinine decrease because of an increase in glomerular filtration rate. BUN and creatinine levels at the high end of normal indicate renal disease in pregnancy.
    ■ Alkaline phosphatase increases markedly.
    ■ Mild proteinuria and glycosuria are normal in pregnancy.
    ■ Electrolytes and liver function tests remain normal.

121. **What cardiovascular and pulmonary changes occur in a normal pregnancy?**
    Normal cardiovascular changes: blood pressure decreases slightly, heart rate increases by 10 to 20 beats/min, stroke volume increases, and cardiac output increases (by up to 50%).
    Normal pulmonary changes: minute ventilation increases because of increased tidal volume, but respiratory rate remains the same or increases only slightly; residual volume and carbon dioxide decrease. Collectively these changes cause the physiologic hyperventilation/ respiratory alkalosis of pregnancy.

122. **What is the average weight gain during pregnancy? What commonly causes weight gain to be more or less?**
    The average weight gain in pregnancy is roughly 28 pounds (12.5 kg). A larger weight gain may mean maternal diabetes. A smaller weight gain may mean hyperemesis gravidarum or psychiatric or major systemic diseases.

123. **Define hyperemesis gravidarum. How do you recognize and treat it?**
    Hyperemesis gravidarum is intractable nausea and vomiting leading to dehydration and possible electrolyte disturbances. It presents in the first trimester, usually in younger patients with their first pregnancy and underlying social stressors or psychiatric problems. Treat with supportive care as well as small, frequent meals and antiemetic medications such as doxylamine, promethazine, or dimenhydrinate (fairly safe in pregnancy). Patients may need intravenous fluids and correction of electrolyte abnormalities.

124. **Define cholestasis of pregnancy. How is it treated?**
    Cholestasis of pregnancy presents with itching (often severe) and/or abnormal liver function tests, usually in the second and third trimester. In rare cases, jaundice may coexist. The only known definitive treatment is delivery, but ursodeoxycholic acid or cholestyramine may help with symptoms.

125. **What is acute fatty liver of pregnancy? How is it treated?**

Acute fatty liver of pregnancy is a more serious disorder than cholestasis. It presents in the third trimester or after delivery and usually progresses to hepatic coma. Treat with intravenous fluids, glucose, and fresh frozen plasma to correct coagulopathies. Vitamin K does not work, because the liver is in temporary failure. If the patient survives with supportive care, liver dysfunction usually resolves on its own with time.

126. **True or false: In terms of surgery, the usual rule of thumb is to treat the disease in a pregnant woman the same as you would treat it in a nonpregnant woman.**

It depends. It definitely is true in the case of an acute surgical abdomen. Pregnant women can develop appendicitis, which may present with right upper quadrant pain due to displacement of the appendix by the pregnant uterus. Just as in nonpregnant patients, a laparotomy or laparoscopy is perfectly appropriate when the diagnosis is unsure and the patient has peritoneal signs.

For semiurgent conditions (e.g., ovarian neoplasm), it is best to wait until the second trimester to perform surgery (when the pregnancy is most stable). Purely elective cases are avoided during pregnancy.

127. **How do you manage fetal malpresentation?**

External cephalic version can be used to rotate the fetus from the breech to the cephalic position. If this fails, the decision must be made whether to attempt vaginal delivery or do a cesarean section. Although under specific guidelines some frank and complete breeches may be delivered vaginally, it is acceptable to do a cesarean section for any breech presentation. With shoulder presentation or incomplete/footling breech, cesarean section is mandatory. For face and brow presentations, watchful waiting is best, because most cases convert to vertex presentations. If they do not convert, do a cesarean section.

128. **What is the "poor man's way" to distinguish between monozygotic and dizygotic twins?**

If the sex or blood type is different, the twins are dizygotic (i.e., fraternal). If the placentas are monochorionic, the twins are monozygotic (i.e., identical). These three simple points differentiate monozygotic from dizygotic twins in 80% of cases. In the remaining 20%, human leukocyte antigen typing studies are required to determine the type of twins.

129. **What are the maternal and fetal complications of multiple gestations?**

Maternal complications include anemia, hypertension, premature labor, postpartum uterine atony, postpartum hemorrhage, and preeclampsia.

Fetal complications include polyhydramnios, malpresentation, placenta previa, abruptio placentae, velamentous cord insertion/vasa previa, premature rupture of the membranes, prematurity, umbilical cord prolapse, IUGR, congenital anomalies, and increased perinatal morbidity and mortality.

The higher the number of fetuses, the higher the risk of most of the conditions mentioned for both mother and offspring.

130. **How are multiple gestations delivered?**

With vertex–vertex presentations of twins (both infants are head first), you can try vaginal delivery for both infants, but with any other twin presentation combination or more than two infants, perform cesarean section.

131. **What is fetal fibronectin? When is a test for this substance useful? Is the test more helpful when positive or negative?**

Fetal fibronectin (an extracellular matrix protein that helps attach the amniotic membranes to the uterine lining) can be detected in the vaginal secretions of some women presenting with signs and symptoms of preterm labor. The test is most helpful when negative between 22 and 34 weeks of gestation, because it indicates a very low likelihood of delivery in the next 2 weeks. Thus, a more conservative, observational approach can be used. When fetal fibronectin is positive in this setting, the woman remains at a higher risk for delivery in the next 2 weeks and a more aggressive approach to tocolysis and fetal lung maturity hastening is typically employed.

CHAPTER 26

ONCOLOGY

1. What are the key differential points for the commonly tested blood dyscrasias?

Type	Age	What to Look for In Case Description/Trigger Words
ALL	Children (peak age: 3–5 yrs)	Pancytopenia (bleeding, fever, anemia), history of radiation therapy, Down syndrome
AML (Fig. 26-1)	> 30 yrs	Pancytopenia (bleeding, fever, anemia), Auer rods, DIC
CML (Fig. 26-2)	30–50 yrs	White blood cell count greater than 50,000, Philadelphia chromosome, blast crisis, splenomegaly
CLL (Fig. 26-3) _SMUDGE CELLS !!!_	> 50 yrs	Male gender, lymphadenopathy, lymphocytosis, infections, smudge cells, splenomegaly
Hairy cell leukemia _⊕TRAP - tartrate resistant acid phosphatase_	Adults	Blood smear (hair-like projections), splenomegaly
Mycosis fungoides/ Sézary syndrome	> 50 yrs	Plaque-like, itchy skin rash that does not improve with treatment, blood smear (cerebriform nuclei known as "butt cells"), Pautrier abscesses in epidermis
Burkitt lymphoma (Fig. 26-4)	Children	Associated with Epstein-Barr virus (in Africa)
CNS B-cell lymphoma	Adults	Seen in patients with HIV infection, AIDS
T-cell leukemia	Adults	Caused by HTLV-1 virus
Hodgkin disease	15–34 yrs	Reed-Sternberg cell, cervical lymphadenopathy, night sweats
Non-Hodgkin lymphoma (Fig. 26-5)	Any age	Small follicular type has best prognosis, large diffuse type has worst; primary tumor may be located in gastrointestinal tract

(continued)

Type	Age	What to Look for in Case Description/Trigger Words
Myelodysplasia/ myelofibrosis	> 50 yrs	Anemia, teardrop cells, "dry tap" on bone marrow biopsy, high MCV and RDW; associated with CML
Multiple myeloma	> 40 yrs	Bence-Jones protein (IgG = 50%, IgA = 25%), osteolytic lesions, high serum calcium
Waldenström macroglobulinemia	> 40 yrs	Hyperviscosity, IgM spike, cold agglutinins (Raynaud phenomenon with cold sensitivity)
Polycythemia vera	> 40 yrs	High hematocrit/hemoglobin, pruritus (especially after hot bath or shower); use phlebotomy
Primary thrombocythemia	> 50 yrs	Platelet count usually greater than 1,000,000; may have bleeding or thrombosis

(handwritten annotation: release of histamine from Basophils. → pointing to pruritus line)

ALL = acute lymphoblastic leukemia; AML = acute myelogenous leukemia; CLL = chronic lymphocytic leukemia; CML = chronic myelogenous leukemia; CNS = central nervous system; DIC = disseminated intravascular coagulation; MCV = mean corpuscular volume; RDW = red cell distribution width.

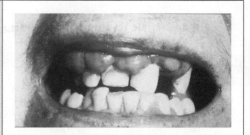

Figure 26-1. Acute myelogenous leukemia (AML), M5 subtype. Leukemic infiltration of the gums is shown, which is classic for the M5 subtype of AML. (From Hoffbrand AV, Pettit JE: Color Atlas of Clinical Hematology, 3rd ed. St. Louis, Mosby, 2000, p 143, with permission.)

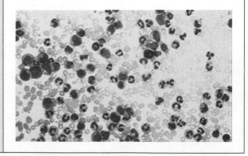

Figure 26-2. Chronic myeloid leukemia (CML). Peripheral smear reveals an excessive number of granulocytic cells in all stages of development. (From Hoffbrand AV, Pettit JE: Color Atlas of Clinical Hematology, 3rd ed. St. Louis, Mosby, 2000, p 169, with permission.)

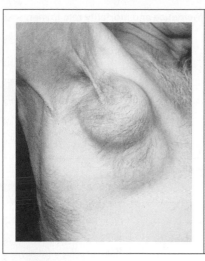

*SMUDGE CELLS!

Figure 26-3. Chronic lymphocytic leukemia (CLL). Massive axillary adenopathy is noted, which was bilateral in this patient and accompanied by other areas of significant palpable adenopathy. (From Hoffbrand AV, Pettit JE: Color Atlas of Clinical Hematology, 3rd ed. St. Louis, Mosby, 2000, p 177, with permission.)

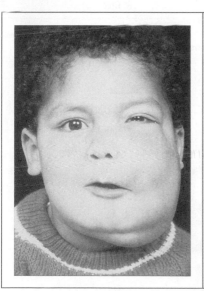

Figure 26-4. Burkitt lymphoma. Characteristic facial swelling, caused by extensive tumor involvement of the mandible and surrounding soft tissues, is shown. (From Hoffbrand AV, Pettit JE: Color Atlas of Clinical Hematology, 3rd ed. St. Louis, Mosby, 2000, p 194, with permission.)

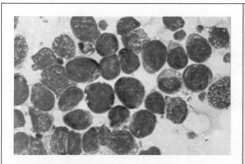

Figure 26-5. Non-Hodgkin lymphoma in an AIDS patient. A fine-needle aspirate of a cervical lymph node reveals lymphoblasts with cytoplasm that was strongly basophilic. (From Hoffbrand AV, Pettit JE: Color Atlas of Clinical Hematology, 3rd ed. St. Louis, Mosby, 2000, p 137, with permission.)

2. **Which cancers have the overall highest incidence and mortality rate in men and women in the United States?**

Overall highest incidence:

Male	Female
1. Prostate	1. Breast
2. Lung	2. Lung
3. Colon	3. Colon

Overall highest mortality rate:

Male	Female
1. Lung	1. Lung
2. Prostate	2. Breast
3. Colon	3. Colon

3. **What are the most common types of cancer in children and young adults (less than age 30 yrs)?**

Leukemia (Fig. 26-6) and lymphoma.

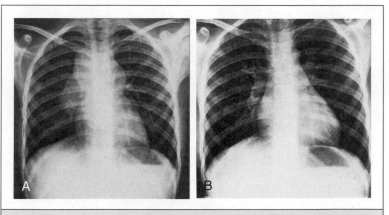

Figure 26-6. Acute lymphoblastic leukemia (ALL) in a 4-year-old boy. **A,** Pretreatment chest x-ray demonstrates upper mediastinal widening caused by thymic involvement. **B,** Chest x-ray taken after chemotherapy reveals disappearance of the thymic mass. ALL is the most curable of the leukemias using currently available therapies. (From Hoffbrand AV, Pettit JE: Color Atlas of Clinical Hematology, 3rd ed. St. Louis, Mosby, 2000, p 143, with permission.)

4. **What is the major risk factor for cancer? What is the major modifiable risk factor for cancer?**
Age is the biggest risk factor (the incidence of cancer in the United States roughly doubles every 5 years after age 25), and smoking is the biggest modifiable risk factor.

5. **What is the most common cancer in most organs?**
   Metastatic cancer (Fig. 26-7). On the Step 2 exam, do *not* assume that the question is looking for the most common primary cancer unless the word "primary" is specified.

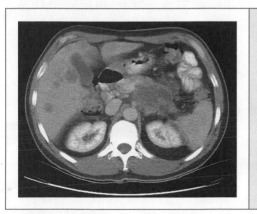

Figure 26-7. Pancreatic carcinoma with liver metastases. Portal venous phase CT shows poorly enhancing liver deposits from a primary mass in the pancreatic body. (From Adam A, et al.: Grainger & Allison's Diagnostic Radiology, 5th ed. Edinburgh, Churchill Livingstone, 2008, Fig. 37-33.)

6. **Metastatic cancer to the spine can cause spinal cord compression. How do you recognize and treat this medical emergency?**
   Spinal cord compression causes local spinal pain and neurologic symptoms (reflex changes, weakness, sensory loss, paralysis, incontinence, urinary retention). In rare cases it may be the first indication of a malignancy. The first step is to start high-dose corticosteroids; then order a magnetic resonance (MRI) scan. The next step is to treat with radiation. Surgical decompression is used if radiation fails or the tumor is known not to be radiosensitive. Prompt intervention is essential, and outcome is closely linked to pretreatment function.

7. **Name the mode of inheritance and types of cancer found in the following conditions:**

Disease/Syndrome	Inheritance	Type of Cancer (In Order of Most Likely)/Other Information
Retinoblastoma	Autosomal dominant	Retinoblastoma, osteogenic sarcoma (later in life)
MEN, type I	Autosomal dominant	Parathyroid, pituitary, pancreas (islet cell tumors)
MEN, type IIa	Autosomal dominant	Thyroid (medullary cancer), parathyroid, pheochromocytoma
MEN, type IIb	Autosomal dominant	Thyroid (medullary cancer), pheochromocytoma, mucosal neuromas
Familial polyposis coli	Autosomal dominant	Hundreds of colon polyps that always become cancer
Gardner syndrome	Autosomal dominant	Familial polyposis plus osteomas and soft tissue tumors
Turcot syndrome	Autosomal dominant	Familial polyposis plus CNS tumors

(continued)

Disease/Syndrome	Inheritance	Type of Cancer (In Order of Most Likely)/Other Information
Peutz-Jeghers syndrome	Autosomal dominant	Look for perioral freckles and multiple non-cancerous GI polyps; increased incidence of noncolon cancer (stomach, breast, ovaries); no increased risk of colon cancer
Neurofibromatosis, type 1 (Fig. 26-8)	Autosomal dominant	Multiple neurofibromas, café-au-lait spots; increased number of pheochromocytomas, bone cysts, Wilms tumor, leukemia
Neurofibromatosis, type 2	Autosomal dominant	Bilateral acoustic neuromas
Tuberous sclerosis	Autosomal dominant	Adenoma sebaceum, seizures, mental retardation, glial nodules in brain; increased renal angiomyolipomas and cardiac rhabdomyomas
Von Hippel-Lindau disease	Autosomal dominant	Hemangioblastomas in cerebellum, renal cell cancer; cysts in liver and/or kidney
Xeroderma pigmentosa	Autosomal recessive	Skin cancer
Albinism	Autosomal recessive	Skin cancer
Down syndrome	Trisomy 21	Leukemia

MEN = multiple endocrine neoplasia; CNS = central nervous system; GI = gastrointestinal.

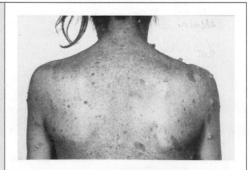

Figure 26-8. Neurofibromatosis. Multiple café-au-lait spots and neurofibromas are present in this woman with a well-established diagnosis. (From du Vivier A: Atlas of Clinical Dermatology, 3rd ed. New York, Churchill Livingstone, 2002, p 474, with permission.)

8. **What other conditions are associated with an increased risk of malignancy?**
Other diseases with an increased incidence of cancer include dermatomyositis, polymyositis, immunodeficiency syndromes, Bloom syndrome, and Fanconi anemia. Breast, ovarian, and colon cancer are well known to have familial tendencies (as well as some other types of cancer), but rarely can a Mendelian inheritance pattern be demonstrated (e.g., BRCA-1 and BRCA-2 account for about 5% of breast cancers).

9. **Cover the right-hand column and specify the major environmental risk factors for the following cancers.**

Cancer Type	Environmental Risk Factors*
Lung	Smoking, asbestos (also nickel, radon, coal, arsenic, chromium, uranium)
Mesothelioma	Asbestos and smoking
Leukemia	Chemotherapy/radiotherapy, other immunosuppressive drugs, benzene
Bladder	Smoking, aniline dyes (rubber and dye industry), schistosomiasis (in immigrants)
Skin	Ultraviolet light exposure (e.g., sun), coal tar, arsenic
Liver	Alcohol, vinyl chloride (liver angiosarcomas), aflatoxins (Africa)
Oral cavity	Smoking, alcohol
Pharynx/larynx	Smoking, alcohol
Esophagus	Smoking, alcohol
Pancreas	Smoking
Renal cell	Smoking
Stomach	Alcohol, nitrosamines/nitrites (from smoked meats and fish)
Clear cell cancer[†]	In utero exposure to diethylstilbestrol (DES)
Colon/rectum	High-fat and low-fiber diet, smoking, alcohol, obesity
Breast	Chest radiation, hormone replacement therapy, alcohol
Cervix	Sex/HPV, smoking, high parity
Thyroid	Childhood neck or chest irradiation, low dietary iodine
Endometrium	Unopposed estrogen stimulation, obesity, tamoxifen, high fat diet
All cancer overall	Smoking (number two is probably alcohol)

*The factor with the greatest impact is listed first.
[†]Of cervix and vagina.

10. **What clinical vignette should make you suspect lung cancer?**
The classic clue is a change in the chronic cough of a smoker. The more pack years of tobacco use, the more suspicious you should be. Patients also may present with hemoptysis, pneumonia, or weight loss. The chest radiograph may show a mass or pleural effusion. Put a needle in the fluid and examine for malignant cells.

11. **How do you diagnose and treat lung cancer?**

As with all cancers, you need a tissue biopsy (e.g., via bronchoscopy, CT-guided biopsy, open lung biopsy) to confirm malignancy and to define the histologic type. Non-small cell lung cancer may be treated with surgery if the cancer remains within the lung parenchyma (i.e., without involvement of the opposite lung, pleura, chest wall, spine, or mediastinal structures). Early metastases of small cell lung cancer make surgery inappropriate. Small cell lung cancer (Figs. 26-9 and 26-10) and extensive non-small cell lung cancer are treated with chemotherapy with or without radiation. Usually a platinum-containing chemotherapy regimen (e.g., cisplatin) is used.

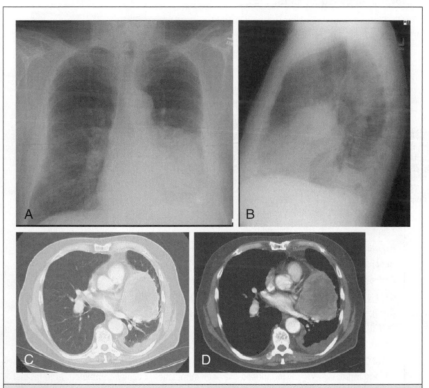

Figure 26-9. Imaging NSCLC. (**A**) Posteroanterior and (**B**) lateral chest radiogram of patients with non-small cell lung cancer which is locally advanced. (**C**) CT imaging using lung and (**D**) mediastinal windows. (From Abeloff M, et al.: Abeloff's Clinical Oncology, 4th ed. Philadelphia, Churchill Livingstone, 2008, Fig. 76-12.)

12. **What consequences can result from an apical (Pancoast) lung cancer?**

Horner syndrome: from invasion of cervical sympathetic chain. Look for unilateral ptosis, miosis, and anhidrosis (no sweating).

Superior vena cava syndrome: due to compression of superior vena cava with impaired venous drainage. Look for edema and plethora (redness) of the neck and face and central nervous system symptoms (headache, visual symptoms, and altered mental status).

Unilateral diaphragm paralysis: from phrenic nerve involvement (apical tumor not required) will result in an elevated hemidiaphragm on chest x-ray

Hoarseness: from recurrent laryngeal nerve involvement (apical tumor not required).

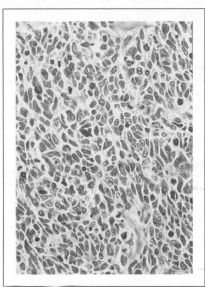

WORST prognosis

Figure 26-10. Small cell lung carcinoma, also known as oat cell carcinoma. The high magnification micrograph reveals the typical small, tightly packed, darkly stained, ovoid tumor cells. This lung cancer subtype has the worst prognosis due to early invasion and metastasis. (From Stevens A, et al.: Wheater's Basic Histopathology, 4th ed. New York, Churchill Livingstone, 2002, p 131, with permission.)

13. **What is a paraneoplastic syndrome? What are the commonly tested paraneoplastic syndromes of lung cancer?**

A paraneoplastic syndrome is a condition caused by a malignancy but not due directly to destruction or invasion by the tumor. Classic examples in lung cancer are as follows:

Cushing syndrome: from production of adrenocorticotropic hormone (histologic type: small cell carcinoma).

Syndrome of inappropriate antidiuretic hormone secretion (SIADH): from production of antidiuretic hormone (histologic type: small cell carcinoma).

Hypercalcemia: from production of parathyroid-like hormone (histologic type: squamous cell carcinoma). SQ CELL

Eaton-Lambert syndrome: myasthenia gravis-like disease from lung cancer that spares the ocular muscles. The muscles become stronger with repetitive stimulation, which is the opposite of myasthenia gravis (histologic type: small cell carcinoma). EMG - muscle contraction improves w stimulation.

14. **How should you manage a patient with a solitary pulmonary nodule on chest radiograph?**

The first step is comparison with previous chest radiographs. If the nodule has remained the same size for more than 2 years, it is very unlikely to be cancer. If no old films are available and the patient is older than 35 years or has more than a 5-year history of smoking, get a CT scan (and possibly a PET scan). If these are not definitely benign, get a biopsy of the nodule (via bronchoscopy or transthoracic needle biopsy, if possible) for tissue diagnosis.

If the patient is younger than 35 years or has no smoking history, the cause is most likely infection (tuberculosis or fungi), hamartoma, or collagen vascular disease. The patient should undergo CT scan and careful observation with follow-up imaging in 3 to 6 months. Investigate for infection if the history is suspicious.

15. **Over the course of their lifetime, how many women in the United States will develop breast cancer?**

Roughly 1 in 8.

16. **What are the risk factors for breast cancer?**

A personal history of breast cancer (major risk factor); female sex; family history in first-degree relatives, age greater than 40 (rare before age 30, incidence steadily increases with age); early menarche, late menopause, late first pregnancy, or nulliparity (more menstrual cycles = higher risk); atypical hyperplasia of the breast; radiation exposure before age 30; inherited gene mutations (e.g., BRCA1); dense breast tissue; high fat diet, diethylstilbestrol exposure; recent oral contraceptive use; combined postmenopausal hormone replacement therapy; alcohol; obesity; and possibly not breastfeeding.

17. **What classic signs and symptoms indicate that a breast mass is cancer until proved otherwise?**

- Fixation of the breast mass to the chest wall or overlying skin
- Satellite nodules or ulcers on the skin
- Lymphedema (peau d'orange) → *inflamm. carcinoma.*
- Matted or fixed axillary lymph nodes
- Inflammatory skin changes (red, hot skin with enlargement of the breast due to inflammatory carcinoma)
- Prolonged unilateral scaling erosion of the nipple with or without discharge (may be Paget disease of the nipple)
- Microcalcifications on mammography
- **Any new breast mass in a postmenopausal woman**

18. **What is the conservative approach to ensure that you do not miss a breast cancer?**

When in doubt, biopsy every palpable breast mass in women over 35 that is not clearly a cyst (ultrasound is needed make the determination), especially if the patient has any of the risk factors mentioned in the previous question. If the Step 2 question does not want you to biopsy the mass, it will give definite clues that the mass is not a cancer (e.g., bilateral lumpy breasts that become symptomatic with every menses and have no dominant mass, patient younger than age 30).

19. **What should you do with a breast mass in a woman under age 30?**

In women under 30, breast cancer is rare. With a discrete breast mass in this age group, you should think of fibroadenoma. Consider ultrasound of the breast and observe the patient over a few menstrual cycles before considering biopsy unless the ultrasound is suspicious. Fibroadenomas are usually roundish, rubbery-feeling, and freely movable.

20. **What is the most common histologic type of breast cancer?**

Invasive (infiltrating) ductal carcinoma (Fig. 26-11) accounts for about 70% of breast cancer.

21. **What is the role of mammography in deciding whether to biopsy a breast mass?**

When a palpable breast mass is detected, the decision to biopsy is made on *clinical* grounds. A mammogram that looks benign should not deter you from doing a biopsy if you are clinically suspicious. On the other hand, a lesion that is detected on mammography and looks suspicious should be biopsied, even if it is not palpable. Needle localization biopsy can be used.

22. **True or false: A mammogram should not be done in women under age 30.**

True in most cases. The breast tissue is too dense for current techniques to be of value. Mammograms in women under age 30 are rarely helpful.

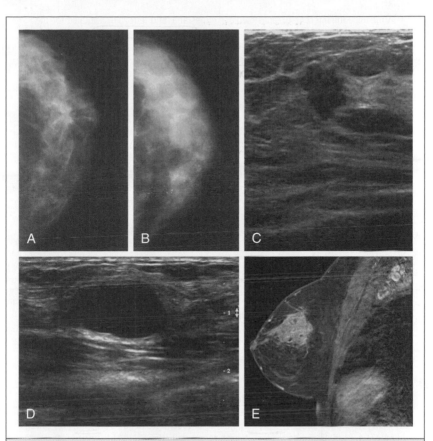

Figure 26-11. Mammographic, ultrasonographic, and MRI findings in breast disease. **A,** Stellate mass in the breast. A density with spiculated borders in combination with distortion of surrounding breast architecture suggests a malignancy. **B,** Clustered microcalcifications. Fine, pleomorphic, and linear calcifications that cluster together suggest the diagnosis of ductal carcinoma in situ. **C,** Ultrasound image of breast cancer. The mass is solid, contains internal echoes, and displays an irregular border. Most malignant lesions are taller than they are wide. **D,** Ultrasound image of a simple cyst. The cyst is round with smooth borders, there is a paucity of internal sound echoes, and there is increased through-transmission of sound with enhanced posterior echoes. **E,** Breast MRI showing gadolinium enhancement of a breast cancer. Rapid and intense gadolinium enhancement reflects increased tumor vascularity. (From Townsend C, et al.: Sabiston Textbook of Surgery, 18th ed. Philadelphia, Saunders, 2008, Fig. 34-6.)

23. **How does tamoxifen affect breast cancer? What other therapies may be used?**
    Tamoxifen (often with endocrine therapy) improves outcomes in premenopausal women with estrogen receptor positive breast cancer. Tamoxifen has also been shown to decrease the risk of breast cancer in women at high risk of developing the disease.

    Raloxifene has also been shown to be as effective as tamoxifen in reducing breast cancer risk in postmenopausal women at increased risk of the disease. However, raloxifene did not reduce the risk of noninvasive breast cancers, such as ductal carcinoma in situ (DCIS) and lobular carcinoma in situ (LCIS). ~ ↓ risk of endometrial carcinoma c̄ raloxifene.

Aromatase inhibitors (e.g., anastrozole, exemestane, and letrozole) are used for the treatment of hormone-sensitive breast cancer in postmenopausal women. Aromatase inhibitors generally are not used in premenopausal women.

Trastuzumab is used after surgery and chemotherapy for HER-2/neu breast cancer and targets the HER-2 protein. *worse prognosis*

24. **True or false: Mastectomy and breast-conserving surgery with radiation are considered equal in efficacy.**
   True. In either case, do an axillary node dissection (or a sentinel node biopsy) to determine spread to the nodes. If nodes are positive, give chemotherapy.

25. **What are the three main risk factors for prostate cancer?**
   Age: prostate cancer is rare in men younger than 40 years old. The incidence increases with age, and about 60% of men older than 80 years have prostate cancer.
   Race: black greater than white greater than Asian.
   Family history: men who have a family history of prostate cancer are more likely to develop the disease at a younger age and to die from it than men who don't have a family history.

26. **How do you recognize prostate cancer on the Step 2 exam?**
   Look for patients over the age of 50 years. Patients often present late, because early prostate cancer is asymptomatic. Look for symptoms typical of benign prostatic hypertrophy (hesitancy, dysuria, frequency) with hematuria and/or elevated prostate-specific antigen (PSA). Look for prostate irregularities (nodules) on rectal exam. Patients also may present with back pain from vertebral metastases, which are osteoblastic.

27. **How is prostate cancer treated?**
   Local prostate cancer is treated with surgery (prostatectomy) or local radiation. With metastases, the patient has several options for hormonal therapy: orchiectomy, gonadotropin-releasing hormone agonist (leuprolide), androgen-receptor antagonist (flutamide), estrogen (diethylstilbestrol), and others (e.g., cyproterone). Radiation therapy is used for local disease or pain from bony metastases; standard chemotherapy is usually ineffective.

28. **List the primary risk factors for colon cancer.**
   Age (incidence begins to increase after age 40; peak incidence between 60 and 75 years)
   Family history (especially with familial polyposis or Gardner, Turcot, Peutz-Jeghers, or Lynch syndrome)
   Inflammatory bowel disease (ulcerative colitis more than Crohn disease, but both are associated with increased risk)
   Low-fiber, high-fat diet

29. **How do patients with colon cancer tend to present?**
   Patients may present with asymptomatic blood in the stool (visible streaks of blood on stool or positive occult blood test). Anemia is classic with right-sided colon cancer. Change in stool caliber ("pencil stool") or frequency (alternating constipation and frequency) is a classic presentation of left-sided colon cancer. Colon cancer is also a common cause of large bowel obstruction in adults. As with any cancer, look for weight loss.

Right - ANEMIA / MELENA - HEMATOCHEZIA   Left - STOOL CALIBER.

30. **What is the rule about occult blood in the stool of a patient over age 40?**
   Occult blood in the stool of a person older than 40 years should be considered colon cancer until proved otherwise. To rule out colon cancer, do a colonoscopy.

31. **How is colon cancer treated?**

Treatment is primarily surgical, with resection of involved bowel. Adjuvant chemotherapy is sometimes given (e.g., 5-fluorouracil with leucovorin; irinotecan; oxaliplatin; cetuximab and panitumumab; or bevacizumab) for lymph node involvement. Distant metastases frequently go to the liver first (as with all gastrointestinal tumors). Surgical resection of a solitary liver metastasis is often attempted. With metastases elsewhere, chemotherapy is the only option, and prognosis is poor.

32. **What is the classic tumor marker for colon cancer? How is it used clinically?**

Carcinoembryonic antigen (CEA) may be elevated with colon cancer, and if a patient is found to have colon cancer, the CEA level is usually measured before surgery. If it is elevated preoperatively (not always), the CEA level should return to normal after surgical removal of the tumor. Periodic monitoring of CEA after surgery may then help to detect recurrence before it is clinically apparent. CEA is *not* used as a screening tool for colon cancer; it is used only to follow known cancer because it is neither sensitive nor specific (can be elevated with other visceral tumors).

→ *Marker of Mucus.*

33. **Describe the classic presentation of pancreatic cancer. How is it treated? What is the cell of origin?**

The classic patient is a smoker in the 40- to 80-year-old range who has lost weight and is jaundiced. Other signs and symptoms include depression, epigastric pain, migratory thrombophlebitis (**Trousseau syndrome,** which also may be seen with other visceral cancers), and a palpable, nontender gallbladder (**Courvoisier sign**). Pancreatic cancer is more common in men than in women, in diabetics than in nondiabetics, and in blacks than in whites. Surgery (Whipple procedure) is rarely curative, and the prognosis is dismal. Chemotherapy is minimally successful at prolonging survival. The cell of origin in pancreatic cancer is ductal epithelium (Fig. 26-12).

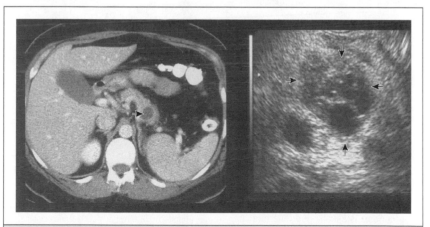

Figure 26-12. A mucinous cystic neoplasm of the tail of the pancreas. The endoscopic ultrasonogram (*right*) demonstrates septa and loculations not seen on the CT scan (*left*) and also allows for sampling of cyst fluid. The arrow on the left panel points to the cystic neoplasm on the CT image, and the arrows on the right image delineate the neoplasm on the ultrasonographic image. (From Feldman M, Friedman L, Brandt L: Sleisenger and Fordtran's Gastrointestinal and Liver Disease, 8th ed. Philadelphia, Saunders, 2006, Fig. 58-11.)

34. **What is the most common islet cell tumor of the pancreas? How is it diagnosed?**

Insulinomas (beta cell tumor) are the most common islet cell tumors. Look for two-thirds of the **Whipple triad:** hypoglycemia (glucose less than 50 mg/dL) and central nervous symptoms due to hypoglycemia (confusion, stupor, loss of consciousness). As a good doctor, you provide the third part of the Whipple triad: administration of glucose to relieve symptoms. Ninety percent of insulinomas are benign; they should be cured with resection, if possible. In your work-up, take a history and check the C-peptide level first to make sure that the patient is not a diabetic who accidentally takes too much insulin or a patient with factitious disorder. C-peptide levels are high with insulinoma and low with the other disorders.

35. **Define Zollinger-Ellison syndrome. What clues point to the diagnosis?**
Zollinger-Ellison syndrome is a gastrinoma that causes acid hypersecretion (gastrin stimulates acid secretion) and peptic ulcer disease. Peptic ulcers are often multiple and resistant to therapy and may be found in unusual locations (distal duodenum or jejunum). More than one-half of these pancreatic islet cell tumors are malignant. Diagnosis is made with an elevated fasting serum gastrin level or a secretin stimulation test.

36. **Name the other two islet cell tumors. What should islet cell tumors make you think about?**
   1. **Glucagonomas** (alpha cell tumor) cause hyperglycemia with high glucagon levels and migratory necrotizing skin erythema.
   2. **VIPomas** (tumors that secrete vasoactive intestinal peptide [VIP]) cause watery diarrhea, hypokalemia, and achlorhydria.
      Watch for multiple endocrine neoplasia (MEN) syndromes in patients with islet cell tumors.

37. **How does ovarian cancer classically present? How are ovarian masses evaluated?**
Female patients classically present late with weight loss, pelvic mass, ascites, and/ or bowel obstruction. Any ovarian enlargement in a postmenopausal female is cancer until proved otherwise. In women of reproductive age, most ovarian enlargements are benign. Ultrasound is a good first test to evaluate an ovarian lesion.

38. **How is ovarian cancer treated? What is the cell of origin? What is the most common type of ovarian cancer?**
Ovarian cancer usually is treated with debulking surgery and chemotherapy. The prognosis is usually poor due to a late presentation. Most ovarian cancers arise from ovarian epithelium. Serous cystadenocarcinoma is the most common type; histopathologic studies classically reveal psammoma bodies. Mucinous cystadenocarcinoma (Fig. 26-13) is also common. When clinicians use the term "ovarian cancer" without a qualifier, they are talking about epithelial malignancies (i.e. cystadenocarcinomas).

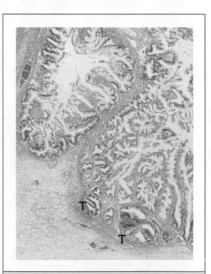

Figure 26-13. Mucinous cystadenocarcinoma of the ovary. Compared to its more common benign counterpart, malignant mucinous tumors demonstrate a greater solid component, smaller cystic spaces, larger and more pleomorphic nuclei, cellular crowding, and increased mitotic activity. In this patient, invasion of tumor cells (T) into the supporting stroma confirms the malignant nature of the tumor. (From Stevens A, et al.: Wheater's Basic Histopathology, 4th ed. New York, Churchill Livingstone, 2002, p 213, with permission.)

39. **List the three commonly tested germ-cell tumors. What clues suggest their presence?**
    1. **Teratoma/dermoid cyst** (most common and most tested type). Look for a description of the tumor to include skin, hair, and/or teeth or bone; it may show up as calcifications on radiograph.
    2. **Sertoli-Leydig cell tumor,** which causes virilization (hirsutism, receding hairline, deepening voice, clitoromegaly).
    3. **Granulosa/theca-cell tumors,** which cause feminization and precocious puberty.
    Female patients with germ cell tumors of the ovary are classically under the age of 30.

40. **What is Meigs syndrome?**
    An ovarian fibroma that causes ascites and right hydrothorax.

41. **What is a Krukenberg tumor?**
    A stomach cancer (or other GI malignancy) with metastases to the ovaries.

42. **What commonly used medication has been shown to reduce the risk of ovarian cancer?**
    Oral contraceptive pills, which also reduce the incidence of endometrial cancer.

43. **What is the best available screening method to reduce the incidence and mortality of cervical cancer?**
    Papanicolaou (Pap) smears. Give all female patients a Pap smear if they are due, even if they present for a totally unrelated complaint. Screening should start approximately three years after the onset of sexual intercourse or age 21, whichever comes first. The frequency of screening depends on whether HPV testing is also being used as well as the patient's age and results of previous Pap smears.

44. **What should you do if a Pap smear is abnormal?**
    The follow-up an abnormal Pap smear depends on the cervical cytologic results. Lower grade lesions may be evaluated with HPV testing and colposcopy/endocervical curettage if needed. Higher grade lesions require colposcopy with biopsy and/or loop electrosurgical excision (LEEP). Invasive cancer requires surgery (at least a hysterectomy) and may include radiation with cisplatin-based chemotherapy.

45. **List the main risk factors for cervical cancer.**
    - Age younger than 20 years old at first coitus, pregnancy, or marriage
    - Multiple sexual partners (role of human papillomavirus and possibly herpes virus)
    - Coitus with a promiscuous partner
    - Smoking
    - Low socioeconomic status
    - High parity (which protects against endometrial and breast cancer)

46. **Where does cervical cancer begin? How does it present? How is it treated?**
    Invasive cervical cancer begins in the transformation zone and usually presents with vaginal bleeding or discharge (postcoital bleeding, intermenstrual spotting, or abnormal menstrual bleeding). Treat with surgery and/or radiation.

47. **What do you need to know about diethylstilbestrol (DES) and cancer?**
    Maternal exposure to DES during pregnancy increases a daughter's risk of developing clear cell cancer of the cervix and/or vagina.

48. What is the rule of thumb for postmenopausal vaginal bleeding?

Postmenopausal vaginal bleeding is cancer until proved otherwise. Endometrial cancer is the most common type to present in this fashion; it is also the fourth most common cancer overall in women. Do an endometrial biopsy (generally preferred) or a transvaginal ultrasound for any woman with postmenopausal bleeding (as well as a Pap smear).

49. List the main risk factors for endometrial cancer.

- Obesity
- Nulliparity
- Late menopause
- Diabetes, hypertension, and gallbladder disease (probably related to obesity)
- Chronic, unopposed estrogen stimulation (e.g., polycystic ovary syndrome, estrogen-secreting neoplasm [granulosa-theca cell tumor], and estrogen replacement therapy without progesterone)

50. What is the most common type of endometrial cancer? How is it treated?

Most uterine cancers are adenocarcinomas and spread by direct extension. Treat with surgery and radiation.

51. What commonly prescribed medication reduces the risk of endometrial cancer?

Oral contraceptive pills, which also decrease the risk for ovarian cancer.

52. Describe the common presentations of brain tumors.

Central nervous system (CNS) tumors are the second most common tumors in children (second to leukemia); be suspicious in this age group. In adults, two-thirds of primary tumors are supratentorial (i.e. above the tentorium cerebelli, a portion of dura that separates the cerebellum from the cerebral hemispheres), whereas in children two-thirds are infratentorial (i.e. lower brainstem or cerebellum [posterior fossa]). In either group, look for new-onset seizures, neurologic deficits or signs of intracranial hypertension (headache, blurred vision, papilledema, nausea, projectile vomiting). In children, also look for hydrocephalus (manifested as an inappropriately increasing head circumference), new clumsiness, ataxia, loss of developmental milestones, or a change in school performance or personality.

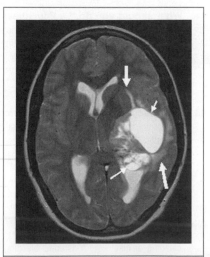

Figure 26-14. A malignant glioma is seen on this T2-weighted MR image demonstrating edema (*large arrows*) and necrosis (uniform high signal regions, *small arrows*). (From Goldman L, Ausiello D: Cecil Medicine, 23rd ed. Philadelphia, Saunders, 2008, Fig. 419-5.)

53. What are the most common histologic types of primary CNS tumors in children and adults? How are primary brain tumors treated?

The most common primary type in adults is glioma (Fig. 26-14). Most gliomas are astrocytomas, which are intraparenchymal and have little or no calcification. The second most common type in adults is meningioma, which often is calcified and is external to the brain substance. In children the most common types are cerebellar astrocytoma (benign pilocytic astrocytoma) and medulloblastoma, followed by ependymoma. Treat with surgical removal (if possible), followed by radiation and/or chemotherapy, depending on the tumor.

54. **Which cancers tend to metastasize to the brain?**
Lung cancer, breast cancer, and melanoma are the most common; together they account for 75% of brain metastases.

55. **What tumor is most likely in a young, obese woman with headaches, papilledema, vomiting, and a negative CT/MR scan?**
A pseudotumor, as in **pseudotumor cerebri.** Pseudotumors are not actual tumors, but reflect idiopathic increased intracranial pressure. Weight loss may help. Repeated lumbar punctures or a CSF shunt may be needed to prevent vision loss.

56. **What tumor should you suspect in an adult with signs of eighth cranial nerve damage and increased intracranial pressure?**
An acoustic neuroma (especially in the setting of neurofibromatosis). Co-involvement of the facial nerve is not uncommon (Fig. 26-15). *type 2.*

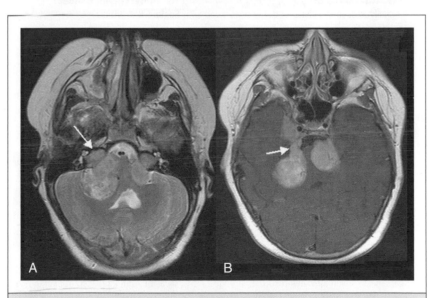

Figure 26-15. Neurofibromatosis type 2 (NF2). **A,** Bilateral cerebellopontine angle masses extending into the internal auditory meati and causing expansion (*arrow*) in a child with NF2 and bilateral acoustic neuromas. **B,** Trigeminal schwannomas extending into the cavernous sinus on the right. The *arrow* indicates the cisternal segment of the right trigeminal nerve. (From Adam A, et al.: Grainger & Allison's Diagnostic Radiology, 5th ed. Edinburgh, Churchill Livingstone, 2008, Fig. 70-24.)

57. **What tumor should you suspect in children with intracranial calcifications on skull radiographs?**
Craniopharyngioma (benign tumors that arise from remnants of the Rathke pouch and grow slowly from birth).

58. **What should you know about testicular cancer?**
It is the most common solid malignancy in adult men younger than 30 years old. The main risk factor is **cryptorchidism**. Transillumination and ultrasound help to distinguish a hydrocele, which is filled with fluid and transilluminates, from cancer, which is solid and does not transilluminate. The most common histologic type is seminoma, which is radiosensitive and highly curable. Use ultrasound to make the diagnosis.

59. **What tumor resembles "a bunch of grapes" coming out of the vagina?**
Sarcoma botryoides, a type of embryonal rhabdomyosarcoma usually seen in children.

60. **What is the classic physical finding of a pituitary tumor? What is the most common type?**
The classic physical finding is **bitemporal hemianopsia.** Order an MR scan of the brain in any patient with this finding. Patients also may have signs and symptoms of increased intracranial pressure. The most common type is a prolactinoma, which is associated with high prolactin levels, galactorrhea, and menstrual or sexual dysfunction. Other types are of pituitary tumors may cause hyperthyroidism, Cushing disease or acromegaly, or they may be nonfunctional (i.e., they do not secrete hormones).

61. **What two points do you need to know about nasopharyngeal cancer?**
It usually is seen in Asians, and it is associated with **Epstein-Barr virus.**

62. **Describe the classic presentation of esophageal cancer. What is the most common cell type?**
The presentation depends on the histologic type. The classic patient with squamous cell carcinoma is a chronic smoker and alcohol drinker between the ages of 40 and 60 years (blacks more than whites) who presents with weight loss, anemia, and the complaint that "my food is sticking," which progresses to dysphagia for liquids. The other cell type is adenocarcinoma, which is typically due to malignant degeneration of Barrett esophagus (columnar metaplasia of esophageal squamous epithelium due to acid reflux); thus patients have a long history of acid reflux and heartburn. Prognosis usually is quite poor in either type due to late presentation. Squamous cell carcinomas used to predominate, but squamous cell carcinoma and adenocarcinoma now occur with almost equal frequency.

63. **What physical and laboratory findings suggest thyroid cancer? What is the most common type of thyroid cancer? What historical point is of concern with thyroid cancer?**
Patients often have a single, stony-hard nodule or mass in the thyroid gland that may be rapidly enlarging. The nodule is "cold" on a nuclear scan (i.e., it fails to take up radioactive tracer). The most common type is papillary thyroid cancer. Other worrisome findings are hoarseness, which indicates recurrent laryngeal nerve invasion, and increased calcitonin level, which indicates the rare medullary thyroid cancer. Patients with medullary thyroid cancer may have a multiple endocrine neoplasia (MEN) syndrome. Historically, irradiation to the head or neck is of concern due to its association with thyroid cancer.

64. **How should you evaluate a thyroid mass for possible malignancy?**
To evaluate a nodule in the thyroid, order thyroid function tests. Thyroid-stimulating hormone (TSH) is the best screening test; "toxic" or functional nodules are unlikely to be cancer. If the TSH is normal, get a fine needle aspiration of the mass. If the TSH is decreased, then order a nuclear scan. A "cold" nodule or area of decreased uptake is more suspicious than a nodule with normal or increased uptake. Ultrasound is also commonly used to help evaluate a thyroid mass. If the history is suspicious (radiation to neck, MEN syndrome, hoarseness, "stony hard" nodule), get a biopsy even if the other tests are normal.

65. **What clinical vignette is suspicious for bladder cancer?**

Persistent, painless hematuria, especially in patients older than 40 years who smoke or work in the rubber or dye industry (exposure to aniline dye). CT scan (Fig. 26-16) to evaluate the upper urinary tract and cystoscopy should be performed to evaluate for potential bladder cancer (as well as other causes of hematuria, including renal cell carcinoma).

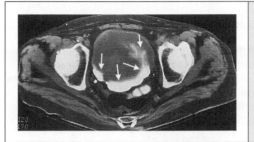

Figure 26-16. CT image shows a large transitional cancer almost completely filling the bladder. Brighter arrows represent the residual bladder lumen. (From Katz DS, Math KR, Groskin SA [eds]: Radiology Secrets. Philadelphia, Hanley & Belfus, 1998, p 195, with permission.)

66. **What increases the risk for hepatocellular cancer of the liver? What is the classic tumor marker for liver cancer?**

The same factors that increase the risk for cirrhosis. The "big three" are alcohol, chronic hepatitis (hepatitis C is now a more likely culprit than hepatitis B), and hemochromatosis. **Alpha-fetoprotein** is often elevated and can be measured postoperatively to detect recurrences. It also is used for screening in high-risk populations (e.g., those with cirrhosis).

67. **How do patients with liver cancer present? How is liver cancer treated?**

Patients often have a history of alcoholism, hepatitis, and/or hemochromatosis or other causes of cirrhosis. They present with weight loss, right upper quadrant pain, and an enlarged liver. Surgery is the only hope for cure. The prognosis is poor.

68. **What other tumors of the liver may appear on the USMLE? What clues suggest their presence?**

Hemangioma: most common primary tumor of the liver; benign and generally left alone. Surgery is done only if symptoms (pain, bleeding) are present.

Hepatic adenoma: benign tumor in women of reproductive age who take **birth control pills.** Stop the birth control pills; the tumor may regress. If not, surgery is usually preferred to prevent hemorrhage and rare malignant transformation.

Cholangiocarcinoma: malignant. Fifty percent of patients have inflammatory bowel disease (especially ulcerative colitis); liver flukes (*Clonorchis* sp.) increase the risk in immigrants.

Angiosarcoma: malignant. Look for industrial exposure to vinyl chloride.

Hepatoblastoma: malignant; the most common primary liver malignancy in children.

69. **What is the significance of adrenal tumors?**

Most are benign, but they may be functional and cause primary hyperaldosteronism (Conn syndrome) or hyperadrenalism (Cushing syndrome). Another possibility is pheochromocytoma, which is associated with intermittent, severe hypertension, mental status changes, headaches, and diaphoresis.

70. **What are the risk factors for stomach cancer? What are the symptoms?**
Risk factors include Asian race, increasing age, smoking history, ingestion of smoked meat, and *Helicobacter pylori* infection. Symptoms and signs include anemia, weight loss, early satiety, abdominal pain, and a nonhealing gastric ulcer. All gastric ulcers must be biopsied to exclude malignancy. Consider follow-up endoscopy to document resolution of an ulcer, though this is somewhat controversial. Be especially suspicious if the question describes a nonhealing ulcer in a patient with weight loss.

71. **What is a Virchow node?**
A Virchow node is a left supraclavicular node enlargement due to the spread of visceral cancer (classically stomach cancer).

72. **What do you need to know about osteosarcomas for the Step 2 exam?**
Osteosarcomas most commonly are seen around the knee in 10- to 30-year-old patients. The classic x-ray finding is a "sunburst" periosteal reaction (Fig. 26-17) in the distal femur or proximal tibia associated with a mass. In older adults, the risk is increased in bones with long-standing Paget disease or osteomyelitis.

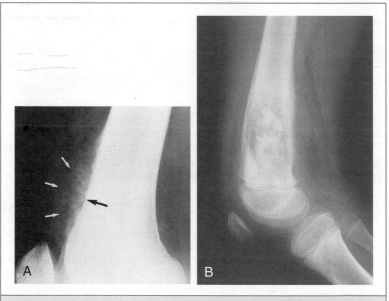

Figure 26-17. Osteogenic sarcoma of the knee. A lateral view of the knee (**A**) in a 19-year-old man shows a sunburst-type periosteal reaction (*arrows*). Knowing that the distal femur is the most common site of osteogenic sarcoma, that periosteal reaction is a feature, and that this patient is a teenager should make osteogenic sarcoma very high on your differential diagnostic list. A destructive central lesion (**B**) is seen here in the distal femur of an 8-year-old girl. (From Mettler F: Essentials of Radiology, 2nd ed. Philadelphia, Saunders, 2004, Fig. 8-113.)

73. **What are the symptoms of carcinoid tumors? Where are they most commonly found?**
Carcinoid tumors secrete serotonin-like products that can cause symptoms, but the liver breaks down serotonin and other vasoactive secretions to make the tumor initially asymptomatic. Once a carcinoid tumor metastasizes to the liver and vasoactive products reach

the systemic circulation, symptoms begin (carcinoid syndrome): episodic cutaneous flushing, abdominal cramps, diarrhea, and right-sided heart valve damage. The most common location is in the small bowel, but carcinoid tumors are also the most common appendiceal tumor (sometimes found at the time of appendectomy in patients with appendicitis).

74. **What lab test detects carcinoid tumors?**
Urinary levels of 5-hydroxyindoleacetic acid (5-HIAA, a serotonin breakdown product) are increased.

75. **What is the classic clinical manifestation of Kaposi sarcoma?**
A rash that does not respond to multiple treatments in an HIV-positive patient. Kaposi sarcoma is a vascular skin tumor that commonly begins as a papule or plaque on the upper body or in the oral cavity. It is highly associated with herpes virus (human herpesvirus-8 [HHV-8]) infection.

76. **What is the main risk factor for skin cancer?**
Ultraviolet light exposure.

77. **Explain the ABCDEs of melanoma. What should you do if they are present?**
The ABCDEs of melanoma are characteristics of a mole that should make you suspicious of malignant transformation: **a**symmetry, **b**orders (irregular), **c**olor (change in color or multiple colors), **d**iameter (lesions greater than 6 mm are more likely to be malignant) and **e**volving changes (lesions that change over time). Do an excisional biopsy of a lesion with any of these characteristics because melanomas commonly metastasize if not caught early. The risk of metastasis correlates most closely with depth of invasion into the skin.

78. **What do you need to know about basal cell and squamous cell skin cancers?**
Both of these cancers usually appear on sun-exposed areas (classically the head and neck area). The classic description of a basal cell cancer is a pearly, umbilicated nodule with telangiectasias; it is extremely common and almost never metastasizes. Squamous cell cancer sometimes metastasizes and often has a red, scaly, inflamed appearance or presents as an area of skin ulceration. Excisional biopsy is appropriate for all suspicious lesions.

79. **How can you differentiate a Wilms tumor from a neuroblastoma?**
Both present as flank masses in children (peak age: around 2 years). Neuroblastomas most commonly arise from the adrenal gland and often contain calcifications, whereas a Wilms tumor arise from the kidney and rarely calcify, thus imaging (CT scan) can usually distinguish the two. In rare cases, neuroblastomas regress spontaneously (for unknown reasons). *Neuroblastoma-adrenal + calcification.*
Wilm's - tumor + no caucification.

80. **What factors increase the risk for oral cancers? Describe the typical appearance.**
Smoking or chewing tobacco and alcohol are the main risk factors for oral cancer; their effect is synergistic. Also look for poor oral hygiene. Lesions often begin as leukoplakia (white patch) or malakoplakia (red patch). Oral hairy leukoplakia can resemble leukoplakia somewhat but is an unrelated condition affecting HIV-positive patients that is associated with the Epstein-Barr virus. The clinical setting should help you distinguish the two.

81. **What are the two major cytologic clues for histiocytosis?**
CD1 positive cells and Birbeck granules (cytoplasmic inclusion bodies that look like tennis rackets; Fig. 26-18).

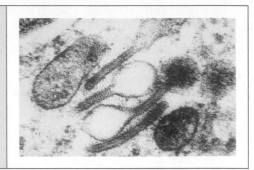

HISTIOCYTOSIS.

Figure 26-18. Birbeck granules. These characteristic racquet-shaped cytoplasmic inclusions are a marker for Langerhans cells of the skin. (From du Vivier A: Atlas of Clinical Dermatology, 3rd ed. New York, Churchill Livingstone, 2002, p 27, with permission.)

82. **What is a unicameral bone cyst? Who gets it? Describe the classic presentation.**

It is an expansile, lytic, well-demarcated benign lesion in the proximal portion of the humerus in children and adolescents. Although benign, it may weaken bone enough to cause a pathologic fracture of the humerus (the classic presentation).

83. **Describe the classic presentation of a retinoblastoma.**

Retinoblastoma classically presents in a child younger than 3 years old with leukocoria (the pupillary red reflex changes to white) and/or unilateral exophthalmos. It may be bilateral in the inherited form.

84. **True or false: All patients with metastatic cancer should be encouraged to receive chemotherapy.**

False. The risks and side effects of chemotherapy can be enormous, and sometimes minimal prolongation of life is achieved. The risks and benefits must be weighed. Patients with cancer (like all other patients) have the right to refuse any treatment. However, watch for and treat depression, even in terminal patients.

85. **Cover the right-hand column and name the cancer(s) associated with the following tumor markers:**

Marker	Cancer(s)
Alpha fetoprotein (AFP)	Liver (hepatocellular carcinoma), gonad (yolk-sac tumors)
Carcinoembryonic antigen (CEA)	Colorectal, lung, breast, ovary, pancreas, thyroid, liver, stomach, bladder, prostate
Prostate specific antigen (PSA)	Prostate
Human chorionic gonadotropin (HCG)	Hydatiform moles, choriocarcinoma, testicular
CA-125	Ovary
S-100	Melanoma
CA 19-9	Pancreas, colorectal
CA 27-29	Breast
CA15-3	Breast

(continued)

Marker	Cancer(s)
Hormone receptors	Breast
HER2	Breast
Beta-2-microglobulin	Multiple myeloma, chronic lymphocytic leukemia (CLL), and some lymphoma
Bladder tumor antigen (BTA)	Bladder
Calcitonin	Medullary thyroid carcinoma

CHAPTER 27

OPHTHALMOLOGY

1. **What is the hallmark of conjunctivitis?**
   Hyperemia of the conjunctival vessels.

2. **Distinguish among allergic, viral, and bacterial conjunctivitis in terms of signs and symptoms and treatment.**

Etiology	Signs and Symptoms	Treatment
Allergic	Itching, bilateral, seasonal, long duration	Vasoconstrictors or topical antihistamines/mast cell stabilizers
Viral*	Preauricular adenopathy, highly contagious (look for affected contacts); clear, watery discharge	Supportive, hand washing to prevent spread
Bacterial	Purulent discharge; classic in neonates	Topical antibiotics ± systemic antibiotics

   *The number-one viral cause is adenovirus.

3. **What are the three common causes of neonatal conjunctivitis?**
   Chemical, *Neisseria gonorrhoeae*, and *Chlamydia trachomatis*.

4. **What causes chemical conjunctivitis? How do you recognize it?**
   Chemical conjunctivitis is caused by the silver nitrate (or erythromycin) drops that are given to all newborns to prevent gonorrhea conjunctivitis. The drops may cause a chemical conjunctivitis (with no purulent discharge) that appears within 12 hours of instilling the drops and resolves within 48 hours. Chemical conjunctivitis is always the best guess if the conjunctivitis happens in the first 24 hours of life.

5. **How can you distinguish gonorrheal from chlamydial conjunctivitis?**
   In cases of suspected **gonorrheal conjunctivitis,** look for symptoms of gonorrhea in the mother. The infant has an extremely purulent discharge starting between 2 and 5 days after birth. Infants who were given prophylactic drops should not develop gonorrheal conjunctivitis. Treatment involves systemic ceftriaxone or cefotaxime.
   In cases of **chlamydial (inclusion) conjunctivitis,** the mother often reports no symptoms. The infant has mild-to-severe conjunctivitis beginning between 5 and 14 days after birth. Oral erythromycin is recommended for chlamydial conjunctivitis or pneumonia; topical therapy for chlamydial conjunctivitis is not effective.

6. **If you forget everything else about neonatal conjunctivitis, what point should you remember to help you distinguish among the three discussed causes?**
The varying time frames during which they present.

7. **True or false: Conjunctivitis frequently causes loss of vision.**
False. Other than transient blurriness (due to tear film debris) that resolves with blinking, conjunctivitis should not affect vision. If vision is affected, think of other, more serious conditions.

8. **Define glaucoma. What are the risk factors for developing it? What are the two general types?**
Glaucoma is best thought of as ocular hypertension (or elevated intraocular pressure, measured with a tonometer); its effects include visual field defects and blindness. The risk factors are age over 40, black race, and positive family history. The two main types are open-angle and closed-angle glaucoma.

9. **Describe the physical findings of open-angle glaucoma. How common is it? How is it treated?**
Open-angle glaucoma causes 90% of the cases of glaucoma; it is painless and does not have acute attacks. The only signs are elevated intraocular pressure (usually 20 to 30 mmHg), a gradually progressive visual field loss, and optic nerve changes (increased cup-to-disc ratio on funduscopic exam). Treatment may involve several different classes of medications, including beta blockers, prostaglandins, alpha adrenergic agonists, carbonic anhydrase inhibitors, cholinergic agonists, as well as laser therapy and surgery.

10. **How does closed-angle glaucoma present? What should you do if you recognize it?**
Closed-angle glaucoma presents with sudden ocular pain, seeing halos around lights, red eye, high intraocular pressure (greater than 30 mmHg), nausea and vomiting, sudden decreased vision, and a fixed, mid-dilated pupil. It is an ophthalmologic emergency. Treat the patient immediately with **pilocarpine,** oral glycerin and/or acetazolamide to break the attack. Definitive surgery (peripheral iridectomy) is used to prevent further attacks. In rare cases, anticholinergic medications can trigger an attack of closed-angle glaucoma in a susceptible, previously untreated patient. Medications do not cause acute attacks in patients with open-angle glaucoma or in patients with surgically treated closed-angle glaucoma.

11. **How do steroids affect the eye?**
Steroids, whether topical or systemic, can cause glaucoma and cataracts. Topical ocular steroids can worsen ocular herpes and fungal infections. For the Step 2 exam, do *not* give topical ocular steroids—especially if the patient has a dendritic corneal ulcer that stains green by fluorescein. Such an ulcer represents herpes.

12. **Define ultraviolet keratitis. How is it treated?**
Exposure to ultraviolet light can cause keratitis (corneal inflammation) with pain, foreign body sensation, red eye, tearing, and decreased vision. Patients have a history of welding, using a tanning bed or sunlamp, or snow-skiing ("snow-blindness"). Treat with an eye patch (for 24 hours) and topical antibiotic. You can reduce pain with an anticholinergic eye drop that causes paralysis of the ciliary muscle (cycloplegia).

13. **What pediatric rheumatologic condition is commonly associated with uveitis?**
Uveitis is common in juvenile rheumatoid arthritis (especially the pauciarticular form). Patients with juvenile rheumatoid arthritis need periodic ophthalmologic examination to check for uveitis.

14. **What is the most common cause of painless, slowly progressive loss of vision?**
Cataracts, especially in the elderly. Treatment is surgical removal of the affected lens(es) and replacement with an artificial lens.

15. **What should cataracts in a neonate suggest?**

Cataracts in a neonate may indicate a TORCH (**t**oxoplasmosis, **o**ther, **r**ubella, **c**ytomegalovirus, and **h**erpes simplex virus) infection or an inherited metabolic disorder (the classic example is galactosemia).

16. **What changes in the retina and fundus are seen in diabetes and hypertension?**

Diabetes is associated with dot-blot hemorrhages, microaneurysms, and neovascularization of the retina. **Hypertension** is associated with arteriolar narrowing, copper/silver wiring, and cotton-wool spots. Papilledema may be seen with severe hypertension and should alert you to the presence of a hypertensive emergency.

17. **What is the most common cause of blindness in patients under and over the age of 55? In black patients?**

In the United States, diabetes is the number-one cause of blindness in younger adults, and senile macular degeneration (look for macular drusen) is the most common cause of blindness in adults over age 55. Glaucoma is the number-one cause of blindness in blacks of any age and the number-three overall cause of blindness in the United States.

18. **Define proliferative diabetic retinopathy. How is it treated? How is nonproliferative diabetic retinopathy treated?**

Proliferative diabetic retinopathy occurs after many years of established diabetes and is defined by the development of neovascularization (new, abnormal growth of vessels in the retina). Treatment involves application of a laser beam to the periphery of the entire retina (**panretinal photocoagulation**). Surgical or medical vitrectomy in used in some cases. Medical therapy for proliferative diabetic retinopathy is investigational but is used in some circumstances. The most promising are the vascular endothelial growth factor (VEGF) inhibitors (bevacizumab, ranibizumab, pegaptanib).

Focal laser treatment is common for nonproliferative (background) retinopathy when macular edema is present; the laser is applied only to the affected area. In severe cases, panretinal photocoagulation may be used. Otherwise, nonproliferative retinopathy is treated supportively—primarily with tight control of blood glucose and follow-up eye exams to watch for development of macular edema or neovascularization.

19. **Distinguish between preorbital (preseptal) and orbital cellulitis.**

Both conditions may present with swollen lids; fever; a history of facial laceration, trauma, insect bite, or sinusitis; and chemosis (edema of the conjunctiva). However, if ophthalmoplegia, proptosis, severe eye pain, or decreased visual acuity is present, the patient has orbital cellulitis (Fig. 27-1). Orbital cellulitis is an ophthalmologic emergency, because it may extend into the skull, causing meningitis, venous thromboses, and/or blindness.

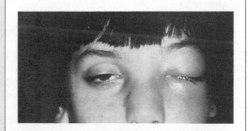

Figure 27-1. A 12-year-old boy with orbital cellulitis. He had a 5-day history of eye pain and progressive swelling and erythema of the eyelids. Anterior and lateral displacement of the globe and impairment of upward gaze were noted when his eyelids were retracted. (From Long S, Pickering L, Prober C: Principles and Practice of Pediatric Infectious Diseases, 3rd ed. Churchill Livingstone, 2008, Fig. 89-8.)

20. What are the common bacterial causes of preorbital and orbital cellulitis? How are they treated?

The most common bugs in both are *Streptococcus pneumoniae, Haemophilus influenzae* type b, and *Staphylococcus aureus* or streptococcal species (in patients with a history of trauma). Treat either condition with blood cultures and administration of broad-spectrum antibiotics until culture results are known. Although preorbital cellulitis may be treated on an outpatient basis with close follow-up, orbital cellulitis requires hospital admission and intravenous antibiotics.

21. What is the key to managing chemical burns to the eye? Which is worse—acid or alkaline burns?

With chemical burns to the eye (acid or alkaline), the key to management is copious irrigation with the closest source of water. The longer you wait, the worse the prognosis. Do not wait to get additional history. Alkali burns have a worse prognosis, because they tend to penetrate more deeply into the eye.

22. Distinguish between a hordeolum (stye) and a chalazion. How are they treated?

A hordeolum is a painful red lump near the lid margin. A chalazion is a painless lump away from the lid margin. Treat both with warm compresses. For chalazions, use intralesional steroid injection or incision and drainage if warm compresses do not work.

23. How do you recognize and treat herpes simplex keratitis?

Herpes simplex keratitis usually begins with conjunctivitis and vesicular lid eruption, then progresses to the classic dendritic keratitis (seen with fluorescein stain). Treat with topical anti-virals (e.g., idoxuridine, trifluridine). Corticosteroids are generally contraindicated with dendritic keratitis, because they may make the condition worse.

24. What findings suggest an ophthalmic herpes zoster infection?

Ophthalmic herpes zoster infection should be suspected in patients with involvement of the tip of the nose (Hutchinson sign) and/or medial eyelid, a typical zoster dermatomal skin rash, and eye complaints. Treat with oral acyclovir. Complications include uveitis, keratitis, and glaucoma.

25. How do you recognize a central retinal artery occlusion? What causes it?

Central retinal artery occlusion presents with sudden (within a few minutes), painless, unilateral loss of vision. The classic funduscopic appearance includes a pale, opaque fundus with a cherry red spot in the fovea (center) of the macula. No satisfactory treatment is available. The most common cause is emboli (from carotid plaque or heart), but watch for temporal arteritis as a cause on the Step 2 exam.

26. Describe the symptoms of temporal arteritis. What should you do if you suspect it?

Temporal arteritis is a vasculitis seen in the elderly. Symptoms include jaw claudication, loss of vision (due to central retinal artery occlusion), tortuous temporal artery (as seen or palpated on exam), markedly elevated erythrocyte sedimentation rate, and coexisting **polymyalgia rheumatica** (in 50%; causes proximal muscle pain and stiffness). If temporal arteritis is suspected in the setting of vision complaints, administer corticosteroids immediately before confirming the diagnosis with a temporal artery biopsy. Withholding treatment until a formal diagnosis can be made may cause the patient to lose vision in the other eye.

27. **How do you recognize central retinal vein occlusion? Describe the cause and treatment.**
Central retinal vein occlusion also presents with sudden (within a few hours), painless, unilateral loss of vision. The classic funduscopic appearance includes distended, tortuous retinal veins, retinal hemorrhages and a congested, edematous fundus. No satisfactory treatment is available. The most common causes are hypertension, diabetes, glaucoma, and increased blood viscosity (e.g., leukemia). Complications are related to neovascularization, which commonly develops and leads to vision loss and glaucoma.

28. **Describe the classic history of a patient with retinal detachment.**
The classic history of a patient with retinal detachment includes a sudden (instant), painless, unilateral loss of vision with "floaters" (little black spots that are seen no matter where the patient looks), and flashes of light. It is sometimes described as a "curtain or veil coming down in front of my eye." This history should prompt immediate referral to an ophthalmologist. Surgery may save the patient's vision by reattaching the retina.

29. **True or false: Cataracts and macular degeneration are common causes of bilateral, painless loss of vision in the elderly.**
True. Although one side may be worse than the other, bilateral complaints are not uncommon. The red reflex typically becomes black with a significant cataract. Those with macular degeneration typically have focal yellow-white deposits called **drusen** in and around the macula on funduscopic exam. Treat cataracts with surgery; most cases (90%) of macular degeneration are the "dry" or nonexudative subtype, which is treated supportively (e.g., magnification aids).

30. **How do optic neuritis and papillitis present? What are the common causes?**
Optic neuritis and papillitis typically present with a fairly quick (over hours to days), painful, unilateral or bilateral loss of vision. The optic disc margins may appear blurred on funduscopic exam with papillitis, just as in papilledema.
Multiple sclerosis (which can also cause internuclear ophthalmoplegia) is a very common cause of optic neuritis, especially in 20- to 40-year-old women. Lyme disease, malignancy and syphilis are other causes.

31. **What causes bitemporal hemianopsia until proved otherwise?**
A pituitary tumor (or other neoplasm) pressing on the optic chiasm.

32. **Use the visual field defect to localize the sight of the brain lesion (Figure 27-2).**

Visual Field Defect	Location of Lesion
Right anopsia (monocular blindness)	Right optic nerve
Bitemporal hemianopsia	Optic chiasm
Left homonymous hemianopsia	Right optic tract
Left upper quadrant anopsia	Right optic radiations in the right temporal lobe
Left lower quadrant anopsia	Right optic radiations in the right parietal lobe
Left homonymous hemianopsia with macular sparing	Right occipital lobe (from posterior cerebral artery occlusion)

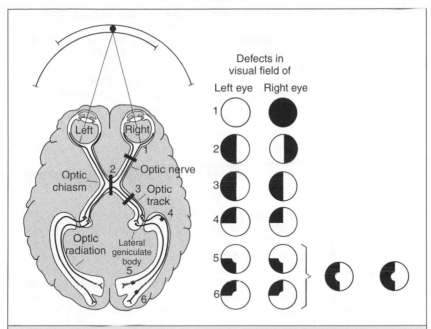

Figure 27-2. Visual field defects produced by lesions at various levels of the visual pathway. **1,** Right optic nerve; **2,** optic chiasm; **3,** optic tract; **4,** Meyer loop; **5,** cuneus; **6,** lingual gyrus; *bracket*, occipital lobe (with macular sparing). (From Berne R: Physiology, 5th ed. Philadelphia, Mosby, 2003, Fig. 8-10.)

33. **What two diseases commonly cause isolated palsies of cranial nerves III, IV, and VI? How do you recognize them?**
Isolated palsies of cranial nerve III, IV, and VI usually are due to vascular complications from diabetes mellitus and hypertension. Symptoms generally resolve on their own within 2 months. In patients over the age of 40 with a history of diabetes or hypertension and no other neurologic deficits or pain, observation is generally all that is required because hypertension and/or diabetes is the most likely cause. If resolution does not occur within 8 weeks, if the patient is under the age of 40, if neither hypertension nor diabetes is present, or if the patient starts to develop pain or other neurologic deficits, order a magnetic resonance (MR) scan of the head to rule out tumor or aneurysm (i.e., benign cause less likely).

34. **What are the physical exam findings of a third cranial nerve palsy? What should you remember when trying to determine the cause?**
With an oculomotor (cranial nerve III) lesion, the eye is down and out, and the patient can move the eye only laterally. If a third cranial nerve palsy is due to benign vascular causes (i.e., hypertension or diabetes), the pupil is normal and close observation is all that is needed, as the condition typically resolves on its own in several weeks. A "blown" (dilated, nonreactive) pupil is a medical emergency. The most likely cause is an aneurysm or tumor. Order an MRI scan and/or a cerebral angiogram.

35. **What are the physical findings in palsies of cranial nerves IV and VI? How do lesions of cranial nerves V and VII affect the eye?**
    With a trochlear (cranial nerve IV) lesion, the affected eye cannot look down when the gaze is medial because of superior oblique muscle paralysis. With an abducens (cranial nerve VI) lesion, the patient cannot look laterally with the affected eye because of lateral rectus muscle paralysis. Cranial nerves V (afferent, sensory limb) and VII (efferent, motor limb) are involved in the corneal blink reflex. Lesions can produce corneal drying, which can be treated with saline eye drops.

36. **What is strabismus? Beyond what age is it abnormal in children?**
    Strabismus is the medical term for a "lazy eye." The affected eye deviates, most commonly inward. Strabismus is normal only if intermittent and during the first 3 months of life; when constant or persistent beyond 3 months it requires ophthalmologic referral to prevent blindness (known as amblyopia) in the affected eye.

37. **Why does blindness develop in patients with strabismus?**
    The visual system is still developing until the age of 7 or 8 years. For this reason, visual screening of both eyes is important in children. If one eye does not see well or is turned outward, the brain cannot fuse the two different images that it sees. Thus, it suppresses the "bad" eye, which does not develop the proper neural connections. This eye will never see well and cannot be corrected with glasses because the problem is neural rather than refractive. This problem is treatable with special glasses or surgery if it is caught in time; the goal of treatment is to allow normal neural connections (and thus vision) to develop.

38. **What is presbyopia? When does it occur?**
    Presbyopia occurs between the ages of 40 and 50 years, when the lens loses its ability to accommodate. Patients then need bifocals or reading glasses for near vision. Presbyopia is a normal part of aging.

CHAPTER 28

ORTHOPEDIC SURGERY

1. **What orthopedic fractures are associated with the highest mortality rate?**
   Pelvic fractures, because patients can bleed to death. If the patient is unstable, consider heroic measures such as military antishock trousers (MAST trousers) and an external fixator.

2. **Why should areas distal to the fracture site be assessed by physical exam?**
   Areas distal to the fracture site should be assessed for neurologic and vascular compromise, either of which may be an emergency.

3. **Distinguish between an open and a closed fracture.**
   With an open (compound) fracture, the skin is broken over the fracture site. In closed fractures the skin is intact over the fracture site.

4. **Explain the difference in management of open and closed fractures.**
   With closed fractures, closed reduction and casting generally can be done. With open fractures, you should give antibiotics with coverage for gram-positive and gram-negative organisms (cefuroxime is appropriate; fluoroquinolones are an alternative). If the patient is at risk for methicillin-resistant *Staphylococcus aureus* (MRSA) infection, add vancomycin. Do surgical debridement, give a tetanus vaccine booster, lavage fresh wounds (if less than 8 hours old), and perform **open reduction and internal fixation** (ORIF). The main risk in open fractures is infection, which usually is not a problem with closed fractures because the skin is intact.

5. **What are the indications for open reduction other than an open fracture?**
   - Intraarticular fractures or articular surface malalignment
   - Nonunion or failed closed reduction
   - Compromise of blood supply
   - Multiple trauma (to allow mobilization at the earliest possible point)
   - Need for perfect reduction to optimize extremity function (e.g., professional athletes)

6. **What type of radiographs should you order if you suspect a fracture?**
   For any suspected fracture, order two views (usually anteroposterior and lateral) of the site, and consider radiographs of the joint above and below the fracture site.

7. **How should you treat a patient with severe pain after trauma and negative x-rays?**
   Treat the patient conservatively. Assume that there is a fracture and have the patient rest the injured area. Splinting may be appropriate for distal extremity injuries. Obtain follow-up radiographs 7 to 14 days after the injury if symptoms persist; many occult fractures will become visible at this time. The exception to waiting is a suspected hip fracture in an elderly person—proceed to CT or MRI of the hip to allow earlier diagnosis and treatment (Fig. 28-1),

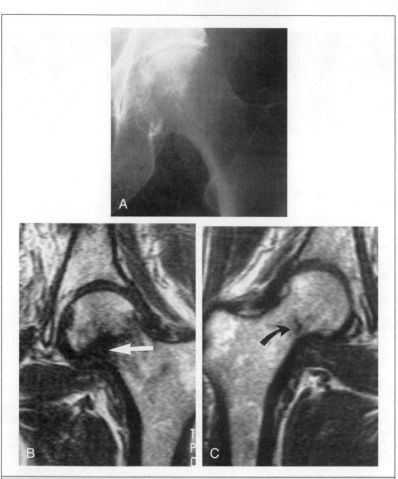

Figure 28-1. Imaging of occult hip fracture. AP radiograph of the **left** hip (**A**) demonstrates no evidence of fracture. Coronal T1-weighted MRI (**B**) clearly shows a well-demarcated line of decreased signal in the subcapital region of the **left** femoral neck consistent with a non-displaced fracture *(arrow)*. MRI of the **right** hip (**C**) shows a subtle medial femoral neck fracture *(curved arrow)* not demonstrated on the conventional radiograph. (From Adam A, et al.: Grainger & Allison's Diagnostic Radiology, 5th ed. Edinburgh, Churchill Livingstone, 2008, Fig. 46-73.)

which decrease operative morbidity and length of hospital stay compared with delayed diagnosis and treatment.

8. **Define compartment syndrome. What is the cause?**
   Compartment syndrome is a problem of muscle compartments, which are limited by the fascia in which they are contained. It is seen in the extremities (most commonly in the calf) when edema or hemorrhage causes swelling inside a muscle compartment. Rising pressure inside the fascial compartment can result in permanent nerve damage and muscle necrosis.

The three common clinical scenarios in which compartment syndrome is seen are fractures (classically midshaft tibial fractures or supracondylar fractures of the humerus in children), burns (especially electrical and circumferential burns), and vascular compromise (or after vascular surgery procedures).

9. **What are the symptoms and signs of compartment syndrome? How is it treated?**
   - Pain (especially pain on passive movement out of proportion to the injury)
   - Paresthesias, hypesthesia, and numbness (decreased sensation and two-point discrimination)
   - Cyanosis or pallor
   - Firm-feeling muscle compartment
   - Paralysis (late, ominous sign)
   - Elevated compartment pressure (greater than 30 to 40 mmHg)

   On the USMLE, the diagnosis of compartment syndrome often has to be made clinically without a pressure reading. Although pulses may be slightly decreased, they usually are palpable (or detectable with Doppler ultrasound). Lack of palpable pulses is an ominous, late sign. Compartment syndrome is an emergency, and quick action can save an otherwise doomed limb. Treatment is immediate fasciotomy; incising the fascial compartment relieves the pressure.

10. **Cover the right-hand columns and specify the motor and sensory functions of the following peripheral nerves. In what common clinical scenarios are they often damaged?**

Nerve	Motor Function	Sensory Function	Clinical Scenario
Radial	Wrist extension (watch for wrist drop)	Back of forearm, back of hand (first 3 digits)	Humeral fracture
Ulnar	Finger abduction (watch for "claw hand")	Front and back of last 2 digits	Elbow dislocation or fracture
Median	Pronation, thumb opposition	Palmar surface of hand (first 3 digits)	Carpal tunnel syndrome, humeral fracture
Axillary	Abduction, lateral rotation	Lateral shoulder	Upper humeral dislocation or fracture
Peroneal	Dorsiflexion, eversion (watch for foot drop)	Dorsal foot and lateral leg	Knee dislocation, fibula fracture

11. **What is the difference between insufficiency stress fracture and fatigue stress fracture? How are stress fractures diagnosed and treated?**
    A stress fracture (Fig. 28-2) is an incomplete or small fracture that develops because of repeated or prolonged forces against the bone. In fatigue fractures, abnormal stresses are applied to normal bones (e.g., overuse injury, as in military recruits or marathon runners). In insufficiency fractures, normal/physiologic stresses are applied to an abnormal bone (e.g., osteoporotic bone). Diagnosis is made using x-rays, with MRI and nuclear medicine

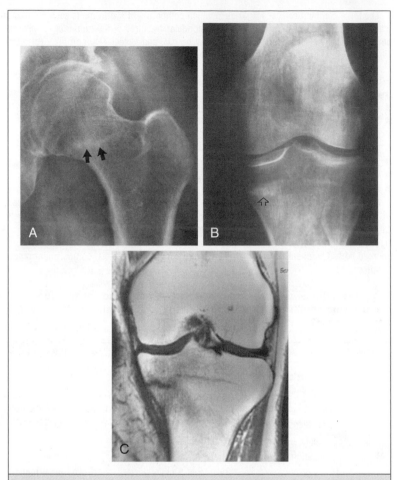

Figure 28-2. A, Stress fracture involving cancellous bone of the subcapital region of the femoral neck has the appearance of a band of sclerosis *(arrows)*. **B,** A more subtle stress fracture at the medial tibial plateau *(open arrow)*. **C,** MRI was ordered to confirm the fracture, clearly showing the low signal fracture line. (From Katz DS, Math KR, Groskin SA [eds]: Radiology Secrets. Philadelphia, Hanley & Belfus, 1998, p 438, with permission.)

scans available if x-rays are negative but strong clinical suspicion remains. The treatment is rest to allow healing and prevent progression to a complete fracture. In the setting of insufficiency fractures, treatment of osteoporosis (e.g., alendronate, calcium, vitamin D) is also needed to help prevent future fractures.

12. **What fracture usually is diagnosed in trauma patients with pain in the anatomic snuff-box?**
    Scaphoid bone fracture (Fig. 28-3), classically after a fall on an outstretched hand.

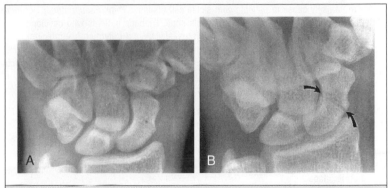

Figure 28-3. Delayed study showing occult scaphoid fracture. **A,** Patient with snuffbox tenderness presents with normal radiograph of the wrist. **B,** A film obtained 10 days later clearly shows the fracture line at the mid-waist of the scaphoid *(curved arrows)*. (From Katz DS, Math KR, Groskin SA [eds]: Radiology Secrets. Philadelphia, Hanley & Belfus, 1998, p 436, with permission.)

13. **What are the most common locations of intervertebral disc herniations? What symptoms do they cause?**
Lumbar disc herniation is a common, often correctable cause of low back pain. The most common location is the L5–S1 disc, which affects the S1 nerve root. Look for decreased ankle jerk, weakness of plantar flexors in the foot, pain from the midgluteal area to the posterior calf, and a positive straight leg-raise test. The second most common location for herniation is the L4–L5 disc, which affects the L5 nerve root. Look for decreased biceps femoris reflex, weakness of foot extensors, and pain in the hip or groin.
  After the lumbar area, the second most common location is the cervical spine. The classic symptom of cervical disc disease is neck pain. Herniation is most common at the C6–C7 disc, which affects the C7 nerve root. Look for decreased triceps reflex/strength and weakness of forearm extension.

14. **How is intervertebral disc herniation diagnosed and treated?**
Diagnosis is made with MRI scan (preferred) or by CT scan or myelography. Conservative treatment, including bed rest and analgesics, usually is tried first, as roughly 90% of cases will resolve with conservative management. Epidural steroid injection may help. Surgery (discectomy) may be required if conservative treatment fails or significant neurologic deficit is present (to prevent permanent nerve damage).

15. **Define Charcot joint. What causes it? How is it managed?**
Charcot joints (neuropathic joints) are seen in patients with diabetes mellitus or other conditions causing peripheral neuropathy (e.g., tertiary syphilis). Lack of proprioception causes gradual arthritis or arthropathy and joint deformity. Patients should get radiographs for any (even minor) trauma because they may not feel even a severe fracture.

16. **What is the most common bacterial cause of osteomyelitis? In what clinical scenarios should you think of other causes?**
Osteomyelitis is caused most commonly by *Staphylococcus aureus*. Think of gram-negative bacteria in immunocompromised patients or intravenous drug abusers. *Salmonella* species

is the most likely cause in patients with sickle cell disease. Think *Pseudomonas aeruginosa* if there is a puncture wound through a tennis shoe. Diabetic patients who develop a "diabetic foot" with subsequent osteomyelitis usually have a polymicrobial infection. Aspirate and biopsy the affected joint or bone, and order a Gram stain, culture, and cell count of the fluid or tissue if osteomyelitis is suspected. Check a serum ESR or C-reactive protein.

17. **Which bacteria are the most common cause of septic arthritis? In what scenario should you think of another cause?**
Septic arthritis is most commonly due to *Staphylococcus aureus,* but in sexually active adults (especially when young and/or promiscuous), suspect *Neisseria gonorrhoeae.* Aspirate the joint, and order a Gram stain, culture, and cell count with differential if infection is suspected.

18. **What is reflex sympathetic dystrophy (RSD)? How do patients present?**
RSD (also known as Sudeck atrophy) is a poorly understood disorder that generally occurs in an extremity and is characterized by pain, swelling and signs of autonomic dysfunction (vasomotor instability with alternating warmth and coolness and/or sweating and dryness of the area). In most (but not all) cases it is post-traumatic in origin. The associated trauma is classically mild, and symptoms may begin days or several weeks after the injury. Patients classically have severe, intermittent pain, often described as burning, with associated temperature changes and sweating during episodes. A minor stimulus (e.g., light touch) may trigger severe pain symptoms. The diagnosis can be confirmed with radiographs or nuclear medicine scan. A presumptive diagnosis is often made in the appropriate setting if a sympathetic nerve block (i.e., injection of local anesthetic into the involved nerve) relieves symptoms. This procedure can be repeated as part of therapy if it is initially successful.

19. **True or false: There is a high incidence of vascular injury with posterior knee dislocations.**
True. Order an angiogram if pulses are asymmetric (i.e., weaker or absent on the affected side) to check for injury.

20. **What is the most common type of bone tumor?**
Metastatic (especially from breast, lung, or prostate cancer).

21. **What is a pathologic fracture? What is the most common cause of a pathologic fracture?**
A pathologic fracture is one that occurs in bone previously weakened by another disease. Osteoporosis (especially in elderly, thin women) is the most common cause, but you should always think about the possibility of malignancy.

22. **To what site is pain from hip inflammation or dislocation/fracture classically referred?**
The knee (especially in children).

23. **Specify age at presentation, epidemiology, symptoms and signs, and treatment for the three classically tested pediatric hip disorders.**

Name	Age	Epidemiology	Symptoms/Signs	Treatment
CHD	At birth	Female, first-borns, breech delivery	Barlow's and Ortolani's signs	Observation, abduction splint, or open or closed reduction
LCPD	4–10 yrs	Short male with delayed bone age	Knee, thigh, groin pain, limp	Orthoses
SCFE	9–13 yrs	Overweight male adolescent	Knee, thigh, groin pain, limp	Surgical pinning

CHD = congenital hip dysplasia; LCPD = Legg-Calvé-Perthes disease; SCFE = slipped capital femoral epiphysis.

Note: All of these conditions may present in an adult as arthritis of the hip.

24. **If you forget everything else about differentiating the three pediatric hip disorders, what historical point will help you the most on the USMLE?**
Age at onset of symptoms.

25. **Define Osgood-Schlatter disease. How is it recognized and treated?**
Osgood-Schlatter disease is osteochondritis of the tibial tubercle. It is often bilateral and usually presents in boys between 10 and 15 years of age. Symptoms and signs include pain, swelling, and tenderness in the knee (remember, the pediatric hip problems above have referred pain in the knee, but no knee swelling or tenderness upon palpation of the knee). Treat with rest, activity restriction, and nonsteroidal anti-inflammatory drugs. Most cases resolve on their own.

26. **How do you check for scoliosis? Who is usually affected? What is the treatment?**
Check for scoliosis by having patients touch their toes while you look at the spine. If scoliosis is present, you will see an abnormal lateral curvature of the spine. Scoliosis usually affects prepubertal girls and is idiopathic. Treat with a brace for anything other than very minor (less than 15 degrees) curvature. If the deformity is severe (e.g., respiratory compromise, rapid progression), surgery should be considered.

27. **What are the common findings with ligament injuries of the knee? How do you distinguish injuries of the anterior cruciate, posterior cruciate, medial collateral, and lateral collateral ligaments on physical exam?**
Ligament injuries in the knee commonly cause pain, joint effusions, instability of the joint, and history of the joint *popping, buckling,* or *locking up.*
■ **Anterior cruciate ligament (ACL)** tears are the most common. Watch for the *anterior* drawer test. The knee is placed in 90° of flexion and pulled forward (like opening a drawer). If the tibia pulls forward more than normal (e.g., more than the unaffected side), the test is positive, and you have an ACL tear.

- **Posterior cruciate ligament (PCL)** tears can be diagnosed with the *posterior* drawer test. Push the tibia back with the knee in 90° of flexion. If the tibia pushes back more than normal, the test is positive and a PCL tear is present.
- **Medial collateral ligament (MCL)** tears are suggested during the *abduction* or *valgus* stress test. With the knee in 30° of flexion, abduct the ankle while holding the knee. If the knee joint abducts to an abnormal degree, the test is positive and a medial compartment injury is present.
- **Lateral collateral ligament (LCL)** tears are suggested during the *adduction* or *varus* stress test. Adduct the ankle while holding the knee. If the knee joint adducts to an abnormal degree, the test is positive, and lateral compartment injury is present.

  MRI (Fig. 28-4) and/or arthroscopy can be used to confirm suspected tears and look for other injuries.

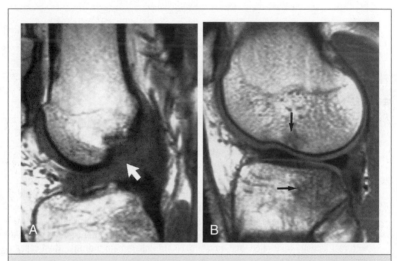

Figure 28-4. MRI appearance of acute ACL rupture. Sagittal T1-weighted MRI of the knee (**A**) demonstrates a mass of intermediate amorphous signal in the expected location of the anterior cruciate ligament *(arrow)*, consistent with a complete tear of the ACL. Further laterally (**B**), low signal in the posterior tibia and lateral femoral condyle represents typical contusions seen in association with ACL injury *(small arrows)*. (From Adam A, et al.: Grainger & Allison's Diagnostic Radiology, 5th ed. Edinburgh, Churchill Livingstone, 2008, Fig. 46-81.)

28. **What are the risk factors for avascular necrosis (AVN)? What is the best test to make the diagnosis?**
   Avascular necrosis describes local intravascular coagulation with subsequent bone ischemia and necrosis of cancellous bone and marrow. Patients present with pain in the affected area. There are many potential causes/associations, including:
   - Trauma (usually in the setting of fracture)
   - Corticosteroid excess (endogenous or iatrogenic)
   - Sickle cell disease or other hemoglobinopathy
   - Alcohol abuse
   - Lupus and other connective tissue disorders
   - Caisson disease (i.e. decompression sickness)

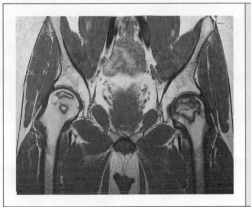

Figure 28-5. Avascular necrosis of the hip. Coronal T1-weighted MR image through both hips confirms the presence of geographic areas of abnormality in both femoral heads which are well demarcated from the adjacent normal bone by a thin rim of low signal material. (From Adam A, et al.: Grainger & Allison's Diagnostic Radiology, 5th ed. Edinburgh, Churchill Livingstone, 2008, Fig. 50-21.)

- Slipped capital femoral epiphysis
- Pancreatitis

The best test to make the diagnosis is MRI (Fig. 28-5), which becomes positive before regular x-rays.

CHAPTER 29

PEDIATRICS

1. Give the average ages at which the following commonly tested milestones are achieved.

Milestone	Age*
Social smile	1–2 mo
Cooing	2–4 mo
While prone, lifts head up 90°	3–4 mo
Rolls front to back	4–5 mo
Voluntary grasp (no release)	5 mo
Stranger anxiety	6–9 mo
Sits with no support	7 mo
Pulls to stand	9 mo
Waves "bye-bye"	10 mo
Voluntary grasp with voluntary release	10 mo
Plays pat-a-cake	9–10 mo
First words	9–12 mo
Imitates others' sounds	9–12 mo
Separation anxiety	12–15 mo
Walks without help	13 mo
Can build tower of 2 cubes	13–15 mo
Understands 1-step commands (no gesture)	15 mo
Good use of cup and spoon	15–18 mo
Can build tower of 6 cubes	2 yr
Runs well	2 yr
Ties shoelaces	5 yr

*Reduce the age of premature infants in the first 2 years for assessing development. For example, for children born after 6 months of gestation, subtract 3 months from their chronologic age. Therefore, they should be expected to perform only at the 6-month-old level when they are 9 months old.

2. True or false: The overall pattern of development is more important than the age at which individual milestones are reached.
   True. The exact age is not as important as the overall pattern in looking for dysfunctional development. When in doubt, use a formal developmental test.

3. **What screening and preventive care measures should be done at every pediatric visit?**
Height, weight, blood pressure, developmental/behavioral assessment, and anticipatory guidance (counseling/discussion about age-appropriate concerns) should be done at every pediatric visit.

4. **True or false: Screening and preventive care are important mainly during a well check-up.**
False. Screening and preventive care are an important part of every encounter with a patient (adult or child). Questions may try to fool you on this point. For example, a mother complains that her 4-year-old child sleeps 11 hours every night. This is normal behavior. The answer to the question, "What should you do next?" may be to give an objective hearing exam, which is a routine screening procedure in a 4-year-old child.

5. **What are the commonly performed screening tests for metabolic and congenital disorders?**
States vary widely in their policies regarding newborn screening. All states screen for hypothyroidism and phenylketonuria at birth; screens must be done within the first month of life. Most states screen for galactosemia and hemoglobinopathies such as sickle cell disease. Some states include screening for homocystinuria, maple syrup urine disease, congenital adrenal hyperplasia, cystic fibrosis, biotinidase deficiency, tyrosinemia, and toxoplasmosis. If any of these screens are positive, the first step is to order a confirmatory test to make sure that the screening test gave you a true-positive result.

6. **What are the frequently tested items under the umbrella of primary prevention using "anticipatory guidance"?**
Tell parents the following:
- Keep the water heater under 110 to 120° F.
- Use car restraints.
- Put the infant to sleep on his or her side or back to help prevent sudden infant death syndrome (SIDS), the most common cause of death in children aged 1 to 12 months.
- Do not use infant walkers because they cause injuries.
- Watch out for small objects, which may be aspirated.
- Do not give cow's milk before 1 year of age.
- Introduce solid foods gradually, starting at 6 months.
- Supervise children in bathtubs and swimming pools.

7. **How often should height, weight, and head circumference be measured? What do they signify?**
Head circumference should be measured at every visit in the first 2 years; height and weight should be measured routinely until adulthood. All three parameters are markers of general well-being; abnormal values may suggest disease.

8. **What if a child has low height, weight, or head circumference compared with peers?**
The pattern of growth along plotted growth curves over time (which you may be asked to interpret) tells you more than any single measurement. If a child has always been low or high compared with peers, generally the pattern is benign. A patient who goes from a normal to an abnormal curve is much more worrisome. Parents commonly bring in a child with delayed physical growth or delayed puberty. You need to know when to reassure and when to do further testing and questioning.

9. **Define failure to thrive. What causes it?**
There is no consensus definition for failure to thrive, but commonly used definitions include a head circumference, height, or weight less than the fifth percentile for age; a weight less than

80% of ideal weight for age; or a weight gain that causes a decrease in two or more major percentage lines on the growth curve. Failure to thrive is due most commonly to psychosocial or functional problems. Watch for signs of neglect and child abuse. Organic causes usually have specific clues to trigger your suspicion.

10. **What conditions are suggested by obesity in children?**
Obesity usually is due to overeating and too little activity (more than 95% of cases). Less than 5% of cases are due to organic causes (e.g., Cushing syndrome, Prader-Willi syndrome).

11. **What conditions should you consider in a child with an abnormal head circumference?**
Increased head circumference may mean hydrocephalus or tumor, whereas decreased head circumference may mean microcephaly (e.g., from congenital TORCH infection). Again, the pattern of head circumference over time (plotted on a growth curve) is most helpful in defining pathology.

12. **How are hearing and vision screened?**
Hearing and vision should be measured objectively at least once by 4 years of age. After the initial screen, measure every few years until adulthood or more often if the history so dictates.

13. **In what situations should you worry about hearing loss?**
■ After a bout of meningitis (hearing loss is the most common neurologic complication)
■ With congenital TORCH (**t**oxoplasmosis, **o**ther [e.g., syphilis, HIV], **r**ubella, **c**ytomegalovirus, **h**erpes simplex) infections
■ With measles or mumps
■ With chronic middle ear effusions or chronic or recurrent otitis media
■ With the use of ototoxic drugs (e.g., aminoglycosides)

14. **What is the red reflex? What should an abnormal reflex suggest?**
Check for loss of the red reflex at birth and routinely thereafter to detect congenital cataracts or ocular tumors. When a penlight is shined at the pupil, you usually see red because of the underlying fundus. If a cataract (or tumor) is present in the eye, the red reflex disappears and you see black (with a cataract) or white (known as leukocoria and classically due to retinoblastoma).

15. **True or false: Before a certain age intermittent strabismus is normal.**
True. It is normal for infants to have occasional ocular misalignment (strabismus) until 3 months of age. After 3 months (or with constant eye deviation), strabismus should be evaluated and managed by an ophthalmologist to prevent possible blindness in the affected eye.

16. **How is screening for anemia done?**
Recommendations for routine screening for anemia (with a complete blood count or hemoglobin/hematocrit) vary and are changing. Hemoglobin or hematocrit measurement is recommended at 12 months of age, but may be required at other times as dictated by history and risk assessment. Recommendations for screening during adolescence vary, but adolescents should be screened at least once. If any risk factors for iron deficiency are present during infancy (prematurity, low birth weight, ingestion of cow's milk before 1 year of age, low dietary intake, low socioeconomic status), screen with a complete blood count or hemoglobin and hematocrit if given the option.

17. **True or false: All children should be given prophylactic iron supplements.**
False. Exclusively breast-fed infants do not require supplementation. All other children should receive supplementation. Start iron supplements in full-term infants at 4 to 6 months of

age and in preterm infants at 2 months of age. Most infant formulas and cereals contain iron, thus separate supplements are usually not required.

18. **How and when do you screen for lead exposure?**
Screening for lead toxicity is controversial. Routine screening is no longer recommended. However, all Medicaid-eligible children must be screened. Consider screening high-risk children (those who live in old buildings, have a sibling or playmate with lead toxicity, eat paint chips, live near a battery recycling plant, or have a parent who works at a battery recycling plant). Screen for lead exposure by doing a serum lead level. If the initial lead level is abnormally high, closer follow-up and intervention are needed. The best first step is to stop the exposure.

19. **True or false: Most children need fluoride supplementation.**
False. Because most water is fluoridated, supplementation is not needed. If, however, a child lives in an area where the water is inadequately fluoridated (rare) or the child is fed exclusively from premixed, ready-to-eat formulas (which use nonfluoridated water), fluoride supplements should be given.

20. **True or false: Breast-fed infants are more likely to require vitamin D supplements than formula-fed infants.**
True. The American Academy of Pediatrics recommends that exclusively and partially breastfed infants receive vitamin D supplements shortly after birth and continue until they are weaned and consume formula or whole milk. Formula-fed infants do not require supplements in the United States because all formulas contain vitamin D supplements.

21. **When should children be screened for tuberculosis?**
Universal screening for tuberculosis is not recommended. There is no need to screen children who have no risk factors. Risk assessment should occur regularly until 2 years of age, then annually. Test those at high risk (family member with tuberculosis, family member with a positive tuberculosis test, a child born in a high-risk country, a child who has traveled to a high-risk country, or a child who has consumed unpasteurized milk or cheese).

22. **True or false: Screening children for renal disease with a urinalysis is not recommended.**
True. However, you should screen for congenital/anatomic abnormalities (e.g., vesicoureteral reflux) after a urinary tract infection in children 2 months to 2 years of age by getting an ultrasound and either voiding cystourethrogram (VCUG) or radionuclide cystogram (RNC). Screening after the age of 2 is more controversial and likely won't be asked on the USMLE.

23. **True or false: Current vaccine recommendations and schedules are always provided on the USMLE.**
False, but because the timing of normal immunizations is being updated constantly, the administration schedule for common vaccines may be provided on the Step 2 exam. Higher yield information relates to special patient populations (e.g., give pneumococcal vaccine to patients with sickle cell disease or splenectomy) and vaccine contraindications (no measles-mumps-rubella or influenza vaccines for egg-allergic patients, no live vaccines for immunocompromised patients).

24. **True or false: Sexually active teenaged girls need screening for chlamydial infection and gonorrhea.**
True.

25. **When should you recommend that a child see a dentist for the first time?**
Around 2 to 3 years of age.

26. **What are the Tanner stages? When do they occur?**
The Tanner stages measure the stages of puberty. Stage 1 is preadolescent, stage 5 is adult. Advancing stages are assigned for testicular and penile growth in boys and breast growth in girls. Both male and female stages also use pubic hair development. The average age of puberty (when a patient first has changes from the preadolescent stage 1) is 10.5 years in girls and 11.5 years in boys. The classic first events of puberty are testicular enlargement in boys and breast development in girls.

27. **Define delayed puberty. What is the most common cause?**
Delayed puberty is defined by a lack of testicular enlargement in boys by age 14 years or a lack of breast development or pubic hair in girls by age 12 years. The most common cause is **constitutional delay,** a normal variant. Watch for parents with a similar history of being "late bloomers." The child's growth curve consistently lags behind that of peers, but the line representing the child's growth curve is parallel to the normal growth curve. Treatment is reassurance only.

28. **What are other causes for delayed puberty?**
Rarely, delayed puberty is due to primary testicular failure (Klinefelter syndrome, cryptorchidism, history of chemotherapy, gonadal dysgenesis) or ovarian failure (Turner syndrome, gonadal dysgenesis). Even more rarely, delayed puberty is due to a hypothalamic/pituitary defect, such as Kallmann syndrome or tumor.

29. **What causes precocious puberty?**
Precocious puberty is usually idiopathic but may be due to the **McCune-Albright syndrome** (in girls), ovarian tumors (granulosa, theca-cell, or gonadoblastoma), testicular tumors (Leydig-cell tumors), central nervous system disease or trauma, adrenal neoplasm, or congenital adrenal hyperplasia, which causes precocious puberty only in boys and usually is due to 21-hydroxylase deficiency.

30. **True or false: If the underlying cause for precocious puberty is uncorrectable or idiopathic after diagnostic work-up, patients should receive treatment.**
True. Most patients are given long-acting gonadotropin-releasing hormone agonists to suppress the progression of puberty. This approach helps to prevent premature epiphyseal closure with short stature.

31. **How are cavernous hemangiomas treated?**
Cavernous hemangiomas are benign vascular tumors that often are first noticed a few days after birth. They tend to increase in size after birth (sometimes becoming quite large) and gradually resolve within the first 2 years of life (Fig. 29-1). The best treatment is to do nothing but observe and follow.

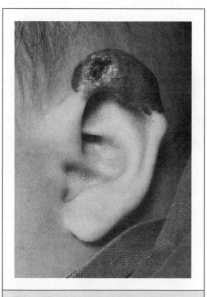

Figure 29-1. Infantile hemangioma. These lesions grow rapidly during the first few months of life once they appear (20% at birth), but they are asymptomatic unless they bleed, become infected, or obstruct a vital structure. Complete resolution is typical before the age of 7, and no treatment is usually required. (From du Vivier A: Atlas of Clinical Dermatology, 3rd ed. New York, Churchill Livingstone, 2002, p 117, with permission.)

32. **Distinguish between caput succedaneum and cephalohematoma. How are these conditions treated?**
Both conditions are noted in newborns after vaginal delivery. Caput succedaneum defines diffuse swelling or edema of the scalp that crosses the midline, is benign, and requires no further investigation or treatment. Cephalohematomas are subperiosteal hemorrhages that are sharply limited by sutures and do not cross the midline. Cephalohematomas are usually benign and self-resolving, but in rare cases they may indicate an underlying skull fracture. Order a radiograph or CT scan to rule out fracture if given the option.

33. **When does the anterior fontanelle usually close? What disorder should you suspect if it fails to close?**
The anterior fontanelle usually is closed by 18 months of age. Delayed closure or an unusually large anterior fontanelle may indicate hypothyroidism, hydrocephalus, rickets, or intrauterine growth retardation.

34. **How many vessels does a normal umbilical cord have? What disorder should you suspect if one of the vessels is absent?**
The umbilical cord is checked at birth for the presence of the normal three vessels: two arteries and one vein. If only one artery is present, consider the possibility of congenital renal malformations.

35. **True or false: Milky-white and possibly blood-tinged vaginal discharge is usually abnormal in the first week of life for a female newborn.**
False. This discharge is usually physiologic and due to maternal hormone withdrawal.

36. **What findings should make you suspect child abuse?**
- Failure to thrive
- Multiple fractures, bruises, or injuries in different stages of healing
- Metaphyseal "bucket handle" or "corner" fractures (Fig. 29-2)
- Shaken baby syndrome (retinal hemorrhages or subdural hematomas with no external signs of trauma)
- Behavioral, emotional, or interactional problems
- Sexually transmitted diseases
- Multiple personality disorder (classically due to sexual abuse)
- Whenever a parent's story does not fit the child's injury

37. **True or false: You do not need proof to report child abuse.**
True. In fact, reporting any suspicion of child abuse is mandatory. You do not need proof and cannot be sued for reporting your suspicion.

38. **True or false: Children have the same range of normal vital signs as adults.**
False. Children have lower blood pressure and higher heart and respiratory rates than adults. In addition, children often have different lab values. For example, a child's hemoglobin/hematocrit value is normally higher at birth and lower throughout childhood compared with an adult. Normal lab value ranges should be provided on the USMLE. In addition, the renal, pulmonary, hepatic, and central nervous systems are not fully mature or functional at birth.

39. **What is an APGAR score? When is it measured?**
The APGAR score is a general measure of well-being in newborns. It is commonly assessed at 1 and 5 minutes after birth if values are normal. If the score is <7, continue to assess every 5 minutes until the infant reaches a score of 7 or more (while resuscitating the child as needed). There are five categories of the APGAR score with a maximal score of 2 points per

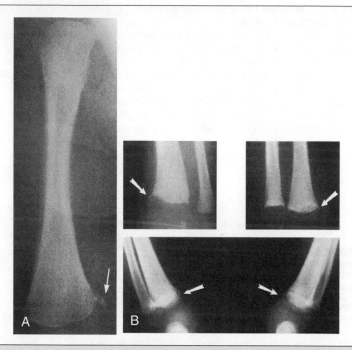

Figure 29-2. Metaphyseal fractures. Radiographs of the right femur (**A**) and both ankles (**B**) of a 2-month-old abused infant demonstrating metaphyseal corner fractures of the distal femur and both distal tibia (*arrows*). The angled tangential view reveals the "bucket handle" appearance of the fracture. (From Adam A, et al.: Grainger & Allison's Diagnostic Radiology, 5th ed. Edinburgh, Churchill Livingstone, 2008, Fig. 68-24.)

category and a possible total of 10 points. Remember the APGAR pneumonic: Appearance (skin color), Pulse (heart rate), Grimace (reflex irritability), Activity (muscle tone), and Respiration (breathing).

Category	Number of Points Given		
	0	1	2
Color	Pale, blue	Body pink, extremities blue	Completely pink
Heart rate	Absent	< 100 beats/min	> 100 beats/min
Reflex irritability*	None	Grimace	Grimace and strong cry, cough, and sneeze
Muscle tone	Limp	Some flexion of extremities	Active motion
Respiratory effort	None	Slow, weak cry	Good, strong cry

*Reflex irritability usually is measured by the infant's response to stimulation of the sole of the foot or a catheter put into the nose.

40. **True or false: The APGAR score is important because it is the first assessment of how a child is doing.**

False. Do not wait until the 1-minute mark to evaluate the infant. You may have to suction or intubate the infant seconds after delivery!

41. **What should you always remember when a question mentions that a child was given aspirin?**

Reye syndrome, which causes encephalopathy and/or liver failure. It usually occurs after aspirin is given for influenza or varicella infection. Use acetaminophen in children to avoid this rare (but often tested) condition.

42. **When should the Moro and palmar grasp reflex disappear?**

By 6 months of age.

CHAPTER 30

PHARMACOLOGY

1. On the USMLE, bizarre, unique, and fatal side effects are tested as well as common side effects of common drugs. Cover the right-hand column and name the side effects of the listed drugs.

Drug	Side Effect(s)
Trazodone	Priapism
Aspirin	Gastrointestinal bleeding, hypersensitivity
Bleomycin	Pulmonary fibrosis
Cyclophosphamide	Hemorrhagic cystitis
Bupropion	Seizures
Isoniazid	Vitamin B_6 deficiency, lupus-like syndrome, liver toxicity
Cyclosporine	Renal toxicity
Penicillins	Anaphylaxis, rash with Epstein-Barr virus
Angiotensin-converting enzyme inhibitors	Cough, angioedema
Demeclocycline	Diabetes insipidus
Lithium	Diabetes insipidus, thyroid dysfunction
Methoxyflurane	Diabetes insipidus
Sulfa drugs	Allergies, kernicterus in neonates
Halothane	Liver necrosis
Local anesthetic	Seizures
Phenytoin	Folate deficiency, teratogen, hirsutism
Vincristine	Peripheral neuropathy
Amiodarone	Thyroid dysfunction, pulmonary toxicity
Valproic acid	Neural tube defects in offspring
Isotretinoin	Terrible teratogen
Thioridazine	Retinal deposits, cardiac toxicity
Heparin	Thrombocytopenia, thrombosis
Vancomycin	Red man's syndrome
Clofibrate	Increased gastrointestinal neoplasms
Tetracyclines	Photosensitivity, teeth staining in children
Quinolones	Teratogens (cartilage damage)
Quinine	Cinchonism (tinnitus, vertigo)
Morphine	Sphincter of Oddi spasm – use morphine in GB cases
Clindamycin	Pseudomembranous colitis (can be caused by any broad-spectrum antibiotic)

(continued)

Drug	Side Effect(s)
Chloramphenicol	Aplastic anemia, gray-baby syndrome
Doxorubicin	Cardiomyopathy
Busulfan	Pulmonary fibrosis
Monoamine oxidase inhibitors	Tyramine crisis (after eating cheese or wine)
Hydralazine	Lupus-like syndrome
Procainamide	Lupus-like syndrome
Minoxidil	Hirsutism
Aminoglycoside	Hearing loss, renal toxicity
Acetaminophen	Liver toxicity (in high doses)
Chlorpropamide	Syndrome of inappropriate antidiuretic hormone (SIADH)
Oxytocin	SIADH
Opiates	SIADH
Didanosine (ddl)	Pancreatitis, peripheral neuropathy
Halogen anesthesia	Malignant hyperthermia
Succinylcholine	Malignant hyperthermia
Zidovudine (AZT)	Bone marrow suppression
Digitalis	Gastrointestinal disorders, vision changes, arrhythmias
Acetazolamide	Metabolic acidosis
Clozapine	Agranulocytosis
Selective serotonin reuptake inhibitors (e.g., fluoxetine)	Anxiety, agitation, insomnia, sexual dysfunction
Warfarin	Necrosis, teratogen
Niacin	Skin flushing, pruritus
HMG CoA reductase inhibitors (e.g., simvastatin)	Liver and muscle toxicity _Myalgias_
Ethambutol	Optic neuritis
Metronidazole	Disulfiram-like reaction with alcohol
Cisplatin	Nephrotoxicity
Methyldopa	Hemolytic anemia (Coombs test-positive)

2. **What are the side effects of diuretics?**
   Thiazide diuretics cause calcium retention, hyperglycemia, hyperuricemia, hyperlipidemia, hyponatremia, hypokalemic metabolic alkalosis, and hypovolemia; because they are sulfa drugs, watch out for sulfa allergy.
   Loop diuretics cause hypokalemic metabolic alkalosis, hypovolemia (more potent than thiazides), ototoxicity, and calcium excretion; with the exception of ethacrynic acid, they also are sulfa drugs.
   Carbonic anhydrase inhibitors cause metabolic acidosis. (_Mountain sickness_)
   Potassium-sparing diuretics (e.g. spironolactone) may cause hyperkalemia.

3. **What are the side effects of beta blockers?**
   Like many antihypertensive agents, beta blockers can cause sedation, depression, and sexual dysfunction. They also cause bradycardia and heart block in susceptible patients and should be avoided in patients with these conditions, as should central-acting calcium channel blockers

(e.g., verapamil and diltiazem). Beta blockers also can precipitate asthmatic attacks and mask the symptoms of hypoglycemia, thus they should be avoided or used with caution in asthmatics and those with COPD. A beta-1 selective beta-blocker (atenolol, metoprolol) or a combined beta and alpha blocker (carvedilol) is preferred if a beta blocker is needed to treat another condition such as heart disease. Use in diabetic patients requires an analysis of the risks and benefits; if other equivalent medications are available, use them instead.

4. **What class of antihypertensive agents is best known for severe, first-dose orthostatic hypotension?**
Alpha$_1$ antagonists.

5. **What antihypertensive is best known for causing depression?**
Methyldopa. Beta blockers may also cause depression.

6. **Cover the right-hand column and give the antidote(s) for overdose or toxic exposure to the drugs in the left-hand column.**

Poison or Medication	Antidote
Acetaminophen	Acetylcysteine
Cholinesterase inhibitors	Atropine, pralidoxime
Quinidine or tricyclic antidepressants	Sodium bicarbonate (cardioprotective)
Iron	Deferoxamine
Digoxin	Normalize potassium and other electrolytes; digoxin antibodies
Methanol/ethylene glycol	Ethanol
Benzodiazepines	Flumazenil
Beta blockers	Glucagon
Lead	Edetate (EDTA); use succimer in children
Iron toxicity	Deferoxamine
Copper or gold	Penicillamine
Opioids	Naloxone
Carbon monoxide	Oxygen (hyperbaric in cases of severe poisoning)
Muscarinic blockers	Physostigmine

7. **If the following medications are given at the same time, what may happen?**

Medications	Possible Effect of Simultaneous Administration
MAO inhibitor plus meperidine	Coma
Aminoglycoside plus loop diuretic	Enhanced ototoxicity
Thiazide plus lithium	Lithium toxicity
MAO inhibitor plus SSRI	Serotonin syndrome (hyperthermia, rigidity, myoclonus and autonomic instability)

MAO = monoamine oxidase; SSRI = serotonin specific reuptake inhibitor.

8. **What prophylactic medication should be given to contacts of a patient with neisserial meningitis?**
Rifampin, ciprofloxacin, ceftriaxone, or azithromycin.

9. **Name three medications that cause hepatic enzyme induction and two that cause hepatic enzyme inhibition.**
Barbiturates, antiepileptics, and rifampin are the classic enzyme inducers; cimetidine, erythromycin and ketoconazole are classic enzyme inhibitors. The end result may be ineffectiveness or toxicity of other administered drugs (e.g., warfarin, oral contraceptives, and antiepileptics).

10. **True or false: If a patient responds to placebo, a psychosomatic condition can be diagnosed.**
False. Response to placebo means only that the patient responded to placebo. Normal people with real diseases often have an improvement in symptoms with a placebo medication or treatment.

11. **Describe the mechanism of action for aspirin and other nonsteroidal anti-inflammatory drugs (NSAIDs). How do they differ?** ASA = irreversible.
Aspirin and other NSAIDs inhibit cyclooxygenase centrally and peripherally, an action that gives them anti-inflammatory, antipyretic, analgesic, and antiplatelet effects. The difference between aspirin and other NSAIDs is that aspirin binds to and inhibits cyclooxygenase *irreversibly*, whereas the cyclooxygenase inhibition of other NSAIDs is reversible. The net result of this difference is in platelets, which cannot make new cyclooxygenase. One dose of aspirin causes antiplatelet effects for the entire life of the platelet, whereas the antiplatelet effects of other NSAIDs last only for several hours.

12. **How is acetaminophen different from aspirin and other NSAIDs?**
Acetaminophen is thought to inhibit cyclooxygenase primarily in the brain; it does not act well in the periphery of the body. Thus it has analgesic and antipyretic effects but no antiplatelet or significant anti-inflammatory effects.

13. **What are the side effects and toxic effects of aspirin?**
Aspirin causes gastrointestinal upset and bleeding; it is the most important preventable risk factor for development of gastric ulcers. Always consider gastrointestinal bleeding and ulcers in any patient taking aspirin. In addition, aspirin can cause renal damage or aggravate gout. Toxic doses of aspirin can cause tinnitus, vertigo, respiratory alkalosis and metabolic acidosis, hyperthermia, coma, and death. Severe overdoses of aspirin can be removed by dialysis.

14. **What are the side effects of non-aspirin NSAIDs?**
NSAIDs also cause gastrointestinal upset, bleeding, and ulcers. Consider gastrointestinal bleeding and ulcer in all patients taking aspirin or other NSAIDs. NSAIDs also may cause renal damage (interstitial nephritis, acute tubular necrosis and/or papillary necrosis), especially in patients who take them chronically and have preexisting renal disease. Phenylbutazone can cause a fatal aplastic anemia/agranulocytosis and should not be used chronically.

15. **What two developments in NSAID therapy may reduce gastrointestinal and bleeding complications?**
New combinations of NSAIDs with prostaglandin E_1 and cyclooxygenase II inhibitors. Normal NSAIDs inhibit type I cyclooxygenase (in addition to type II), which is thought to be the main culprit in causing gastrointestinal problems. Prostaglandin E_1 protects the stomach by

supplying what NSAIDs take away. Cyclooxygenase II (COX-2) inhibitors avoid the problem altogether, but may not be as protective against GI bleeding as initially thought. Two of the three COX-2 inhibitors initially approved in the United States have been removed from the marked due to adverse cardiovascular effects.

16. **What happens with an overdose of acetaminophen?**

High doses of acetaminophen cause liver toxicity due to depletion of glutathione. Treat with **acetylcysteine** to decrease liver injury.

17. **What age group should not be given aspirin? What finding on physical exam is a contraindication to aspirin use?**

Children younger than 15 years of age (especially with a fever or viral infection) should not be given aspirin because of concern about causing Reye syndrome. Do not give aspirin to people with **nasal polyps** because hypersensitivity reactions involving an asthmatic attack are extremely common. People with asthma may have an asthma attack after aspirin even in the absence of nasal polyps.

18. **What is the relationship between aspirin and myocardial infarction?**

Low-dose aspirin has been proved to be of benefit in reducing the risk of myocardial infarction in both patients who have had a previous myocardial infarction and patients with stable or unstable angina who have not had an infarction. The 2008 American College of Chest Physicians (ACCP) clinical practice guidelines on antithrombotic and thrombolytic therapy recommends that all patients with chronic stable angina or other clinical or laboratory evidence of coronary artery disease receive aspirin indefinitely. There is strong medical literature support for the net benefit of aspirin for the primary prevention of first myocardial infarction in individuals at moderate to high risk. Aspirin is recommended in all diabetics with cardiovascular disease and for primary prevention in diabetics with one or more risk factors (e.g., age greater than 40 years, cigarette smoking, hypertension, hyperlipidemia, obesity, albuminuria, or family history of cardiovascular disease). The risks of aspirin prophylaxis may outweigh the benefits in patients with a history of liver disease, kidney disease, peptic ulcer disease or gastrointestinal bleeding, poorly controlled hypertension, or a bleeding disorder.

19. **Discuss the relationship between aspirin and strokes.**

Low-dose aspirin is of proven benefit in reducing strokes in patients with transient ischemic attacks (TIAs) and/or known carotid artery stenosis. That having been said, the risks may outweigh the benefits, as mentioned in the question above, especially in patients with uncontrolled hypertension, which, coupled with aspirin, can increase the risk of a hemorrhagic stroke.

20. **True or false: Patients should be given an aspirin as soon as possible in the emergency department for a suspected myocardial infarction or unstable angina.**

True, but beware the patient who presents with chest pain and ends up having an aortic dissection (aspirin should be avoided in such patients).

21. **True or false: In the setting of an acute neurologic deficit, you should give aspirin before ordering brain imaging.**

False. When patients present with an acute neurologic deficit, you do not know whether they are having a stroke or TIA. TIA is a retrospective diagnosis made once the symptoms clear. First you should order a computed tomography (CT) scan or MRI to rule out hemorrhagic stroke and potentially locate an area of infarct, which is a contraindication to aspirin. If the CT scan is negative for blood, the patient should be given aspirin 325 mg within 24 to 48 hours of TIA or stroke onset.

CHAPTER 31

PREVENTIVE MEDICINE

1. **Cover all but the left-hand column, and give the appropriate screening recommendations. Although other guidelines for cancer screening are in clinical use, the recommendations from the American Cancer Society (below) are a good guideline to use for the USMLE.**

Cancer	Procedure	Age	Frequency
Colorectal	Colonoscopy or	> 50 yrs for all studies	Every 10 years
	Flexible sigmoidoscopy or		Every 5 years
	Double contrast barium enema or		Every 5 years
	CT colonography or		Every 5 years
	Fecal occult blood test or		Annually
	Fecal immunochemical test or		Annually
	Stool DNA test		Interval uncertain
Colon, prostate	Digital rectal exam	> 40 yrs	Annually
Prostate	Prostate specific antigen test	> 50 yrs*	Controversial, but offer annually
Cervical	Pap smear	Within 3 years of onset of sexual activity or age 21, whichever comes first	If conventional Pap test is used, test annually; every 2–3 years for women ≥ 30 who have had three negative cytology tests. If Pap and HPV testing are used, then every 3 years if HPV negative and cytology negative.

(continued)

Cancer	Procedure	Age	Frequency
Gynecologic	Pelvic examination	21–64 yrs	Annually. Every 2–3 yrs after 3 normal exams.
		> 65 yrs	Annually. When to stop is not clearly established.
Endometrial	Endometrial biopsy	Menopause	No recommendation for routine screening.
Breast	Breast self-examination	> 20 yrs	Benefits and limitations should be discussed, but breast self examination is no longer recommended by the American Cancer Society.
Breast	Physical exam by doctor	20–40 yrs	Every 3 yrs
		> 40 yrs	Annually
Breast	Mammography	> 40 yrs	Annually
Lung	Sputum, chest x-ray, CT scan		Testing is not recommended for asymptomatic individuals, even if they are high-risk.

*Start at age 45 in African Americans and at age 40 for patients with a first degree relative diagnosed at an early age.

2. **True or false: Tumor markers are generally not used for cancer screening.**
True. Prostate-specific antigen is the exception to this rule. Alpha-fetoprotein (liver and testicular cancer), carcinoembryonic antigen (CEA), CA-125 and other serum markers are not appropriate for screening the general population. However, look for abnormal lab values to show up in questions as a clue to diagnosis.

3. **True or false: Urinalysis should not be used to screen the general population for bladder cancer.**
True. Screening with urinalysis for urinary tract cancer (which causes hematuria) is not recommended. However, look for persistent, painless hematuria as a clue that urinary tract cancer may be present.

4. **Cover the right-hand column and give the indications for each of the following vaccines in adults.**

Vaccine	Which Adults Should Receive and Other Information
Hepatitis B	Adolescents though 18 years of age and adults at increased risk of hepatitis B virus infection (children are vaccinated as well)
Influenza	Anyone who wants to reduce their chances of getting the flu can get vaccinated. It is recommended for people who are at high risk of having serious flu complications or people who live with or care for people at high risk for serious complications. People who should get vaccinated each year are children ages 6 months to 18 years, women who will be pregnant during the flu season, people who are immunosuppressed, adults ages 50 and over, people with chronic medical conditions (pulmonary, cardiovascular, renal, hepatic, hematologic, or metabolic disorders including diabetes), people who live in nursing homes and other long-term care facilities, health-care personnel, household contacts and caregivers of children younger than 5 years old and adults over age 50, and household contacts and caregivers for those at high risk of serious flu complications.
Pneumococcus	All adults 65 years of age and older; people ages 2 to 64 years with chronic cardiovascular disease, chronic pulmonary disease, or diabetes mellitus; people ages 2 to 64 years with functional or anatomic asplenia; people ages 2 to 64 years with alcoholism, chronic liver disease, or cerebrospinal fluid leak
Rubella	All women of child-bearing age who lack immunity or history of immunization. Do not give to pregnant women. Women should avoid pregnancy for 4 weeks after the vaccine. Also give to health care workers (to protect pregnant women's unborn children). Give to susceptible adolescents and adults without evidence of rubella immunity. Do not give to immunocompromised patients (except HIV-positive patients).
Tetanus	All people should be given a tetanus booster every 10 years. Give tetanus prophylaxis for any wound if vaccination history is unknown or patient has received less than 3 total doses. Give tetanus booster in people with full vaccination history if more than 5 years have passed since last dose for all wounds other than clean, minor wounds (including burns). Give tetanus immunoglobulin with vaccine for patients with unknown/incomplete vaccination and unclean or major wounds. Adults (ages 11 to 64) should receive a single dose of DTaP to replace a single dose of Td if they received their last dose of Td 10 or more years earlier. Adults who have or anticipate having close

(continued)

Vaccine	Which Adults Should Receive and Other Information
	contact with an infant younger than 12 months old should receive a single dose of DTaP. When possible, women should receive DTaP before conception. Pregnant women should receive DTaP in the immediate postpartum period. Healthcare workers should receive DTaP. DTaP is preferred to Td if prophylaxis is indicated for a wound. Adults 65 years of age and older should get Td (not DTaP) every 10 years.

5. **Define the following rates that are commonly seen on the USMLE.**

Rate	Definition
Birth rate	Live births/1000 population
Fertility rate	Live births/1000 population of women aged 15 to 45 years
Death rate	Deaths/1000 population
Neonatal mortality rate	Neonatal deaths (first 28 days of life)/1000 live births
Perinatal mortality rate	Neonatal deaths + stillbirths/1000 total births
Infant mortality rate	Deaths (from 0 to 1 year old)/1000 live births
Maternal mortality rate	Maternal pregnancy-related deaths (deaths while pregnant or in the first 42 days after delivery)/100,000 live births

6. **Define stillbirth.**
A stillbirth (fetal death) is defined as a prenatal or natal (during delivery) death after 20 weeks of gestation.

7. **Name the major cause of neonatal mortality. What is the neonatal mortality rate in the United States?**
The major cause of neonatal mortality is prematurity. The neonatal mortality rate in the United States is roughly 6/1000 (higher in blacks).

8. **List the top three causes of infant mortality in the United States.**
■ Congenital abnormalities
■ Prematurity/low birth weight
■ Sudden infant death syndrome

9. **List the top three causes of maternal mortality in the United States.**
■ Pulmonary embolus
■ Hypertension/pregnancy-induced hypertension (preeclampsia/eclampsia)
■ Hemorrhage
The rate increases with age and is higher among black women.

10. **What is the basic difference between Medicare and Medicaid?**

    Medicare is health insurance for people who are eligible for Social Security (primarily people older than 65 years as well as permanently or totally disabled people and people with end-stage renal disease). Nursing home fees are paid by Medicare only for a short time after a hospital admission; then they are paid by the patient. If the patient has no money, the state usually pays.

    Medicaid covers the indigent and poor who are deemed eligible according to the criteria of individual states.

CHAPTER 32

PSYCHIATRY

1. **What are the five main diagnostic criteria for schizophrenia?**
   1. Delusions
   2. Hallucinations
   3. Disorganized speech
   4. Grossly disorganized or catatonic behavior
   5. Negative symptoms (i.e., flat affect, avolition)

2. **Why is the duration of symptoms important with psychosis?**
   The time frame is important because, given the exact same symptoms, a patient is given one of three different diagnoses based only on their duration:
   - Less than 1 month = acute psychotic disorder
   - 1 to 6 months = schizophreniform disorder
   - More than 6 months = schizophrenia

3. **List the positive symptoms of schizophrenia.**
   - Delusions
   - Bizarre behavior
   - Hallucinations
   - Thought disorder (e.g., tangentiality, clanging)
   These symptoms respond well to all currently used antipsychotics.

4. **List the negative symptoms of schizophrenia.**
   - Flat affect
   - Anhedonia
   - Alogia (no speech)
   - Poor attention
   - Avolition (apathy) – unable to feel emotion
   These symptoms respond poorly to traditional antipsychotics (e.g., haloperidol) but may respond to "atypical" agents like risperidone, olanzapine, aripiprazole, paliperidone, quetiapine, or ziprasidone.

5. **What features of schizophrenia suggest a poor prognosis?**
   - Poor premorbid functioning (most important)
   - Family history of schizophrenia
   - Early onset
   - Negative symptoms
   - No precipitating factors
   - Poor support system
   - Single, divorced, or widowed status

6. **What features suggest a good prognosis?**
   - Good premorbid functioning (most important)
   - Family history of mood disorders

- Late onset
- Positive symptoms
- Obvious precipitating factors
- Good support system
- Married status

7. **What is the difference in age of onset for schizophrenia in males and females?**
The typical age of onset is 15 to 25 years for males (look for someone going to college and deteriorating) and 25 to 35 years for females.

8. **True or false: Roughly 1% of the population has schizophrenia in almost every country in the world.**
True.

9. **True or false: In the United States, most schizophrenic people are born in the summer months.**
False. Most schizophrenic patients in the United States are born in the winter (reason unknown).

10. **Roughly what percentage of patients with schizophrenia commit suicide?**
In the United States, roughly 10% of patients with schizophrenia eventually commit suicide (a past attempt is the best predictor of eventual success).

11. **True or false: Psychosocial treatment has been shown to improve outcome in schizophrenia.**
True. Antipsychotic medications are the mainstay of therapy, but psychosocial treatment has been shown to improve outcome. Medications are needed first, but the best treatment (as in most psychiatric illnesses) is medications plus therapy.

12. **Differentiate among the classes of antipsychotics drugs.**

	High Potency	Low Potency	Atypical Agents*
Prototype drug	Haloperidol	Chlorpromazine	Risperidone, olanzapine, aripiprazole, paliperidone, quetiapine, ziprasidone
EPS side effects	High incidence	Low incidence	Low incidence
ANS side effects[†]	Low incidence	High incidence	Medium incidence
Positive symptoms	Works well	Works well	Works well
Negative symptoms	Works poorly	Works poorly	Works fairly well

EPS = extrapyramidal system; ANS = autonomic nervous system.
*Atypical, newer antipsychotics are generally first-line treatment and maintenance therapy due to reduced extrapyramidal side effects and efficacy with negative symptoms. Choose them over older agents.
[†]ANS side effects include anticholinergic effects (dry mouth, urinary retention, blurry vision, mydriasis), alpha₁ blockade (orthostatic hypotension), and antihistamine effects (sedation).

13. **What are the four commonly tested extrapyramidal side effects of antipsychotics?**

Acute dystonias, akathisia, parkinsonism, and tardive dyskinesia.

14. **Define acute dystonia. How is it treated?**

Acute dystonia is an extrapyramidal movement disorder that occurs in the first few hours or days of treatment. Patients develop muscle spasms or stiffness (e.g., torticollis, trismus), tongue protrusions and twisting, opisthotonos, and/or oculogyric crisis (forced sustained deviation of the head and eyes). Acute dystonia is most common in young men. Treat with antihistamines (e.g., diphenhydramine) or anticholinergics (e.g., benztropine, trihexyphenidyl).

15. **Define akathisia.**

Akathisia occurs in the first few days of treatment. The patient has a subjective feeling of restlessness and may pace constantly, alternate sitting and standing, and be unable to sit still. Beta blockers can be tried for treatment.

16. **Describe the relationship between antipsychotics and parkinsonism.**

Parkinsonism usually occurs in patients taking antipsychotics within the first few months of treatment. Parkinsonism is thought to develop because of dopamine depletion whereas psychosis is thought to develop because of too much dopamine in the brain (a gross oversimplification). Thus, antipsychotics create an iatrogenic lowering of effective dopamine in the brain by blocking dopamine receptors. The patient develops stiffness, cogwheel rigidity, shuffling gait, mask-like facies, and drooling. Parkinsonism is most common in older women. Treat with antihistamines (e.g., diphenhydramine) or anticholinergics (e.g., benztropine, trihexyphenidyl).

17. **Define tardive dyskinesia. When does it occur?**

Tardive dyskinesia appears after years of treatment with antipsychotics. Most commonly, the patient develops perioral movements (darting, protruding movements of the tongue, chewing, grimacing, and puckering). The patient also may have involuntary, choreoathetoid movements of the head, limbs and trunk. There is no known treatment for tardive dyskinesia. If you are asked to make a choice when the patient develops tardive dyskinesia, discontinue the current antipsychotic and consider switching to a second generation agent (e.g., clozapine, risperidone).

18. **What is neuroleptic malignant syndrome? How do you recognize and treat it?**

Neuroleptic malignant syndrome is a life-threatening condition that can occur at any time during antipsychotic treatment. Patients classically develop rigidity, mutism, obtundation, agitation, high fever (up to 107° F), very high levels of creatine phosphokinase (more than 10 times the normal range), sweating, and myoglobinuria. Treat first by discontinuing the antipsychotic; then give supportive care for fever and potential renal shutdown due to myoglobinuria (primarily IV fluids). Lastly, consider dantrolene (just as in malignant hyperthermia, which is thought to be a similar condition). muscle relaxer

19. **Describe the relationship between antipsychotics and prolactin.**

Dopamine blockade causes increases in prolactin levels because dopamine is a prolactin-inhibiting factor in the tuberoinfundibular tract of the brain. The end result may be high serum prolactin levels, resulting in **galactorrhea** and impotence, menstrual dysfunction, and/or decreased libido.

20. **What are the classic side effects of thioridazine, chlorpromazine, and clozapine?**
    - Thioridazine: retinal pigment deposits
    - Clozapine: agranulocytosis (white blood cell counts must be monitored)
    - Chlorpromazine: jaundice and photosensitivity

21. **What are the side effects of the atypical antipsychotics?** *Ziprasidone/ aripiprazole - least likely to cause metabolic syn*
    - Olanzapine: weight gain, sedation, hypotension, dry mouth.
    - Quetiapine: sedation, orthostatic hypotension, akathisia, weight gain, dry mouth
    - Ziprasidone: nausea, weakness, mild QT prolongation
    - Aripiprazole: headache, nausea, akathisia, tremor, constipation
    - Paliperidone: parkinsonism, dystonia, dyskinesia, akathisia, QT prolongation *EPS Sx*
    - Clozapine: orthostatic hypotension, weight gain, metabolic syndrome, sedation, constipation, *agranulocytosis*

22. **Define bipolar disorder. What are the classic symptoms?**
    Mania is the only criterion required for a diagnosis of bipolar disorder, but a history of or future episodes of depression are classically present. Classic symptoms of mania include decreased need for sleep, pressured speech, sexual promiscuity, shopping sprees, and an exaggerated self-importance or delusions of grandeur. Look for initial onset between 16 and 30 years old.
    DIG FAST

23. **How is bipolar disorder treated?**
    Both lithium and valproic acid are mood stabilizers and first-line agents. Typical antipsychotics (haloperidol) atypical antipsychotics (risperidone, quetiapine, clozapine, ziprasidone, and aripiprazole), carbamazepine, and gabapentin are second line agents. Antipsychotics or antidepressants may be needed if the patient becomes psychotic or depressed; use at the same time as the mood stabilizer.

24. **What are the side effects of lithium, valproic acid, and carbamazepine?**
    - Lithium: renal dysfunction (diabetes insipidus), thyroid dysfunction, tremor, and central nervous system (CNS) effects at toxic levels *acne*
    - Valproic acid: liver dysfunction
    - Carbamazepine: bone marrow suppression

25. **Define bipolar II disorder and cyclothymia.**
    Bipolar II disorder is hypomania (mild mania without psychosis that does not cause occupational dysfunction) plus major depression. Cyclothymia is at least 2 years of hypomania alternating with depressed mood, but there are *no* full-blown episodes of mania or major depression.
    Bipolar 1 = mood + hypomania

26. **List the major risk factors for suicide.**
    - Age greater than 45 years
    - Prior psychiatric history
    - Alcohol or substance abuse
    - Depression
    - History of rage or violence
    - Recent loss or separation
    - Prior suicide attempts
    - Loss of health
    - Male gender (men commit suicide three times more often than women, but women attempt it four times more often than men)
    - Unemployed or retired status
    - Single, widowed, or divorced status

27. **What is the best predictor of future suicide?**
A past attempt.

28. **True or false: Be careful in asking about suicide because you may plant the idea in the patient's head.**
False. Always ask a patient about suicidal thoughts; it does not make them more likely to commit suicide. If necessary, you should temporarily hospitalize an acutely suicidal patient against his or her will.

29. **True or false: When patients are just emerging from a deep depression, they are at an increased risk of suicide.**
True. When the antidepressant begins to work, the patient gets a little more energy—possibly just enough to carry out a suicide plan.

30. **True or false: The highest suicide rates are in people aged 15 to 24 years.**
False. Suicide rates are rising most rapidly in 15 to 24 year olds, but the greatest absolute risk is in people over age the age of 65. *2nd mcc death 15-24*

31. **True or false: Patients with depression often do not complain about it directly.**
True. Patients often do not come out and say, "I'm depressed." You must watch for the clues: change in sleep habits (classically insomnia), vague somatic complaints, anxiety, low energy or fatigue, change in appetite (classically decreased appetite), poor concentration, psychomotor retardation, and/or anhedonia (loss of pleasure). The history may or may not reveal obvious precipitating factors, such as loss of loved one, divorce or separation, unemployment or retirement, or chronic or debilitating disease. *SIG E CAPS*

32. **How do you treat depression?**
As with most psychiatric illnesses, the treatment of choice is both medications (antidepressants) and psychotherapy. The combination is more effective than medications alone. Serotonin-specific reuptake inhibitors (SSRIs) usually are the preferred first-line agents. Other options include serotonin-norepinephrine reuptake inhibitors (SNRIs), and the tricyclic antidepressants. Bupropion and mirtazapine have unique modes of action. *Wellbutrin Remeron*

33. **Is depression more common in males or females?**
Depression is more common in females.

34. **What is an adjustment disorder with depressed mood?**
A diagnosis that you must be able to distinguish from major depression. With adjustment disorder, a patient goes through a normal life experience (e.g., relationship break-up, failing grade, loss of job) but does not handle it well. There is marked distress that is in excess of what would be expected from exposure to the stressor or causes significant impairment in social or occupational functioning. Although patients may have a depressed mood, they do not meet the criteria for full-blown major depression. For example, a woman divorces her husband, seems to cry a lot for the next few weeks, and leaves work early on most days. Or a high-school boy doesn't make the basketball team and mopes around the house, crying and not wanting to go to school or out with his friends for a few weeks.

35. **Define dysthymia.**
Dysthymia is a depressed mood on most days for more than 2 years without episodes of major depression, mania/hypomania, or psychosis. *Will have same sx → varying levels of severity.*

36. **True or false: Antidepressants can trigger mania or hypomania.**
True—especially in bipolar patients.

37. How do tricyclic antidepressants work? What are their side effects?

Tricyclic antidepressants (e.g., nortriptyline, amitriptyline) prevent reuptake of norepinephrine and serotonin. They also block alpha-adrenergic receptors (watch for orthostatic hypotension, dizziness, or falls) and muscarinic receptors (watch for anticholinergic effects, such as dry mouth, blurred vision, constipation, and urinary retention), cause sedation (antihistamine effect), and lower the seizure threshold (especially bupropion, which technically is not a tricyclic). Tricyclic antidepressants are dangerous in overdose primarily because of **cardiac arrhythmias**, which may respond to bicarbonate.

38. How do selective serotonin reuptake inhibitors (SSRIs) work? Why are they preferred over tricyclics?

SSRIs (e.g., fluoxetine, citalopram, paroxetine, sertraline, fluvoxamine, and escitalopram) prevent reuptake of serotonin only. They have less serious side effects (insomnia, anorexia, jitteriness, headache, sexual dysfunction) and are not dangerous with overdose. Tricyclics used to be the number-one cause of prescription drug overdose in the United States.

39. How do serotonin-norepinephrine reuptake inhibitors (SNRIs) work?

SNRIs (e.g., venlafaxine, duloxetine, desvenlafaxine) prevent reuptake of serotonin and norepinephrine. The side effects of SNRIs are similar to those of SSRIs but also include noradrenergic symptoms, such as sweating and dizziness.

40. What are monoamine oxidase (MAO) inhibitors? Describe their side effects.

MAO inhibitors (e.g., phenelzine, tranylcypromine) are older medications that are not used as first-line agents for treatment of depression. They may be good for atypical depression (look for hypersomnia and hyperphagia—the opposite of classic depression) that fails to respond to other agents. When patients taking MAO inhibitors eat tyramine-containing foods (especially wine and cheese), they may get a hypertensive crisis. Do *not* give MAO inhibitors at the same time as SSRIs or meperidine; severe reactions can occur, possibly even death.

41. What is the most notorious side effect of trazodone?

Priapism (persistent, painful erection in the absence of sexual desire that may lead to permanent impotence if not treated).

42. Distinguish between normal grief and pathologic grief (i.e., depression).

Initial grief after a loss (e.g., death of a loved one) may include a state of shock, feeling of numbness or bewilderment, distress, crying, sleep disturbances, decreased appetite, difficulty in concentrating, weight loss, and guilt (survivor guilt) for up to 1 year—in other words, the same symptoms as depression. It is normal to have an illusion or hallucination about the deceased, but a normal grieving person knows that it is an illusion, whereas a depressed person believes that it is real. Intense yearning (even years after the death) and even searching for the deceased are normal. Feelings of worthlessness, psychomotor retardation, and suicidal ideation are not signs of normal grief; they are signs of depression.

43. How do you recognize and treat panic disorder?

Panic disorder classically affects 20- to 40-year-old patients, who often think that they are dying or having a heart attack, although in fact they are healthy and have a negative work-up for organic disease. Patients often hyperventilate and are extremely anxious. Remember the association between panic disorder and agoraphobia (fear of leaving the house). Treat with SSRIs (e.g., fluoxetine), which are favored over benzodiazepines.

44. What is generalized anxiety disorder? How is it treated?

Patients with generalized anxiety disorder worry about everything (e.g., career, family, future, relationships, and money) at the same time. Symptoms are not as dramatic as in panic disorder; the patient is simply a severe worrier. Treat with cognitive behavioral therapy and medications: buspirone (nonaddictive, nonsedating but slow onset of action), SSRIs (especially if depressive symptoms coexist), or benzodiazepines (addictive, sedating).

45. Give the classic examples of simple phobias. How are they treated?
Classic examples of simple phobias include fear of needles, blood products, animals, and heights. Treat with behavioral therapy, including flooding (sudden, intense exposure to feared object without chance for escape), systematic desensitization (gradual increase in intensity and type of exposure until the person is comfortable with intense exposure to feared object), and biofeedback (control autonomic variables like heart rate during anxiety-inducing maneuvers).

46. What is social phobia?
Social phobia, also known as social anxiety disorder, is a specific type of simple phobia (fear of social situations) that is best treated with behavioral therapy. Beta blockers may be used before a public appearance that cannot be avoided to reduce symptoms and SSRIs are increasingly being used as a primary treatment, though SNRIs and benzodiazepines also may be used.

don't use BB in asthma, COPD.

47. How do you recognize and treat posttraumatic stress disorder?
Look for someone who has been through a life-threatening event (e.g., war, severe accident, rape) repeatedly experiences the event (nightmares, flashbacks), and tries to avoid thinking about it. As a result, patients have depression or poor concentration. Treat with peer group therapy; if you have to choose a medication, use an antidepressant, usually an SSRI.

eye movement desens. EMDR.

48. True or false: Homosexuality is not considered a psychiatric disorder.
True. Homosexuality and homosexual experimentation are not considered a disease at any age; they are normal variants. Having kinky fantasies and occasionally doing kinky things (a man wearing women's underwear, mild foot fetish) also are considered normal.

49. Explain the concept of somatoform disorders.
A patient with somatoform disorder experiences psychiatric stress and expresses it through physical symptoms. Patients do not do so on purpose. *unconscious*

Somatoform / conversion d/o

50. Describe the four major somatoform disorders.
Somatization disorder: the patient has multiple different complaints in multiple different organ systems over many years and has had extensive work-ups in the past.
Conversion disorder: the patient has an obvious precipitating factor (e.g., fight with boyfriend), then develops unexplainable neurologic symptoms (e.g., blindness, stocking-glove numbness).
Hypochondriasis: the patient continues to believe that he or she has a disease despite extensive negative work-up. *fear of having ds.*
Body dysmorphic disorder: the patient is preoccupied with an imagined physical defect; for example, a teenager who thinks that his or her nose is too big when it is normal size.

51. How are somatoform disorders treated?
Treat all somatoform disorders with frequent return visits to the clinic and/or psychotherapy. Screen for and treat any coexisting depression.

52. Distinguish among somatoform disorders, factitious disorders, and malingering.
In **somatoform disorders,** the patient does not intentionally create symptoms (unconscious process). In **factitious disorders,** patients intentionally create an illness or symptoms (e.g., they inject insulin to create hypoglycemia) and subject themselves to procedures in

order to assume the role of a patient (no financial or other secondary gain). In **malingering,** patients intentionally create their illness for secondary gain (e.g., money, release from work or jail).

53. **How do you recognize dissociative fugue (also called psychogenic fugue or fugue state)?**
Dissociative fugue is a reversible amnesia for personal identity including the memories, personality, and other identifying characteristics of individuality. It usually involves unplanned travel or wandering. There is complete amnesia for the fugue episode. The classic patient develops amnesia, travels, and assumes a new identity, but does remember the event upon returning.

54. **What psychiatric disorder is most likely to be associated with childhood sexual abuse?**
Multiple personality disorder (now known as dissociative identity disorder).

55. **Define personality disorders.**
Personality disorders are lifelong disorders that affect the way in which a person interacts with the world. Look for a history dating back to childhood or teenage years. No real treatment is available, although psychotherapy can be tried.

56. **Give a one- or two-sentence description of each of the following ten personality disorders below.**
Paranoid: Patients are paranoid and think that everyone (friends, too) is out to get them; they often start law suits.
Schizoid: Patients are classic loners who have no friends and no interest in having friends.
Schizotypal: Patients have bizarre beliefs (cults, superstition, or illusions) and manner of speaking but no psychosis.
Avoidant: Patients have no friends but want them; they avoid others out of fear of criticism and rejection (inferiority complex).
Histrionic: Patients are overly dramatic, attention-seeking, and inappropriately seductive; they must be the center of attention.
Narcissistic: Patients are egocentric, lack empathy, and use others for their own gain; they have a sense of entitlement.
Antisocial: The most frequently tested personality disorder. Patients have long criminal records (e.g., con men) and tortured animals or set fires as children. A history of pediatric conduct disorder is required for this diagnosis. Patients are aggressive and do not pay their bills or support their children. They are liars and have no remorse or conscience. Antisocial personality disorder has a strong association with alcoholism, drug abuse, and somatization disorder. Most patients are male.
Borderline: Patients have unstable moods, behaviors, relationships (many are bisexual), and self-image. Look for splitting; that is, people are all good or all bad and may frequently change categories. Other clues include suicide attempts, micropsychotic episodes (2 minutes of psychosis), impulsiveness, and constant crisis.
Dependent: Patients cannot be or do anything alone. A wife may stay with her abusive husband despite continued abuse.
Obsessive-compulsive: Patients are obsessed with rules, perfection, and organization. They may seem anal-retentive and stubborn. Rules are more important than objectives. Affect is restricted. Money is a frequent concern and is often hoarded.

57. **Define obsessive-compulsive disorder. How is it treated?**
Obsessive-compulsive disorder describes patients with recurrent thoughts or impulses (obsessions) or recurrent behaviors or actions (compulsions) that cause marked dysfunction

in their occupational and/or interpersonal lives. It is not the same as obsessive-compulsive personality disorder. Look for washing rituals (washing of hands 30 times per day) or checking rituals (checking to see if the door is locked 30 times per day). The onset usually is in adolescence or early adulthood. Treat with SSRIs or clomipramine and psychotherapy. Behavioral therapy (e.g., flooding) also may be effective.

58. **True or false: Some psychiatric patients can be hospitalized against their will.**

True. Patients can be hospitalized against their will if they are a danger to themselves (suicidal or unable to take care of themselves) or others (homicidal).

59. **Describe the hallmark findings of narcolepsy. How is it treated?**

Narcolepsy is a sleep disorder characterized by daytime sleepiness in spite of a normal daily sleep regimen. Patients have decreased latency for rapid-eye-movement (REM) sleep (patients go into REM as soon as they fall asleep); cataplexy (random loss of muscle tone that causes patients to fall down); and hallucinations as they awaken (hypnopompic) or fall asleep (hypnagogic). Treat with modafinil (a non-amphetamine stimulant), methylphenidate, or amphetamines.

60. **What is the difference between objective and subjective psychological tests?**

Objective tests are generally multiple-choice tests that are scored by a computer; the classic example is the IQ test. **Subjective tests** have no "right" answers and are scored by the test-giver (the classic example is the Rorschach test).

61. **Characterize each of the following psychological tests as objective or subjective and briefly describe its use:**

Name of Test	Description
Stanford-Binet	Objective IQ test for adults
Wechsler Intelligence Scale for Children	Objective IQ test for children (4–17 years old)
Rorschach test	Subjective test in which patients describe what they see in an inkblot
Thematic Apperception Test	Subjective test in which the patient describes what is going on in a cartoon drawing of people
Beck Depression Inventory	Objective test to look for depression
Minnesota Multiphasic Personality Inventory	Objective test to measure personality type
Halstead-Reitan Battery	Objective test used to determine the location and effects of specific brain lesions
Luria-Nebraska Neuropsychological Battery	Objective test that assesses many cognitive functions as well as cerebral dominance (left or right)

Note: Psychological tests can be used to aid in a difficult diagnosis; they are not used or needed for a straightforward case.

Blessed questionnaire – for family members about depression

62. **True or false: Roughly 85% of cases of mental retardation are mild.**
True. Patients with mild mental retardation can have a reasonable level of independence, with assistance or guidance during periods of stress.

63. **What are the common causes of mental retardation?**
Although mental retardation is usually idiopathic, look for fetal alcohol syndrome (the number-one preventable cause of mental retardation), Down syndrome (number-one overall known cause of mental retardation), and fragile X syndrome (in males).

64. **How do you recognize autism?**
Autism usually starts at a very young age. Look for impaired social interaction (isolative, unaware of surroundings), impaired verbal and nonverbal communication (strange words, babbling, repetition), and restricted activities and interests (head banging, strange movements). Autism can be thought of as a spectrum of disorders in which patients may range from very highly functioning (e.g., Asperger syndrome) to severely mentally retarded. Most individuals with autism manifest some degree of mental retardation, which typically is moderate in severity.
No single cause has been identified for the development of autism. Genetic origins are suspected by twin studies and an increased incidence among siblings. Possible contributing factors include fetal alcohol exposure, infections (congenital rubella infection), other perinatal factors, or immunologic causes.

65. **What is a learning disorder?**
Learning disorders describe isolated impairment in math, reading, writing, speech, language, or coordination. All other skills are normal; no mental retardation is present (e.g., "Johnny just can't do math").

66. **Define conduct disorder. With what adult disorder is it associated?**
Conduct disorder is the pediatric form of **antisocial personality disorder.** Look for fire setting, cruelty to animals, lying, stealing, and/or fighting. As adults, patients often have antisocial disorder. **Note:** Conduct disorder as a child is required for a diagnosis of antisocial personality disorder in adults.

67. **Define attention-deficit/hyperactivity disorder (ADHD)**
As the name implies, patients are hyperactive and have short attention spans. ADHD is more common in males than females. Look for a fidgety child who is impulsive and cannot pay attention, but is not cruel. Treat with stimulants (paradoxical calming effect) such as methylphenidate (Ritalin) or an amphetamine, either of which may cause insomnia, abdominal pain, anorexia, weight loss, and growth suppression.

68. **Describe the behavior of a child who has oppositional-defiant disorder.**
The child displays negative, hostile, and defiant behavior toward authority figures (e.g., parents, teachers). He or she is a pain in the butt around adults but behaves normally around peers and is not a cruel, lying criminal.

69. **Give the classic description of children with separation anxiety disorder.**
Affected children refuse to go to school. Basically, they think that something will happen to them or their parents if they separate. They will do anything to avoid separation (e.g., stomach ache, headache, temper tantrum).

70. **How do you recognize anorexia?**
Classic is a female adolescent who is a good athlete or student with a perfectionistic personality. Three criteria are required for the diagnosis: (1) body weight at least 15% below

normal; (2) intense fear of gaining weight or "feeling fat" despite emaciation; and (3) amenorrhea. Roughly 10% to 15% of patients die from complications of starvation or coexisting bulimia (electrolyte imbalances, cardiac arrhythmias, infections). Though more "positive" therapies are preferred, patients sometimes need to be hospitalized against their wills for intravenous nutrition. Roughly one-half of patients with anorexia also have bulimia.

SSRI's, Behavioral tx, Olanzapine (refractory)

71. **Define bulimia. What are the classic findings of the mouth and fingers?**
Bulimic patients have binge-eating episodes, during which they feel a lack of control, and then engage in purging behavior (vomiting, laxatives, exercise, fasting). Those affected are typically normal weight or overweight (unless coexisting anorexia is present) adolescent females. Patients may require hospitalization for electrolyte disturbances. Classic findings include eroded tooth enamel due to frequent vomiting and eroded skin over the knuckles from putting fingers in the throat.

72. **Describe Tourette syndrome. How is it treated?** *motor + vocal tics*
Tourette syndrome is a motor tic disorder (eye-blinking, grunting, throat-clearing, grimacing, barking, or shoulder shrugging) that is exacerbated by stress and remits during activity or sleep. Although part of the classic description, coprolalia (swearing) affects only 10% to 30% of patients. Males are affected more often than females. Of interest, Tourette syndrome can be caused or unmasked by the use of stimulants (e.g., for presumed ADHD). Antipsychotics (haloperidol) can be used if the symptoms are severe. Tourette syndrome tends to be a life-long problem. *tx: atypical anti-psychotic, pimozide, clonidine* *Pimozide*

73. **True or false: A diagnosis of encopresis or enuresis cannot be made before a certain age.**
True. Encopresis is normal until age 4 and enuresis is normal until age 5. This diagnostic point is obviously important when the parent complains, because both are normal findings in a 3-year-old child. Rule out physical problems (e.g., Hirschsprung disease, urinary tract infection), then treat with behavioral therapy ("gold-star for being good" charts, alarms, biofeedback). Desmopressin and imipramine may be used for refractory cases of enuresis.

74. **True or false: Depression in children frequently presents as an irritable rather than a depressed mood.**
True.

75. **What are the three leading causes of death in adolescents?**
Accidents, homicide, and suicide. Together they cause about 75% of teenage deaths.

76. **What is the most commonly abused illicit drug? Describe its effects on users.**
Marijuana. Watch for a teenager who listens to rock music, has red eyes, and acts "weird." Other symptoms include amotivational syndrome (chronic use results in laziness and lack of motivation), time distortion, and "munchies" (eating binges during intoxication). No physical symptoms have been reported with withdrawal, but psychological cravings may be present. Marijuana is not dangerous in overdose (although patients may experience temporary dysphoria) and is a controversial teratogen (evidence weak).

77. **What symptoms are associated with cocaine intoxication? Cocaine withdrawal?**
Cocaine causes sympathetic stimulation (insomnia, tachycardia, mydriasis, hypertension, sweating) with hyperalertness and possible paranoia, aggressiveness, delirium, psychosis, or formications ("cocaine bugs"; patients think that bugs are crawling on them). Overdose can be fatal as a result of arrhythmia, myocardial infarction, seizure, or stroke. On withdrawal the patient is sleepy, hungry (vs. anorexic with intoxication), and irritable with possible severe

depression. Cocaine withdrawal is not dangerous, but psychological cravings usually are severe. Cocaine is teratogenic, causing vascular disruptions in the fetus.

78. **Describe the symptoms of amphetamine intoxication.**
Amphetamines are longer acting and associated more commonly with psychotic symptoms (patients may appear to be full-blown schizophrenics), but basically their effects are similar to those of cocaine.

79. **Describe the effects of opioids. What symptoms are seen in withdrawal?**
Heroin and other opioids cause euphoria, analgesia, drowsiness, miosis, constipation, and CNS depression. Overdoses can be fatal because of respiratory depression, which should be treated with naloxone. Because the drug often is taken intravenously, associated morbidity and mortality include endocarditis, HIV infection, hepatitis, cellulitis, and talc damage. Withdrawal is not life-threatening, but patients act as though they are going to die. Symptoms include gooseflesh, diarrhea, insomnia, and abdominal cramping, and pain. Methadone or buprenorphine can be used to reduce acute withdrawal symptoms. *clonidine also*

80. **How do you recognize intoxication with lysergic acid diethylamide (LSD) or hallucinogenic mushrooms?**
Symptoms of intoxication with LSD or mushrooms include hallucinations (usually visual vs. auditory in schizophrenia), mydriasis, tachycardia, diaphoresis, and perception and mood disturbances. Neither is dangerous in overdose—unless the patient thinks that he or she can fly and jumps out a window. No withdrawal symptoms or teratogenic effects have been reported. Users may experience "flashbacks" (brief feelings of being on the drug again even though none was taken) months to years later or a "bad trip" (acute panic reaction or dysphoria), which should be treated with reassurance or a benzodiazepine or antipsychotic, if needed.

81. **What about phencyclidine (PCP) intoxication?** *horizontal nystagmus*
PCP intoxication causes LSD/mushroom symptoms plus confusion, agitation, and aggressive behavior. Also look for vertical and/or horizontal nystagmus, possible schizophrenic-like symptoms (e.g., paranoia, auditory hallucinations, disorganized behavior and speech). Overdose can be fatal because of convulsions, coma, and respiratory arrest. Treat with supportive care and urine acidification to hasten elimination. No withdrawal symptoms have been reported.

82. **Describe the symptoms and signs of inhalant intoxication. Who is likely to abuse inhalants?**
Inhalant intoxication (e.g., gasoline, glue, varnish remover) causes euphoria, dizziness, slurred speech, a feeling of floating, ataxia, or a sense of heightened power. It usually is seen in younger teenagers (11 to 15 years old), because these substances are cheap, legal to buy, and readily available. Inhalants can be fatal in overdose as a result of respiratory depression, cardiac arrhythmias, or asphyxiation and may cause severe permanent sequelae (CNS, liver or kidney toxicity, peripheral neuropathy). There is no known withdrawal syndrome.

tx = abstinence

83. **True or false: Benzodiazepines and barbiturates can be fatal in overdose but not in withdrawal.**
False. Both can be fatal in overdose and withdrawal.

84. **Describe the symptoms and signs of benzodiazepine or barbiturate intoxication.**
Benzodiazepines and barbiturates cause sedation and drowsiness as well as disinhibition and reduced anxiety. They can be fatal in overdose as a result of respiratory depression;

treat overdoses of a benzodiazepine with **flumazenil.** In withdrawal, death may result from seizures and/or cardiovascular collapse. Treat withdrawal on an inpatient basis with a long-acting benzodiazepine, and gradually taper the dose over several days. Benzodiazepines and barbiturates are especially dangerous when mixed with alcohol because all three are CNS depressants. *respiratory depressants*

85. **What are the symptoms of caffeine withdrawal?**
Headaches and fatigue.

86. **What is the basic rule of thumb about the difference in symptoms between intoxication and withdrawal for the same drug?**
The symptoms are usually the opposite of each other. For example, stimulants (e.g., cocaine, amphetamines) cause insomnia with intoxication and hypersomnolence in withdrawal, whereas depressants (e.g., alcohol, benzodiazepines, and barbiturates) cause sedation with intoxication and insomnia in withdrawal.

1. **Describe the difference between obstructive and restrictive pulmonary disease on pulmonary function testing.**

   In chronic obstructive pulmonary disease (COPD), the functional expiratory volume in one second divided by the total forced vital capacity (FEV_1/FVC) is less than normal (the normal value [0.75 to 0.80] should be given in the question). In restrictive lung disease, FEV_1/FVC is often normal. FEV_1 may be equal in both conditions, but the ratio of FEV_1/FVC is always different.

2. **What causes emphysema?**

   Emphysema is almost always due to smoking (even second-hand smoke). If you have a young person with minimal smoke exposure (fewer than 5 years), then think of alpha$_1$-antitrypsin deficiency.

3. **How do you recognize and treat asthma?**

   Watch for chronic wheezing in "allergic" children with a family history of asthma or allergies. In the acute setting, treat with beta$_2$ agonists. Use steroids if the attack is severe or does not respond to beta$_2$ agonists. Inhaled glucocorticoids, long-acting beta-agonists, leukotriene modifiers (zafirlukast, zileuton), and cromolyn are prophylactic agents and are not used for acute attacks. Phosphodiesterase inhibitors (theophylline, aminophylline) are older agents that are now infrequently used. Do *not* prescribe beta blockers for asthmatics or patients with COPD; they block the beta$_2$ receptors that are needed to open the airways.

4. **What is a common cause of wheezing in children under age 2 years?**

   Respiratory syncytial virus (RSV) infection, which classically occurs in the winter and causes a fever. Asthma also may be the cause but usually is associated with a chronic history.

5. **What should you think if a patient with acute asthma stops hyperventilating or has a normal carbon dioxide (CO_2) level?**

   Beware the asthmatic who is no longer hyperventilating or whose CO_2 is normal or rising. The patient should be hyperventilating, which causes low CO_2. If the patient seems calm or sleepy, do *not* assume that he or she is "okay." Such patients probably are crashing; they need an immediate arterial blood gas analysis and possible intubation. Fatigue alone is sufficient reason to intubate. Remember also that any patient with COPD may normally live with a higher CO_2 and lower oxygen (O_2) level. Treat the patient, not the lab value. If the patient is asymptomatic and talking to you, the lab value should not cause panic.

6. **When should you intubate?**

   As a rough rule of thumb, think about intubation in any patient whose CO_2 is more than 50 mmHg or whose O_2 is less than 50 mmHg, especially if the pH in either situation is less than 7.30 while the patient is breathing room air. Usually, unless the patient is crashing rapidly, a trial of oxygen by nasal cannula or face mask is given first. If it does not work or if the patient becomes too tired (use of accessory muscles is a good clue to the work of breathing), intubate. Clinical correlation is always required; patients with chronic lung disease may be asymptomatic at lab value levels that seem to defy reason. Alternatively, lab values may look great, but if the patient is becoming tired from increased work of breathing, intubation may be needed.

7. **What should you do if a patient has a solitary pulmonary nodule on chest radiograph?**
The first step is to compare the current film with old films (if available). If the lesion has not changed in more than 2 to 3 years, it is very likely to be benign. A nodule that has increased in size on serial imaging should be biopsied or excised. CT scans are used to evaluate and follow a solitary pulmonary nodule. A nodule that has a low probability of being malignant can be followed with serial CT scans. PET scan is used to evaluate intermediate probability nodules. A nodule that has a high probability of being malignant should be excised.

8. **What classic clues on the Step 2 exam point to the cause of a solitary pulmonary nodule?**
■ Immigrant: think of tuberculosis; do a skin test.
■ Southwest United States exposure: think of *Coccidioides immitis*
■ Cave explorer, exposure to bird droppings or Ohio/Mississippi River valleys (Midwest): think of histoplasmosis.
■ Smoker over the age of 50: think of lung cancer; order bronchoscopy and biopsy.
■ Person under 40 with none of the previous: think of hamartoma.

9. **What should you know about pulmonary function in the setting of surgery?**
A baseline chest radiograph is not part of the standard preoperative evaluation, but is often used for patients over age 60 or patients with known pulmonary or cardiovascular disease. Preoperative pulmonary function testing is somewhat controversial, and the question probably will not appear on Step 2. Overall, the best indicator of possible postoperative pulmonary complications is preoperative pulmonary function. The best way to reduce pulmonary complications postoperatively is to **stop smoking** preoperatively, especially if it is stopped at least 8 weeks prior to surgery. Aggressive pulmonary toilet, incentive spirometry, minimal narcotics, and early ambulation help to prevent or minimize postoperative pulmonary complications. Lastly, remember that the most common cause of a postoperative fever in the first 24 hours is atelectasis.

10. **How do you recognize and treat adult respiratory distress syndrome (ARDS)?** $PaO_2/FiO_2 < 200$ $PCWP < 18$
ARDS results from acute lung injury and causes noncardiogenic pulmonary edema, respiratory distress, and hypoxemia. Common causes are sepsis, major trauma, pancreatitis, shock, near- drowning, and drug overdose. Look for ARDS to develop within 24 to 48 hours of the initial insult. The classic patient has mottled/cyanotic skin, intercostal retractions, rales or rhonchi, and no improvement of hypoxia with oxygen administration. Radiographs show pulmonary edema with a normal cardiac silhouette (no cardiomegaly). Treat with intubation, mechanical ventilation with high percentage oxygen, and positive end-expiratory pressure (PEEP), while addressing the underlying cause (if possible).

11. **How is pneumonia diagnosed?**
The diagnosis of pneumonia usually is based on clinical findings (rales or rhonchi, fever) plus elevated white blood cell count and an abnormal chest radiograph consistent with pneumonia. Sputum and/or blood cultures usually are obtained before empiric antibiotic therapy is begun.

12. **What is the difference between typical and atypical pneumonia?**
Typical pneumonia is usually caused by bacteria such as *Streptococcus pneumoniae* or *Staphylococcus aureus*, the most common causes of pneumonia. Atypical pneumonia may be caused by influenza virus, *Mycoplasma, Chlamydia* spp., *Legionella, Haemophilus,* or adenovirus.

	Typical Pneumonia	Atypical Pneumonia
Prodrome	Short (< 2 days)	Long (> 3 days) (headache, malaise, body aches)
Fever	High (> 102° F)	Low (< 102° F)
Age	> 40 yrs	< 40 yrs
Chest radiograph	One distinct lobe involved	Diffuse or multilobe involvement
Bug	*Streptococcus pneumoniae*	Many (*Haemophilus, Mycoplasma, Chlamydia* spp.)
Antibiotic*	Ceftriaxone, broad-spectrum	Macrolides (e.g., azithromycin), doxycycline, or fluoroquinolone (e.g., levofloxacin)

*Avoid the temptation to pull out the "bigger-gun" antibiotics (very wide spectrum, potent) unless the patient is crashing or unstable.

13. **What are the classic clinical clues on Step 2 for the different causative bugs in pneumonia?**
College student: think of *Mycoplasma* sp. (look for cold agglutinins) or *Chlamydia* sp.
   Alcoholic: think of *Klebsiella* sp. ("currant jelly" sputum), *Staphylococcus aureus,* other enteric bugs (aspiration).
   Cystic fibrosis: think of *Pseudomonas* sp. or *Staphylococcus aureus.*
   Immigrant: think of tuberculosis.
   COPD: think of *Haemophilus influenzae, Moraxella* sp.
   Known tuberculosis with pulmonary cavitation: think of *Aspergillus* sp.
   Silicosis (metal, granite, pottery workers): think of tuberculosis.
   Exposure to air conditioner or aerosolized water: *Legionella* sp.
   HIV/AIDS: think of *Pneumocystis carinii* or cytomegalovirus (if you are shown koilocytosis).
   Exposure to bird droppings: think of *Chlamydia psittaci* or histoplasmosis.
   Child less than 1 year old: think of RSV.
   Child 2 to 5 years old: think of parainfluenza (croup).

14. **What should you suspect if a child has recurrent pneumonias?**
If the pneumonia always occurs in the same spot (especially the right middle and/or right lower lobe), it most likely is due to foreign body aspiration. Remember that a foreign body is most likely to go down the right mainstem bronchus. This diagnosis should be considered especially if the child has no other signs of immunodeficiency (e.g., other types of infections, symptoms of cystic fibrosis) before or during the episodes. If immunodeficiency is the cause of recurrent pneumonias, the child should have a history of chronic bilateral lung problems and other types of infection.

15. **What is "round" pneumonia?**

Pneumonia may appear round, typically in children, which causes it to simulate a mass. In such cases involving children, assume pneumonia and treat appropriately. A follow-up x-ray can be obtained to confirm resolution, which is not usually required in children, who almost never develop lung malignancies. In an adult, a round pneumonia should be viewed with suspicion (more likely to be a malignancy) and further work-up with a CT scan is typically employed.

16. **Why should you get a follow-up chest x-ray in all people over age 40 who develop pneumonia?**

A follow-up chest x-ray is routine in those over 40 who develop pneumonia to make sure it clears after appropriate antibiotic treatment. If pneumonia does not clear by 4 to 6 weeks, suspect something other than bacterial pneumonia. The classic culprit is malignancy, specifically, **bronchoalveolar carcinoma,** which is a subtype of adenocarcinoma (Fig. 33-1). In addition, recurrent pneumonias in the same location in an adult may be due to an endobronchial mass, whether benign or malignant.

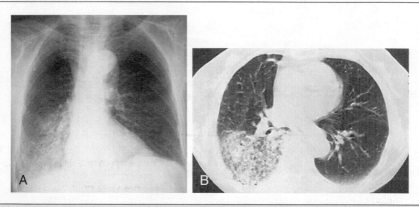

Figure 33-1. Consolidation in the right lower lobe, seen on front chest radiograph (**A**) and CT (**B**), progressed despite antibiotic therapy. Biopsy proved bronchoalveolar carcinoma. (From Katz DS, Math KR, Groskin SA [eds]: Radiology Secrets. Philadelphia, Hanley & Belfus, 1998, p 80, with permission.)

17. **What should you know about infant respiratory distress syndrome?**

Infant respiratory distress syndrome is due to atelectasis from a deficiency of surfactant; it is seen almost exclusively in premature infants and infants of diabetic mothers. Look for rapid, labored respirations, substernal retractions, cyanosis, grunting, and/or nasal flaring. Arterial blood gas shows hypoxemia and hypercarbia; radiograph shows diffuse atelectasis (described as diffuse, granular infiltrates). Treat with oxygen, give surfactant, and intubate if necessary. Complications include intraventricular hemorrhage and pneumothorax or bronchopulmonary dysplasia (complications of acute or chronic mechanical ventilation).

18. **What prenatal tests help to determine whether respiratory distress syndrome will occur?**

Measurement of amniotic fluid in the pregnant mother can determine whether the fetus is producing adequate surfactant. A lecithin-to-sphingomyelin ratio greater than 2:1 or the presence of **phosphatidylglycerol** in the amniotic fluid indicates fetal lung maturity and a low likelihood of infant respiratory distress syndrome. The fluorescence polarization test reflects the ratio of surfactant to albumin in amniotic fluid, and is a direct measurement of surfactant concentration. An elevated ratio indicates fetal lung maturity.

19. **Define diaphragmatic hernia. How is it recognized clinically?**
A defect in the diaphragm allows bowel to herniate into the chest. Diaphragmatic hernia is mentioned in the pulmonary section because it presents with respiratory difficulty, not GI problems. Herniated bowel pushes on the developing lung and causes lung hypoplasia on the affected side. Look for a scaphoid abdomen and bowel sounds in the chest. Herniated bowel can be seen on the chest radiograph; 90% are left-sided.

20. **How do you recognize and diagnose a tracheoesophageal fistula? How is it treated?**
The most common type (85% of cases) of tracheoesophageal fistula is an esophagus with a blind pouch proximally and a fistula between a bronchus/carina and the distal esophagus. Look for a neonate with excessive oral secretions, coughing or cyanosis with attempted feedings, abdominal distention, and aspiration pneumonia. The diagnosis is made by the inability to pass a nasogastric tube; alternatively, an injection of air via a nasogastric tube under x-ray (i.e., fluoroscopy) shows only the proximal esophagus. Treatment is early surgical correction.

21. **What is the most common lethal genetic disease in Caucasians? How do you recognize it?**
Cystic fibrosis, which is an autosomal recessive disease. Always suspect cystic fibrosis in pediatric patients with rectal prolapse, meconium ileus, esophageal varices, or recurrent pulmonary infections or failure to thrive. The classic complaint from the mother is a "salty-tasting" baby. Patients also commonly have pancreatic insufficiency and infertility (98% of affected males and 50% of females); they also may develop cor pulmonale (right-heart failure).

22. **How is cystic fibrosis diagnosed and treated?**
Diagnosis is made by an abnormal increase in the electrolytes of the patient's sweat (sodium and chloride) and/or DNA testing. Treat with chest physical therapy, annual influenza vaccine, fat-soluble vitamin supplements, pancreatic enzyme replacement, bronchodilators, dornase alfa, and aggressive treatment of infections with antibiotics that cover *Staphylococcus, Haemophilus influenzae,* and *Pseudomonas* spp.

23. **What should you do if a patient has a pleural effusion?**
If you do not know the cause of the effusion (Fig. 33-2), consider thoracocentesis to examine the fluid in an attempt to determine its etiology. Common tests ordered on pleural fluid include Gram stain, culture and sensitivity testing (including tuberculosis culture), cell count with differential, glucose (low with infection), protein (high in infection), cytology (to look for malignancy), amylase (if pancreatitis is a suspected cause of effusion), triglycerides (if a chylous effusion is suspected), albumin, and lactate dehydrogenase (last two tests help to determine whether the fluid is an exudate or transudate).

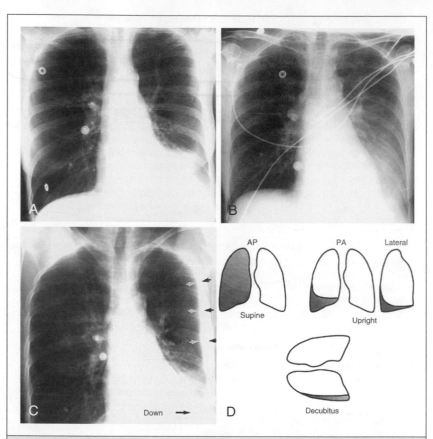

Figure 33-2. The appearance of pleural effusions depends on patient position. On an upright posteroanterior chest x-ray (**A**), a large left pleural effusion obscures the left hemidiaphragm, the left costophrenic angle, and the left cardiac border. On a supine anteroposterior view (**B**), the fluid runs posteriorly, causing a diffuse opacity over the lower two thirds of the left lung while the left hemidiaphragm remains obscured. This can easily mimic left lower lobe infiltrate or left lower lobe atelectasis. With a left lateral decubitus view (**C**), the left side of the patient is dependent, and the pleural effusion can be seen to be freely moving and layering (*arrows*) along the lateral chest wall. These findings are shown diagrammatically as well for a right pleural effusion (**D**). (From Mettler F: Essentials of Radiology, 2nd ed. Philadelphia, Saunders, 2004, Fig. 3-80.)

CHAPTER 34

RADIOLOGY

1. **Cover the right-hand columns and specify what imaging study you should order for the following conditions.**

Condition	Screening (or only) Test to Order	Confirmatory Test	Comments
Skull fracture (depressed)	CT scan		
Head trauma	CT without contrast		
Intracranial hemorrhage	CT without contrast		
Acute stroke	CT without contrast	MRI of brain without contrast	
Multiple sclerosis	MRI of brain with and without contrast		
Brain tumor	CT or MRI with contrast		
Pneumonia	Chest x-ray		
Chest trauma	Chest x-ray	CT scan with contrast	
Chest mass	Chest x-ray	CT scan with contrast	
Hemoptysis	Chest x-ray	Bronchoscopy or CT scan with contrast	
Pulmonary embolism	Ventilation/perfusion scan (nuclear scan) or CT with contrast	Pulmonary arteriogram	
Aortic aneurysm/ Dissection	Ultrasound (US) or CT with contrast (preferred if dissection is suspected)	Angiogram	
Aortic tear (trauma)	CT with contrast	Angiogram	
Carotid stenosis	Duplex ultrasound or MRA	Angiogram	

(continued)

Condition	Screening (or only) Test to Order	Confirmatory Test	Comments
Esophageal obstruction	Barium x-ray or endoscopy	Endoscopy	
Esophageal tear	Gastrografin x-ray or endoscopy	Endoscopy	
Bowel perforation	Abdominal x-ray	CT scan or laparoscopy	
Hematemesis	Endoscopy		
Peptic ulcer disease	Upper GI series or endoscopy	Endoscopy	
Abdominal trauma	CT scan with contrast	Laparoscopy	
Abdominal abscess	CT scan with contrast		
Cholelithiasis	Ultrasound (US)		
Choledocholithiasis	US	ERCP or MRCP	
Cholecystitis	US	Nuclear hepatobiliary study (HIDA scan)	
Intestinal obstruction	Abdominal x-ray (AXR)	CT scan with contrast	
Appendicitis	CT scan with contrast or appendiceal CT scan with rectal contrast or CT scan with contrast or US	Laparoscopy	
Nephrolithiasis	CT scan without contrast (test of choice), or AXR, or intravenous pyelogram (IVP)		
Ovarian pathology	US		
Diverticulitis	CT scan with contrast		No endoscopy or barium enema acutely
Upper GI bleeding*	Upper GI series or endoscopy	Endoscopy	
Lower GI bleeding*	Barium enema or endoscopy	Endoscopy	

(continued)

Condition	Screening (or only) Test to Order	Confirmatory Test	Comments
Unknown GI bleeding*	Nuclear medicine bleeding study		For brisk bleed, angiography or laparotomy
Hydronephrosis	US or CT scan		
Hematuria (persistent)	CT scan with contrast	Cytoscopy or CT scan with contrast	
Fibroid uterus	US	MRI	
Pelvic mass (female)	US	CT with contrast or laparoscopy	
Bone metastases	Bone scan		Plain x-rays for multiple myeloma
Pregnancy evaluation	US (transvaginal detects sooner than transabdominal)		First get beta-HCG
Fracture	X-ray		CT scan without contrast can help evaluate complex fractures
Osteomyclitis	X-ray	Bone scan and/or MRI with contrast	
Arthritis	X-ray	MRI	
Pyloric stenosis	US, upper GI series second choice		
Meckel diverticulum	Meckel scan (nuclear medicine)		

MRA = magnetic resonance angiogram (an MRI test); ERCP = endoscopic retrograde cholangiopancreatography; MRCP = magnetic resonance cholangiopancreatography; HIDA = hepato-iminodiacetic acid; HCG = human chorionic gonadotropin.
*For brisk bleeds, endoscopy is preferred. For occult bleeding, barium study or endoscopy can be used. An "unknown" GI bleed means that initial tests failed to localize the bleed and that the patient is still actively bleeding.

Note: With suspected GI perforation, do not use barium (it may cause a chemical peritonitis); use water-soluble contrast (e.g., Gastrografin).

CHAPTER 35

RHEUMATOLOGY

1. **What is the most common form of arthritis?**
   Osteoarthritis (at least 75% of cases), which is also called "degenerative" joint disease (Fig. 35-1).

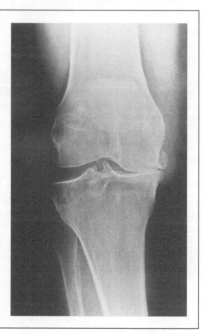

Figure 35-1. Degenerative joint disease of the knee. Significant joint space narrowing at the medial compartment of the knee is combined with osteophyte formation at the medial tibial plateau and femoral condyle. The joint space narrowing results in varus alignment at the knee (normal = slight valgus alignment). (From Katz DS, Math KR, Groskin SA [eds]: Radiology Secrets. Philadelphia, Hanley & Belfus, 1998, p 271, with permission.)

2. **If the cause of arthritis is in doubt, what should you do?**
   When in doubt, or if you suspect something other than osteoarthritis, perform an x-ray of and aspirate fluid from the affected joint. Examine the fluid for cell count and differential, glucose, bacteria (Gram stain and culture), and crystals.

3. **How do you distinguish among the common causes of arthritis?**

	OA	RA	Gout	Pseudogout	Septic
Usual age/sex	Older adults	Women 20 to 45 yrs	Older men	Older adults	Any age
Classic joints	DIP, PIP, hip, knee	PIP, MCP, wrist	Big toe	Knees, elbows	Knee

(continued)

	OA	RA	Gout	Pseudogout	Septic
Joint fluid WBC	< 2,000	> 2,000	> 2,000	> 2,000	> 50,000
% Neutrophils	< 25%	> 50%	> 50%	> 50%	> 75%

OA = osteoarthritis; RA = rheumatoid arthritis; DIP = distal interphalangeal joints; PIP = proximal interphalangeal joints; MCP = metacarpophalangeal joints; WBC = white blood cells.

4. **What other clues point to a diagnosis of osteoarthritis?**
   Osteoarthritis typically occurs in those over the age of 40 and has few signs of inflammation on exam, thus the joints are not hot, red, or tender like in the other four types of arthritis above. Look for Heberden nodes (visible and palpable distal interphalangeal [DIP] joint osteophytes) and Bouchard nodes (proximal interphalangeal [PIP] joint osteophytes), worsening of symptoms after use and in the evening, bony spurs, and increasing incidence with age. Treat with weight reduction and as-needed nonsteroidal anti-inflammatory drugs (NSAIDs) or acetaminophen.

5. **What clues point to a diagnosis of rheumatoid arthritis?**
   Rheumatoid arthritis often causes systemic symptoms (fever, malaise, subcutaneous nodules, pericarditis or pleural effusion, uveitis), prolonged morning stiffness, and swan neck and boutonnière deformities. The diagnosis is often made by an elevated sedimentation rate or C-reactive protein and positive rheumatoid factor, which is present in most adults but often negative in children. Radiographs and MRI can also support the diagnosis. General treatment strategies reflect the fact that the destruction of affected joints due to inflammation occurs early in the course of rheumatoid arthritis. The patient should be offered treatment with disease modifying antirheumatic drugs (DMARDs) as soon as possible after the onset of disease. Escalate the intensity of treatment until synovitis and inflammation have improved.
   There are five general classes of medications used for the treatment of rheumatoid arthritis, with DMARDs forming the backbone of treatment. Treatment options include the following: analgesics (from acetaminophen to narcotics), nonsteroidal anti-inflammatory drugs (NSAIDs), glucocorticoids, nonbiologic DMARDs (methotrexate, sulfasalazine, leflunomide, hydroxychloroquine, and minocycline), and biologic DMARDs. Biologic DMARDs include tumor necrosis factor (TNF) inhibitors (etanercept, infliximab, and adalimumab), an interleukin-1 receptor antagonist (anakinra), a monoclonal antibody (rituximab), and biologic response modifiers (abatacept).

6. **What clues point to a diagnosis of gout?**
   Gout classically begins with podagra (gout in the big toe). Also look for high uric acid levels (not always present), tophi (subcutaneous uric acid deposits that look like punched-out lesions on bone radiographs), **needle-shaped crystals** in joint fluid with **negative birefringence,** and male gender (more commonly affected than female gender). Alcohol and protein-rich foods may precipitate an attack. Colchicine or NSAIDs (but *not* aspirin, which causes decreased excretion of uric acid by the kidney) are used for acute attacks. For maintenance therapy, high fluid intake, alkalinization of the urine, and/or allopurinol or probenecid (neither drug is for acute attacks) may be used.

7. **What causes pseudogout? How is it diagnosed?**
   Pseudogout is caused by deposition of calcium pyrophosphate crystals into joints. Look for **rhomboid crystals** with **weakly positive birefringence** (vs. negative birefringence with gout crystals).

8. **What clues point to a diagnosis of septic arthritis? What are the common causes?**

In septic arthritis, Gram stain usually reveals bacteria in the synovial fluid. *Staphylococcus aureus* is the most common organism except in sexually active young adults, in whom the most common bug is *Neisseria gonorrhoeae.* Do blood cultures in addition to joint cultures, because the bug usually reaches the joint via the hematogenous route. Also do urethral swabs and cultures in appropriate patients.

9. **Name some other causes of arthritis.**
   - Prior trauma
   - Lupus and other collagen vascular diseases (e.g., scleroderma)
   - Psoriasis
   - Inflammatory bowel disease
   - Lyme disease
   - Ankylosing spondylitis
   - Reiter syndrome
   - Lyme disease
   - Hemophilia
   - Paget disease
   - Hemochromatosis, Wilson disease
   - Neuropathy (i.e., Charcot joint)

10. **True or false: Psoriasis can cause an arthritis that resembles osteoarthritis.**

False. The arthritis resembles rheumatoid arthritis. On the Step 2 exam, look for psoriatic skin lesions to make an easy diagnosis (Fig. 35-2). The arthritis usually affects the hands and feet and though it resembles rheumatoid arthritis, the rheumatoid factor is negative. NSAIDs are first-line therapy. Other treatments include methotrexate, PUVA, retinoic acid derivatives, cyclosporine, sulfasalazine, azathioprine, and antimalarials.

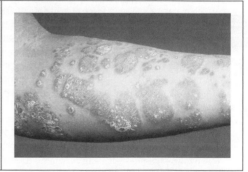

Figure 35-2. Psoriasis. The limbs are usually affected, as shown. Lesions are typically clearly delineated, deep red in color, and have a silvery scale. (From du Vivier A: Atlas of Clinical Dermatology, 3rd ed. New York, Churchill Livingstone, 2002, p 71, with permission.)

11. **Describe the hallmarks of ankylosing spondylitis.**

Ankylosing spondylitis is associated with human leukocyte antigen B27 (**HLA-B27**). Most often a 20- to 40-year-old man with a positive family history presents with back pain and morning stiffness. Patients may assume a bent-over posture. The sacroiliac joints are primarily affected, and radiographs may reveal a **"bamboo" spine** (Fig. 35-3). Patients have other autoimmune type symptoms, such as fever, elevations in erythrocyte sedimentation rate and C-reactive protein, and anemia. Some develop uveitis. Treat with NSAIDs, methotrexate, sulfasalazine, or tumor necrosis factor (TNF) antagonists (etanercept, infliximab, adalimumab).

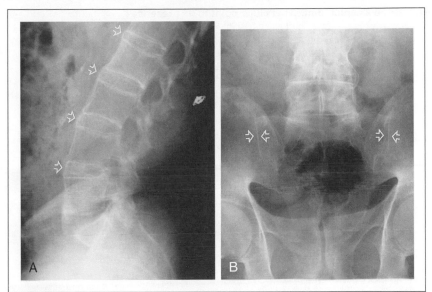

Figure 35-3. Ankylosing spondylitis. A lateral view of the lumbar spine (**A**) demonstrates calcific bridging across the disk spaces (*arrows*), causing the typical "bamboo spine" appearance. **B,** Anteroposterior view of the pelvis shows that the sacroiliac joints (*arrows*) are not easily visualized due to fusion of both sacroiliac joints. (From Mettler F: Essentials of Radiology, 2nd ed. Philadelphia, Saunders, 2004, Fig. 8-39.)

12. How do you recognize Reiter syndrome as the cause of arthritis?
Reiter syndrome also is associated with HLA-B27. The classic triad of symptoms consists of **urethritis** (due to chlamydial infection), **conjunctivitis,** and **arthritis** (*"can't pee, can't see, can't climb a tree"*). Reiter syndrome may also follow enteric bacterial infections. Superficial oral and penile ulcers are common. Diagnose and treat the sexually transmitted disease, and use NSAIDs for arthritis. Also treat the patient's sexual partners.

13. Why do patients with hemophilia get arthritis?
Recurrent hemarthroses (bleeding into the joints), which can cause a debilitating arthritis. Treatment is with acetaminophen. Avoid aspirin and other NSAIDs due to bleeding concern.

14. What clues point to Lyme disease as the cause of arthritis?
Look for a history of a tick bite or hiking in the woods, **erythema chronicum migrans** rash, and migratory arthritis (later). Treat *Borrelia burgdorferi,* the causative bacteria of Lyme disease, with doxycycline, amoxicillin, or cefuroxime. Avoid doxycycline in children under the age of 8 years and in pregnant or lactating women.

15. True or false: One of the major Jones criteria for the diagnosis of rheumatic fever is arthritis.
True. Migratory polyarthritis is one of the major Jones criteria. Look for a history of strep throat.

16. Why do patients with sickle cell disease often have arthritis?
Patients frequently experience arthralgias (pain) from ischemic sickle crises, but the classic cause of arthritis is avascular necrosis (e.g., hip arthritis from avascular necrosis of the femoral head).

17. **Define Charcot joint. What clues point to its presence?**
A Charcot joint is seen most commonly in diabetes but also occurs in other neuropathies. A lack of sensation causes the patient to overuse or misuse joints, which become deformed and painful. The best treatment is prevention. After even seemingly mild trauma, patients with neuropathy in the area of the trauma need radiographs to rule out fractures.

18. **What about lupus erythematosus and other autoimmune disorders as a cause of arthritis?**
With lupus erythematosus, inflammatory bowel disease, and other autoimmune diseases, symptoms of the primary disease help make these diagnoses on the USMLE exam.

19. **How do hemochromatosis and Wilson disease cause arthritis?**
Via deposition of excessive iron (hemochromatosis) or copper (Wilson disease) into the joints.

20. **What generalized systemic signs of inflammation may suggest an autoimmune disorder?**
Systemic signs and symptoms of inflammation include elevations in erythrocyte sedimentation rate and C-reactive protein, fever, anemia of chronic disease, fatigue, and weight loss. If these symptoms are present in a woman of reproductive age, you should consider the possibility of an autoimmune disease.

21. **Describe the hallmarks of systemic lupus erythematosus (SLE).**
SLE can cause malar rash, discoid rash, photosensitivity, kidney damage, arthritis, pericarditis and pleuritis, positive **antinuclear antibody (ANA),** positive anti-Smith antibody, positive syphilis results (on the Venereal Disease Research Laboratory and rapid plasmin reagin screening tests), positive lupus anticoagulant, blood disorders (thrombocytopenia, leukopenia, anemia, or pancytopenia), neurologic disturbances (depression, psychosis, seizures), and oral ulcers. Any of these may be presenting symptoms. Use the ANA titer as a screening test, and confirm with the **anti-Smith antibody** test. Treat with NSAIDs, hydroxychloroquine, corticosteroids, or immunosuppressive agents (methotrexate, cyclophosphamide, azathioprine, or mycophenolate).

22. **Describe the hallmarks of scleroderma.**
Scleroderma (also known as progressive systemic sclerosis) classically presents with **CREST** symptoms (**c**alcinosis, **R**aynaud phenomenon, **e**sophageal dysmotility with dysphagia, **s**clerodactyly, and **t**elangiectasia), heartburn, and mask-like, leathery facies. Use the ANA test for screening; confirm the diagnosis with the **anticentromere antibody** test (for CREST symptoms only) and the **antitopoisomerase antibody** (for full-blown scleroderma). Treatment depends on the symptoms, but often includes corticosteroids and/or methotrexate.

23. **What are the hallmarks of Sjögren syndrome?**
Sjögren syndrome causes dry eyes (keratoconjunctivitis sicca) and dry mouth (xerostomia) and often is associated with other autoimmune diseases. Treat with eye drops and good oral hygiene.

24. **What are the signs and symptoms of dermatomyositis?**
Dermatomyositis causes polymyositis (see question 29) plus skin involvement (a **heliotrope rash around the eyes** with associated periorbital edema is classic). Patients usually have trouble rising from a chair or climbing steps because of the effects on proximal muscles. Muscle enzymes are elevated, and electromyography is irregular. Muscle biopsy establishes the diagnosis. Affected patients have an increased incidence of malignancy.

25. **With what is polyarteritis nodosa associated? How is it diagnosed?**
Polyarteritis nodosa is a type of vasculitis classically associated with hepatitis B infection and cryoglobulinemia. Patients present with fever, abdominal pain, weight loss, renal disturbances, and/or peripheral neuropathies. Lab abnormalities include elevations in erythrocyte sedimentation rate and C-reactive protein, leukocytosis, anemia, and hematuria or proteinuria. Patients often have a positive **antineutrophil cytoplasmic antibody (ANCA)** titer. The vasculitis involves medium-sized vessels. Biopsy of an affected organ is the gold standard for diagnosis.

26. **Describe the usual presentation of Kawasaki disease. How is it treated?**
Kawasaki disease usually affects children younger than 5 years; it is more common in Japanese and female children. Patients present with truncal rash, high fever (which lasts longer than 5 days), conjunctival injection, cervical lymphadenopathy, strawberry tongue, late skin desquamation of palms and soles, and/or arthritis. Patients may develop coronary vessel vasculitis and subsequent aneurysms, which may thrombose and cause a myocardial infarction. Kawasaki disease should be suspected in any child who has a heart attack. Treat during the acute stage with aspirin and intravenous immunoglobulins to reduce the risk of coronary aneurysm.

27. **How does Takayasu arteritis present?**
Takayasu arteritis tends to affect Asian women between the ages of 15 and 30 years. It is called the "pulseless disease" because you may not be able to feel the pulse or measure blood pressure on the affected side. The vasculitis affects the aortic arch and its branches. Carotid involvement may cause neurologic signs or stroke, and congestive heart failure is not uncommon. Angiogram shows the characteristic lesions. Treat with steroids.

28. **How do you recognize Behçet syndrome on the Step 2 exam?**
Behçet syndrome classically presents in young men in their 20s with painful oral and genital ulcers. Patients also may have uveitis, arthritis, and other skin lesions (especially erythema nodosum). Steroids are the mainstay of therapy.

29. **How do you distinguish among fibromyalgia, polymyositis, and polymyalgia rheumatica?**

	Fibromyalgia	Polymyositis	Polymyalgia Rheumatica
Classic age/ sex	Young adult women	Female aged 40–60 yrs	Female > age 50 yrs
Location	Various	Proximal muscles	Pectoral and pelvic girdles, neck
ESR	Normal	Elevated	Markedly elevated (often > 100)
EMG/biopsy	Normal	Abnormal	Normal
Classic findings	Anxiety, stress, insomnia, point tenderness over affected muscles	Elevated CPK, abnormal EMG/ biopsy, higher risk of cancer	Temporal arteritis, great response to steroids, very high ESR, elderly patients

(continued)

	Fibromyalgia	Polymyositis	Polymyalgia Rheumatica
Treatment	Antidepressants, NSAIDs, pregabalin, rest	Steroids	Steroids

ESR = erythrocyte sedimentation rate; CPK = creatine phosphokinase; EMG = electromyography.

30. **Give the basic facts of Paget disease. How is it linked with cancer?**

In Paget disease, bone is broken down and regenerated, often simultaneously. It usually is seen in persons over 40 years old and is more common in men. Often it is discovered in an asymptomatic patient through a radiograph. Classic cases involve the pelvis and skull; watch for a person who has had to buy larger-sized hats. Patients may complain of bone pain, arthritis, or hearing loss. **Alkaline phosphatase** is markedly elevated in the presence of normal calcium and phosphorus levels. The risk of osteosarcoma is increased in affected bones. The main treatment is the antiresorptive agents (e.g., zoledronic acid, alendronate, risedronate, pamidronate).

31. **If a pediatric patient has uveitis and an inflammatory arthritis, but the rheumatoid factor is negative, what disease should you suspect?**

Rheumatoid arthritis. The rheumatoid factor is often negative in the pauciarticular variant. Affected patients commonly develop uveitis.

CHAPTER 36

SHOCK

1. **Define shock.**
   Shock is a state in which blood flow to and perfusion of peripheral tissues is inadequate to sustain life. Although they are not included in a rigid definition of shock, for board purposes hypotension and oliguria or anuria are associated findings. Tachycardia is also usually present.

2. **List the five primary clinical types of shock.**
   Hypovolemic, cardiogenic, septic, anaphylactic, and neurogenic.

3. **What should you do if a patient is in shock?**
   Keep the patient alive with the ABCs (airways, breathing, and circulation) while you try to figure out the cause of the shock. Give oxygen and fluids while you are thinking unless the patient is in congestive heart failure. If congestive heart failure is present, avoid fluids.

4. **How should fluids be given if a patient is in shock?**
   Many patients in shock need fluid. The standard intravenous bolus is 10 to 20 mL/kg of normal saline or lactated Ringer solution; infuse 1 to 2 liters as fast as it will go. Then reassess the patient to determine whether the bolus helped; positive signs include increases in blood pressure and urine output. Do *not* be afraid to give a second bolus if the first bolus leads to no improvement. Of course, you should watch for fluid overload, which may cause congestive heart failure. Make sure that no bilateral crackles can be heard on lung exam. Place a Foley catheter to ensure accurate monitoring of urine output.

5. **What should you do if fluid challenges fail to raise the blood pressure?**
   Use invasive hemodynamic monitoring (i.e., Swan-Ganz catheter) to help determine the cause of the shock and to guide therapeutic decisions.

6. **What are the classic parameters of each type of shock?**

Type of Shock	CO	PCWP	SVR	SVO$_2$
Septic (early)	**High**	Low	Low	**High**
Hypovolemic*	Low	Low	**High**	Low
Cardiogenic	Low	**High**	High	Low
Neurogenic	Low	Low	**Low**	Low

CO = cardiac output; PCWP = pulmonary capillary wedge pressure; SVR = systemic vascular resistance; SVO$_2$ = systemic venous oxygen saturation.
*Also the parameters for late septic shock.

With **anaphylactic shock,** the cause is usually obvious because of a temporal relation to a common culprit (see question 11).

7. **Specify the usual findings in patients with neurogenic shock.**

Patients usually have a history of severe central nervous system trauma or hemorrhage and flushed skin. The heart rate may be normal.

8. **How do you recognize septic shock?**

Look for fever, leukocytosis (unless the patient is on chemotherapy or has an immunosuppressive condition such as AIDS), skin that is flushed and warm to the touch, and extremes of age. Start broad-spectrum antibiotics after "pan-culturing" (blood, sputum, and urine cultures plus others as dictated by history).

9. **What clues suggest cardiogenic shock?**

Look for a history of myocardial infarction, congestive heart failure, or chest pain. Assess patients for risk factors for coronary artery disease. Most patients have cold, clammy skin and look pale. Distended neck veins and pulmonary congestion (as demonstrated by physical exam and/or chest radiograph) are usually present.

10. **How do you recognize hypovolemic shock?**

Look for a history of fluid loss (hemorrhage, diarrhea, vomiting, sweating, use of diuretics, inability to drink water). Patients have cold, clammy skin and look pale. Fluid loss may be internal, as with a ruptured abdominal or thoracic aortic aneurysm and obstruction or infarction of the spleen, pancreas, or bowel. The postoperative state also may lead to hypovolemic shock. Patients usually have orthostatic hypotension, tachycardia, sunken eyes, tenting of skin, and sunken fontanelle (young children).

11. **What clues suggest anaphylactic shock?**

Look for a history of recent exposure to the common culprits: bee stings, peanuts, shellfish, penicillins, sulfa drugs, or any new medication. Treat with **epinephrine** and fluids. Administer oxygen, and intubate if necessary. A tracheostomy or cricothyroidotomy should be performed if laryngeal edema prevents intubation. Antihistamines are helpful primarily when the reaction is mild. Use corticosteroids when the reaction is prolonged or severe, but note that they are not first-line drugs in the treatment of anaphylaxis. Monitor all patients for at least 6 hours after the initial reaction.

12. **What clues suggest pulmonary embolus as a cause of shock?**

Look for deep venous thrombosis (positive **Homan sign** with painful, swollen leg) or risk factors for deep venous thrombosis. Remember the **Virchow triad:** endothelial damage, stasis, and hypercoagulable state. Watch for postoperative status (especially after orthopedic or pelvic surgery) or a history of recent delivery (amniotic fluid embolus) or bone fractures (fat emboli). Patients classically have chest pain, tachypnea, shortness of breath, right-axis shift on EKG, and positive ventilation/perfusion scan or CT pulmonary angiography. Heparin or a low-molecular weight heparin should be administered to prevent further clotting and emboli.

13. **How do you recognize pericardial tamponade as a cause of shock?**

Look for a history of a stab wound in the left chest and distended neck veins. Do pericardiocentesis emergently in the setting of shock.

14. **Explain toxic shock syndrome.**

Toxic shock syndrome usually presents in a woman of reproductive age who leaves her tampon in place too long. Look for skin desquamation. It is caused by a *Staphylococcus aureus* toxin.

15. **What clues suggest Addison disease as a cause of shock?**
Patients usually have a history of steroid use, hyperkalemia, and hyponatremia. Treat with steroids.

16. **What is the most important point to remember if a patient is in shock?**
The ABCs. Patients in shock often need heroic measures to survive and are among the exceptions to the "wait-and-see" and "be conservative" rules that are usually favored by USMLE examiners. Intubate at the drop of a hat, do not feed the patient, and avoid narcotics if possible. Mental status changes are often an important clue to impending doom. Also monitor the EKG, vital signs, Swan-Ganz parameters, urine output, arterial blood gas, and hemoglobin/hematocrit.

17. **Discuss the use of dobutamine, dopamine, norepinephrine, and isoproterenol to support blood pressure in the setting of shock.**
Dobutamine is a beta$_1$ agonist used to increase cardiac output by increasing contractility; it is the intensive-care equivalent of digoxin.

Dopamine affects dopamine receptors at low doses and results in selective vasodilation (the traditional use for renal perfusion is questionable). At higher doses, its beta$_1$ agonist effects increase contractility. At the highest doses, dopamine has alpha$_1$ agonist effects and causes vasoconstriction.

Norepinephrine is used for its alpha$_1$ agonist effects, but it also has beta$_1$ effects. It is given primarily to patients with hypotension to increase peripheral resistance so that perfusion to vital organs can be maintained.

Isoproterenol is a beta$_1$ agonist that has chronotropic effects (may help in cases of bradycardia) and causes vasodilation. As such, its use in hypotensive patients is limited.

18. **What about the use of phenylephrine, epinephrine, and milrinone in the setting of shock?**
Phenylephrine is used for its alpha$_1$ agonist effects; it is similar to norepinephrine but has no beta effects.

Epinephrine is used in patients with cardiac arrest and anaphylaxis for its alpha and beta effects.

Milrinone and **amrinone** are phosphodiesterase inhibitors. They are used in patients with refractory heart failure (they are not first-line agents) because they have a positive inotropic effect via potentiation of cyclic adenosine monophosphate (cAMP), but they cannot be used in hypotensive patients.

CHAPTER 37

SMOKING

1. **Does smoking really deserve its own chapter in this book?**
   Smoking is the single most significant source of preventable morbidity and premature death in the United States. This is a recurrent theme on the boards, so whenever you are not sure which risk factor to choose to reduce morbidity or mortality, smoking is a safe guess.

2. **How is smoking related to heart disease?**
   Smoking is the best risk factor to eliminate for prevention of deaths related to heart disease; it is responsible for 30% to 45% of such deaths in the United States. This risk is decreased by 50% within 1 year of quitting, and by 15 years after quitting, the risk is the same as someone who has never smoked.

3. **What cancers are more likely in smokers?**
   Smoking increases the risk for cancers of the lung (smoking causes 85-90% of cases), oral cavity (90% of cases), esophagus (70-80% of cases), larynx, pharynx, bladder (30-50% of cases), kidney (20-30%), pancreas (20-25%), cervix, stomach, colon, and rectum.

4. **Describe the effect of smoking on the lung.**
   Lung cancer and chronic obstructive pulmonary disease (emphysema, chronic bronchitis, and bronchiectasis) are due to smoking. Emphysema almost always results from smoking; if the patient is very young or has no smoking history, you should consider **alpha$_1$-antitrypsin deficiency.** Although the changes of emphysema are irreversible, the risk of death still decreases if the patient stops smoking.

5. **What about second-hand smoke?**
   Second-hand smoke has been proved to be a risk factor for lung cancer and other lung disease. The risk increases linearly with increasing exposure. When parents smoke, their exposed children are at an increased risk for asthma and upper respiratory infections, including otitis media.

6. **What other bad things does smoking do?**
   Smoking retards the healing of peptic ulcer disease, and cessation stops the development of **Buerger disease** (Raynaud symptoms in a young male smoker). Smoking by a pregnant woman increases the risk of low birth weight, prematurity, spontaneous abortion, stillbirth, and infant mortality. Cessation of smoking preoperatively is the best way to decrease the risk of postoperative pulmonary complications, especially if it is stopped at least 8 weeks before surgery.

7. **True or false: Women who smoke cannot take birth control pills.**
   True—if the woman is over the age of 35 years and smokes or is younger than 35 and smokes 15 or more cigarettes per day. The risk of thromboembolism is increased sharply in women who smoke and take birth control pills. Postmenopausal women, however, can take estrogen therapy regardless of smoking status.

8. **So what is the bottom line for the boards?**
   Smoking is a very dangerous habit that should be avoided.

CHAPTER 38

UROLOGY

1. **Cover the right-hand columns and specify the classic differences between testicular torsion and epididymitis. What imaging test can diagnose and distinguish these two conditions?**

	Testicular Torsion	Epididymitis
Age	Under 30 yrs (usually prepubertal)	Over 30 yrs*
Appearance	Testis may be elevated into the inguinal canal; swelling	Swollen testis, overlying erythema, urethral discharge/urethritis, prostatitis
Prehn sign	Pain stays the same or worsens	Pain decreases with testicular elevation
Treatment	Immediate surgery to salvage testis; surgical orchiopexy for both testes	Antibiotics*

*In men younger than 50 years, epididymitis is commonly due to sexually transmitted disease (chlamydial infection and gonorrhea). Treat accordingly. In men over age 50, epididymitis is commonly due to urinary tract infection (e.g., *Escherichia coli*). Treat with trimethoprim-sulfamethoxazole or ciprofloxacin.

Ultrasound is the diagnostic test of choice in the setting of testicular/scrotal pain. It can easily differentiate between these two conditions as well as visualize testicular tumors (which sometimes present with pain, although classically they are painless).

2. **How does testicular cancer usually present? Describe the major risk factors, histology, and treatment.**
Testicular cancer usually presents as a painless testicular mass in a young man (15 to 35 years old). The main risk factor is cryptorchidism. Roughly 90% are germ cell tumors; the most common type is **seminoma.** Testicular cancer generally is treated with orchiectomy and radiation; if disease is widespread, use chemotherapy. Alpha-fetoprotein is a marker for yolk sac tumors; human chorionic gonadotropin is a marker for choriocarcinoma. Leydig cell tumors may secrete androgens and cause precocious puberty.

3. **How is renal cell carcinoma diagnosed and treated?**
Painless hematuria (gross or microscopic) is the most typical presenting sign. Patients rarely present with the classic triad of hematuria, flank pain, and a palpable flank mass. CT scan (preferred over intravenous pyelography) is a good initial diagnostic test (Fig. 38-1). Treatment for disease confined to the kidney or with extension limited to renal vein invasion (classic)

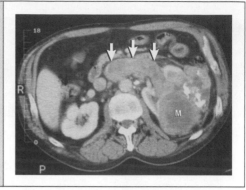

Figure 38-1. Renal cell carcinoma. A computed tomography (CT) scan at the mid portion of the kidneys (A) demonstrates a large left renal mass (M) that extends into the renal vein and into the inferior vena cava (*arrows*). (From Mettler F: Essentials of Radiology, 2nd ed. Philadelphia, Saunders, 2004, Fig. 7-25.)

is surgical resection. With other organ invasion or distant metastatic disease (usually to lung or bone), immunotherapy (e.g., interleukin-2) is the preferred treatment.

4. **What is the classic cause of orchitis? How is it treated? Does it usually cause infertility?**
   Mumps can cause orchitis, which classically presents with a painful, swollen testis in a postpubertal male. The best treatment is prevention (immunization against the mumps virus). Mumps orchitis rarely causes sterility because it is usually unilateral. Epididymo-orchitis is more common and typically due to spread from adjacent bacterial epididymitis.

5. **What are the symptoms and sequelae of benign prostatic hypertrophy (BPH)?**
   BPH can cause urinary hesitancy, intermittency, terminal dribbling, decreased size and force of the urinary stream, sensation of incomplete emptying, nocturia, urgency, dysuria, and frequency. It may result in acute urinary retention, urinary tract infections, hydronephrosis, and even kidney damage or failure in severe cases.

6. **How is BPH treated?**
   Medical therapy, which is started when the patient becomes symptomatic, includes alpha$_1$ blockers (e.g., prazosin, terazosin, or doxazosin), 5-alpha-reductase inhibitors (finasteride, dutasteride), antiandrogens, and gonadotropin-releasing hormone analogs. Transurethral resection of the prostate (TURP) is used for more advanced cases, especially with repeated urinary tract infections, urosepsis, urinary retention, and/or hydronephrosis or kidney damage due to reflux. Open surgical prostatectomy is used in some patients, but is associated with a higher complication rate.

7. **How do you recognize and manage acute urinary retention?**
   Acute urinary retention generally presents with abdominal pain; palpation of a full, distended bladder on abdominal exam; a history of BPH in men; and a lack of urination in the past 24 hours or longer. The first step is to empty the bladder. If you cannot pass a regular Foley catheter, consider the use of a larger catheter with a firm Coude tip, or alternatively do a suprapubic tap to drain the bladder. Then address the underlying cause—usually BPH, which in this setting is generally treated with TURP.

8. **What are the common causes of impotence?**
   Impotence is caused most commonly by vascular problems and atherosclerosis. Medications are also a common culprit (especially antihypertensive and antidepressant agents). Diabetes can cause impotence through vascular (increased atherosclerosis) or neurogenic (diabetic

autonomic neuropathy) compromise. Patients undergoing dialysis are often impotent. Remember "**p**oint and **s**hoot": **p**arasympathetics mediate erection; **s**ympathetics mediate ejaculation.

The history often gives you a clue if the cause of impotence is psychogenic. Look for a normal pattern of nocturnal erections, selective dysfunction (the patient has normal erections when masturbating but not with his partner), and a history of stress, anxiety, or fear.

9. **What are the signs of urethral injury?**
Usually urethral injury occurs in the context of pelvic trauma. The four hallmark warning signs are a boggy, movable prostate on exam, blood at the urethral meatus, severe pelvic fracture, and scrotal/perineal ecchymosis.

10. **True or false: Urethral injury is a contraindication to passing a Foley catheter.**
True. Always look for the four warning signs of urethral injury. If even one of these signs is present, do not attempt to pass a Foley catheter. Order a retrograde urethrogram to rule out urethral injury in this setting (Fig. 38-2).

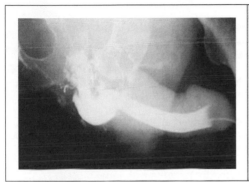

Figure 38-2. Retrograde urethrogram in pelvic fracture patient demonstrates complete disruption of posterior urethra. (From Wein A, et al.: Campbell-Walsh Urology, 9th ed. Philadelphia, Saunders, 2007, Fig. 83-10.)

11. **Distinguish between hydrocele and varicocele.**
A **hydrocele** represents a remnant of the processus vaginalis (remember embryology?) and transilluminates. It generally causes no symptoms and needs no treatment. A **varicocele** is a dilatation of the pampiniform venous plexus ("bag of worms," usually on the left). It does not transilluminate, disappears in the supine position, and becomes prominent with standing or the Valsalva maneuver. Varicoceles may cause infertility or pain; in either case, they can be treated surgically.

12. **Describe the classic findings of nephrolithiasis.**
Nephrolithiasis (kidney stones) can cause severe flank pain that often radiates to the groin and is colicky in nature. It may cause hematuria (gross or microscopic), and usually an abdominal radiograph reveals the stone (85% of stones are radiopaque). A noncontrast helical CT scan is the diagnostic test of choice.

13. **What are the different types of stones? What causes them?**
Roughly 75% to 85% of stones contain calcium. Look for hypercalcemia (usually due to hyperparathyroidism) or small bowel bypass, which increases oxalate absorption and thus calcium stone formation. Roughly 10% to 15% of stones are struvite (magnesium-ammonium-phosphate) stones, which are caused by urinary tract infection (usually with *Proteus* species). The classic example is the staghorn calculus (a stone that fill the entire

calyceal system). About 5% to 10% of stones are uric acid. Look for gout or leukemia. The remaining 1% to 3% are cystine stones, which suggest hereditary cystinuria.

14. **How is nephrolithiasis treated?**

The cornerstones of nephrolithiasis treatment are large amounts of fluid hydration, narcotics for pain, and observation, because most stones pass spontaneously. Stones less than or equal to 4 mm in diameter pass spontaneously. Stones 4 to 10 mm in diameter may or may not pass. Spontaneous passage is unlikely with stones greater than or equal to 10 mm in diameter. If a stone does not pass, treat with lithotripsy, uteroscopy with stone retrieval, or open surgery (last resort).

15. **Define cryptorchidism. When does it occur?**

Cryptorchidism is arrested descent of the testicle(s) between the renal area and the scrotum. The more premature the infant, the greater the likelihood of cryptorchidism. Many arrested testes eventually descend on their own within the first year. Intramuscular hCG may be used to induce testicular descent. After 1 year, surgical intervention (orchiopexy) is warranted in an attempt to preserve fertility as well as to facilitate future testicular exams. Affected testes have an increased risk for testicular cancer.

16. **True or false: It is important to place abdominal testes in the scrotum surgically to decrease the risk of cancer.**

False. Cryptorchidism is a major risk factor for testicular cancer (40 times increased risk), but bringing the testis into the scrotum probably does not alter the increased risk. The higher the testicle is found (the further away from the scrotum), the higher the risk of developing testicular cancer and the lower the likelihood of retaining fertility.

17. **Where do the left and right ovarian/testicular veins drain?**

The right ovarian/testicular vein drains into the inferior vena cava, whereas the left ovarian/testicular vein drains into the left renal vein.

18. **When is kidney transplant considered for patients with renal disease?**

Kidney transplant is an option for patients with end-stage renal disease (creatinine clearance less than 10 to 15 mg/min), unless they have active infections or other life-threatening conditions (e.g., AIDS, malignancy). Lupus erythematosus and diabetes are not contraindications to transplantation.

19. **Who makes the best donor for patients who need a kidney transplant?**

Living, related donors are best (siblings or parents), especially when human leukocyte antigens (HLA) are similar, but cadaveric kidneys are more commonly used because of availability. Before transplant, perform ABO blood typing and lymphocytotoxic (HLA) cross-matching to ensure a reasonable chance at success.

20. **Describe unacceptable kidney donors.**

Unacceptable kidney donors include newborns (most centers set an age less than 18 years as an exclusion criterion) and patients with a history of generalized or intraabdominal sepsis, malignancy, or any disease with possible renal involvement (e.g., diabetes, hypertension, lupus erythematosus).

21. **Where is the transplanted kidney placed? What happens to the native kidneys?**

A transplanted kidney is placed in the iliac fossa or pelvis (for easy biopsy access in case of later problems as well as for technical reasons). Usually the recipient's kidneys are left in place to reduce the morbidity of the surgery.

22. **What are the three basic types of rejection with kidney transplantation?**
Hyperacute, acute, and chronic.

23. **What causes hyperacute rejection? What is the classic clinical description?**
Hyperacute rejection is due to preformed cytotoxic antibodies against the donor kidney; it occurs with ABO blood-type mismatch as well as other preformed antibodies. In the classic clinical description, the surgery is completed, the vascular clamps are released to allow blood flow, and the transplanted kidney quickly turns bluish-black. Treat by removing the kidney.

24. **What causes acute rejection? How does it present? How is it treated?**
Acute rejection is T-cell–mediated. It presents *days to weeks* after the transplant with fever, oliguria, weight gain, tenderness and enlargement of the graft, hypertension, and/or laboratory derangements. Increases in creatinine are more reliable than increases in blood urea nitrogen. Treatment involves pulse corticosteroids, anti T-cell antibody therapies, (polyclonal antibodies, OKT3), other antibody therapies (basiliximab, daclizumab) and other immunosuppressants (tacrolimus, mycophenolate, cyclosporine). **Accelerated rejection** occurs over the *first few days* and is thought to reflect reactivation of previously sensitized T cells.

25. **What causes chronic rejection? How does it present? How is it treated?**
Chronic rejection can be T-cell– or antibody-mediated. This late cause (months to years after transplant) of renal deterioration presents with gradual decline in kidney function, proteinuria, and hypertension. Treatment is supportive and not effective, but the graft may last several years before it gives out completely. A new kidney can be transplanted if this occurs.

26. **Discuss the mechanism of action of the commonly used immunosuppressant drugs in transplant medicine.**
- Steroids inhibit interleukin-1 production.
- Methotrexate is a folic acid antagonist, but precise mechanism in immunosuppression is unclear.
- Cyclosporine inhibits interleukin-2 production.
- Tacrolimus inhibits signaling through the T-cell receptor.
- Mycophenolate prevents T-cell activation.
- Azathioprine is an antineoplastic that is cleaved into mercaptopurine and inhibits DNA/RNA synthesis (which causes decreased production of B cells and T cells).
- Antithymocyte globulin is an antibody against T cells.
- OKT3 is an antibody to the CD3 receptor on T cells.
- Thalidomide: mechanism of action is not known.
- Hydroxychloroquine interferes with antigen presentation.
- Basiliximab is a monoclonal antibody against the interleukin-2 receptor.
- Daclizumab is a monoclonal antibody against the interleukin-2 receptor.

27. **How do you distinguish the nephrotoxicity of cyclosporine from rejection?**
Cyclosporine is a well-known cause of nephrotoxicity that can be difficult to distinguish from graft rejection clinically. When in doubt, a percutaneous needle biopsy of the graft should be done if the patient is taking cyclosporine, because in most cases the two can be distinguished histologically. Renal ultrasound also helps. Practically speaking, if you increase the immunosuppressive dose, acute rejection should decrease, whereas cyclosporine toxicity stays the same or worsens.

28. **What risks are associated with immunosuppression?**
Immunosuppression carries the risk of infection (with common as well as strange bugs that infect patients with AIDS) and an increased risk of cancer (especially lymphomas and epithelial cell cancers).

29. **Define epispadias and hypospadias. How are they treated?**
Both are congenital penile anomalies. In **hypospadias** the urethra opens on the dorsal (under) side of the penis (Fig. 38-3). In **epispadias** the urethra opens on the ventral (top) side of the penis. Epispadias is associated with exstrophy of the bladder. Both are treated with surgical correction.

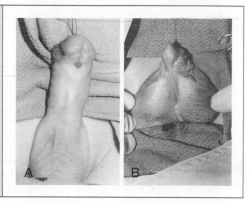

Figure 38-3. A, Distal hypospadias. **B,** Severe proximal hypospadias in the midscrotal area. (From Resnick MJ, Novick AC: Urology Secrets, 2nd ed. Philadelphia, Hanley & Belfus, 1999, with permission.)

30. **Define Potter syndrome. With what is it associated?**
Potter syndrome is bilateral renal agenesis, which causes oligohydramnios in utero (because the fetus swallows fluid but cannot excrete it). It is also associated with limb deformities, abnormal facies, and hypoplasia of the lungs. It is incompatible with life because of the severe associated lung hypoplasia.

CHAPTER 39

VASCULAR SURGERY

1. **What clues suggest carotid stenosis? How is it diagnosed?**

   The classic presentation of carotid stenosis is a transient ischemic attack—especially amaurosis fugax, which is the sudden onset of transient, unilateral blindness, sometimes described as a "shade pulled over one eye." Physical exam may reveal a carotid bruit. Ultrasound of the carotid arteries (duplex scan of the carotids) is used to diagnose and quantify the degree of stenosis.

2. **How is carotid stenosis managed?**

   If the stenosis is **70% to 99%** and symptoms are present, patients usually are advised to undergo carotid endarterectomy for the best long-term prognosis—if their state of health allows them to tolerate the surgery. Patients should not undergo carotid endarterectomy after a stroke that leaves them severely disabled, but small, nondisabling strokes are not contraindications to surgery. Carotid endarterectomy should not be performed during a transient ischemic attack or stroke in evolution. Surgery is always done electively, not on an emergent basis.

   If the stenosis is **less than 50%,** whether the patient has symptoms or not, do not advise carotid endarterectomy. Treat with daily aspirin and/or clopidogrel instead. Between 50% and 70% stenosis, treatment is controversial (unlikely to be asked on USMLE) and depends on degree of symptoms, type of plaque and experience of local surgeons. The role of carotid angioplasty and carotid stenting in carotid stenosis is not yet defined. Carotid endarterectomy remains the treatment of choice for suitable carotid stenosis.

3. **What is the most common cause of death during vascular surgery?**

   Myocardial infarction, regardless of the procedure performed. Peripheral vascular and aortic disease are generalized markers for atherosclerosis, and almost all patients have significant coronary artery disease. Always evaluate patients for modifiable and treatable atherosclerosis risk factors (i.e., cholesterol, hypertension, smoking, diabetes).

4. **What are the classic findings in a patient with an abdominal aortic aneurysm? How is it evaluated?**

   Abdominal aortic aneurysm (Fig. 39-1) classically presents as a pulsatile abdominal mass that may cause abdominal pain. If pain is present, rupture/leak of the aneurysm should be suspected, although an unruptured aneurysm may cause some degree of pain. Ultrasound or computed tomography (CT) scan is used for initial evaluation and diagnostic confirmation in stable patients, as well as for serial monitoring.

5. **How is an abdominal aortic aneurysm managed? What clues indicate that the aneurysm has ruptured?**

   If the aneurysm is smaller than 5 cm, you can follow it with serial ultrasound examinations to ensure that it is not enlarging. These smaller aneurysms should be managed with risk factor reduction (smoking cessation and treatment of hypertension and dyslipidemia). If the aneurysm is larger than 5 cm (or if you are told that it is enlarging rapidly), surgical correction should be advised if the patient can tolerate the surgery.

A **pulsatile abdominal mass plus hypotension** equals emergent laparotomy for a presumed ruptured aneurysm, which carries a mortality rate of roughly 90%. The management of an abdominal aortic aneurysm dissection depends upon the location of the dissection. Patients who survive the initial tear typically present with a severe sharp or tearing sensation in the back or chest. Acute dissections involving the ascending aorta are considered surgical emergencies. Dissections confined to the descending aorta are treated medically unless the dissection progresses or continues to bleed.

6. **Define Leriche syndrome. For what is it a marker?**
   Leriche syndrome is the combination of claudication in the buttocks, buttock atrophy, and impotence in men due to aortoiliac occlusive disease. Most patients need an aortoiliac bypass graft.

7. **Define claudication. What are the associated physical findings?**
   Claudication is pain, usually in the lower extremity, brought on by exercise and relieved by rest. It occurs with severe atherosclerotic disease and is the equivalent of angina for the extremities. Associated physical findings include cyanosis (with dependent rubor), atrophic changes (thickened nails, loss of hair, shiny skin), decreased temperature, and decreased (or absent) distal pulses.

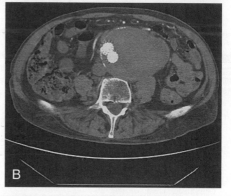

Figure 39-1. Cross sectional CT image (**A**) of an 11-cm abdominal aortic aneurysm. **B,** CT image 3 months after endovascular repair. Note the thrombosed aneurysm and patent limbs of the stent-graft. (From Townsend C, et al.: Sabiston Textbook of Surgery, 18th ed. Philadelphia, Saunders, 2008, Fig. 65-4.)

8. **How are patients with claudication managed?**
   The best treatment is conservative: cessation of smoking, exercise, and good control of cholesterol, diabetes, smoking and hypertension. Antiplatelet agents are warranted in patients with claudication. Aspirin is preferred, but clopidogrel may be used for patients who cannot tolerate aspirin. Cilostazol may be used for the treatment of intermittent claudication. Beta blockers may worsen claudication (as a result of $beta_2$ receptor blockade), but benefits may outweigh the risks in some patients (e.g., prior myocardial infarction). If claudication progresses to rest pain (forefoot pain, generally at night, which is classically relieved by hanging the foot over the edge of the bed) or interferes with lifestyle or work obligations, perform diagnostic angiography and use angioplasty or surgical revascularization procedure for treatment. Because claudication and peripheral vascular disease are generalized markers for atherosclerosis, check for other atherosclerosis risk factors.

9. **What is the probable cause of severe, sudden onset of foot pain in patients with no previous history of foot pain, trauma, or associated chronic physical findings?**

   This scenario may indicate an embolus (look for atrial fibrillation; the pulse may be absent in the affected area) or compartment syndrome (common after revascularization procedures).

10. **Describe the classic presentation of chronic mesenteric ischemia.**

    The classic patient has a long history of postprandial abdominal pain (also known as intestinal angina; eating is "exercise" for the intestines), which causes "fear" of food and extensive weight loss. This diagnosis is difficult because, like all atherosclerotic disease, it presents in patients over 40, who have other conditions that may cause the same problem (e.g., peptic ulcer disease, pancreatic cancer, stomach cancer). Look for a history of extensive atherosclerosis (previous myocardial infarctions or strokes, known coronary artery disease or peripheral vascular disease, multiple risk factors), abdominal bruit, hemoccult-positive stool, and lack of jaundice (jaundice suggests pancreatic cancer). Most patients get a CT scan of the abdomen; negative results raise the suspicion of ischemia. Diagnosis can be made with an angiogram of the mesenteric vessels (mesenteric duplex ultrasonography is emerging as a diagnostic tool, and contrast-enhanced magnetic resonance angiography is being studied). Patients are treated with surgical revascularization because of the risks of bowel infarction and malnutrition.

11. **How does an acute bowel infarction present?**

    Classically, a patient with a history of extensive atherosclerosis or multiple atherosclerosis risk factors presents with abdominal pain or tenderness, bloody diarrhea, and possibly peritoneal signs (e.g., rebound tenderness, guarding). Watch for "thumbprinting" (thickened bowel walls that resemble thumb prints) on abdominal radiographs. Patients also may have tachycardia, hypotension, and/or shock.

12. **What causes arteriovenous fistulas and pseudoaneurysms in the extremities? How do you recognize them?**

    Penetrating trauma in an extremity or iatrogenic catheter damage may be followed by the development of an arteriovenous fistula or pseudoaneurysm. Watch for bruits over the area or a palpable pulsatile mass. Small fistulas can be left alone, but other patients require surgical or angiographic intervention.

13. **What are the signs and symptoms of venous insufficiency? How is it treated?**

    Venous insufficiency generally occurs in the lower extremities. Patients may have a history of deep venous thrombosis, varicose veins, and/or positive swelling in the extremity with pain, fatigability, or heaviness. Symptoms are relieved by elevating the extremity. Patients also may have increased skin pigmentation around the ankles with possible skin breakdown and ulceration.

    Treatment is at first conservative, including elastic compression stockings, elevation with minimal standing, and treatment of ulcers with cleaning, wet-to-dry dressings, and antibiotics, if cellulitis occurs.

14. **True or false: A superficial palpable cord is a fairly specific sign of deep venous thrombosis.**

    False. A superficial palpable cord usually represents superficial thrombophlebitis.

15. **Describe the usual history of a patient with superficial thrombophlebitis. How is it treated?**

    Patients often have a history of varicose veins and present with localized leg pain with superficial cord-like induration, reddish discoloration, and mild fever. Superficial thrombophlebitis is not a significant risk factor for pulmonary embolus, and patients do not need anticoagulation. Treatment is usually conservative, including nonsteroidal anti-inflammatory drugs and warm compresses. The condition generally subsides on its own within a few days. A thrombectomy under local anesthesia can be done for severe or nonresolving symptoms.

16. **Define subclavian steal syndrome. What symptoms does it cause? How is it treated?**

The subclavian steal syndrome is usually due to left subclavian artery obstruction proximal to the vertebral artery origin. To perfuse an exercising arm, blood is "stolen" from the vertebrobasilar system; that is, it flows backward into the distal subclavian artery instead of forward into the brainstem. Patients present with central nervous system symptoms (e.g., syncope, vertigo, confusion, ataxia, dysarthria) and upper extremity claudication during exercise. Treat with surgical bypass.

17. **What are the symptoms of thoracic outlet syndrome? How is it treated?**

Thoracic outlet obstruction refers to symptoms caused by obstruction of the nerves or blood vessels that serve the arm as the neurovascular bundle passes from the thoracocervical region to the axilla. Affected patients have upper extremity paresthesias (nerve impingement), weakness, cold temperature (arterial compromise), edema, and/or venous distention (venous compromise). The absence of central nervous system symptoms helps to differentiate this condition from subclavian steal syndrome. Causes include cervical ribs (ribs arising from a cervical vertebrae that are usually asymptomatic but may compromise subclavian blood flow) or muscular hypertrophy (classic in young male weight lifters). Treat with surgical intervention (e.g., cervical rib resection). TOBIN !

CHAPTER 40

VITAMINS AND MINERALS

1. Specify the signs and symptoms of the various vitamin deficiencies and toxicities.

Vitamin	Deficiency	Toxicity
A	Night blindness, scaly rash, xerophthalmia (dry eyes), Bitot spots (debris on conjunctiva); increased infections	Pseudotumor cerebri, bone thickening, teratogenic
C	Scurvy (hemorrhages/skin petechiae, bone, gums; loose teeth; gingivitis), poor wound healing, hyperkeratotic hair follicles, bone pain (from periosteal hemorrhages)	
D	Rickets, osteomalacia, hypocalcemia	Hypercalcemia, nausea, renal toxicity
E	Anemia, peripheral neuropathy, ataxia	Necrotizing enterocolitis (infants)
K	Hemorrhage, prolonged prothrombin time	Hemolysis (kernicterus)
B_1 (thiamine)	Wet beriberi (high-output cardiac failure), dry beriberi (peripheral neuropathy), Wernicke and Korsakoff syndromes	
B_2 (riboflavin)	Angular stomatitis, dermatitis	
B_3 (niacin)	Pellagra (dementia, dermatitis, diarrhea), stomatitis	
B_6 (pyridoxine)	Peripheral neuropathy, stomatitis, convulsions in infants, microcytic anemia, seborrheic dermatitis	Peripheral neuropathy (only B vitamin with toxicity)
B_{12} (cobalamin)	Megaloblastic anemia *plus* neurologic symptoms	
Folic acid	Megaloblastic anemia *without* neurologic symptoms	

[handwritten annotation:] ophthalmoplegia, confabulations, ataxia

2. **Specify the signs and symptoms of the various mineral deficiencies and toxicities.**

Mineral	Deficiency	Toxicity
Iron	Microcytic anemia, koilonychia (spoon-shaped fingernails)	Hemochromatosis
Iodine	Goiter, cretinism, hypothyroidism	Myxedema
Fluoride	Dental caries (cavities)	Fluorosis with mottling of teeth and bone exostoses
Zinc	Hypogeusia (decreased taste), rash, slow wound healing	
Copper	Menkes syndrome (X-linked; kinky hair, mental retardation)	Wilson disease
Selenium	Cardiomyopathy and muscle pain	Loss of hair and nails
Manganese		"Manganese madness" in miners of ore (behavioral changes/psychosis)
Chromium	Impaired glucose tolerance	

3. **What are the fat-soluble vitamins? In what general category of patients are they deficient?**
   Vitamins A, D, E, and K are fat-soluble. Deficiency of any of these vitamins may be due to malabsorption (e.g., cystic fibrosis, cirrhosis, celiac disease, duodenal bypass, bile-duct obstruction, pancreatic insufficiency, chronic giardiasis). In such patients, parenteral supplements are required if high-dose oral supplements fail.

4. **What vitamin, mineral, and electrolyte deficiencies are classically seen in alcoholics?**
   Any can be seen, but watch especially for folate, thiamine, phosphorus, and magnesium deficiencies.

5. **What is the most common cause of vitamin B_{12} deficiency?**
   Pernicious anemia, in which antiparietal cell antibodies destroy the ability to secrete intrinsic factor. Conditions associated with pernicious anemia include hypothyroidism, type I diabetes, and vitiligo (Fig. 40-1). The Schilling test is used to diagnose the cause of B_{12} deficiency. Removal of the ileum and the tapeworm *Diphyllobothrium latum* are exotic causes of B_{12} deficiency.

6. **What is the classic iatrogenic cause of vitamin B_6 deficiency?**
   Prolonged therapy with isoniazid (especially in young people). Many clinicians automatically give pyridoxine supplements to patients who start isoniazid therapy for tuberculosis.

7. **Which medications may cause folate deficiency?**
   Anticonvulsants (especially phenytoin), methotrexate, and trimethoprim.

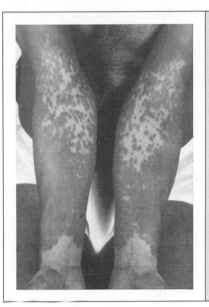

Figure 40-1. Vitiligo. Patches of depigmentation typically appear totally white, are well defined, have convex borders, and are of varying sizes. Symmetry, as shown in the figure, is typical. Half of patients develop the condition before the age of 20. On histology, there is an absence of melanocytes and melanin and antimelanocyte or antityrosinase antibodies are present. Close biologic relatives have a significantly increased (roughly fourfold) risk. (From du Vivier A: Atlas of Clinical Dermatology, 3rd ed. New York, Churchill Livingstone, 2002, p 659, with permission.)

8. **Which vitamin is a known teratogen?**

   Vitamin A. Female patients taking one of the vitamin A analogs (e.g., isotretinoin) as treatment for acne must have a negative pregnancy test before the medication is started and should be counseled about the risks of teratogenicity. Some form of birth control should be used, and periodic pregnancy tests should be offered.

9. **Which vitamin should be taken by all sexually active women of reproductive age?**

   Folate, which reduces the risk of neural tube defects in the fetus. The maximal benefit often occurs before the woman knows that she is pregnant.

10. **What are the physical findings of rickets (vitamin D deficiency in children)?**
    - Craniotabes (poorly mineralized skull; bones feel like a ping-pong ball)
    - Rachitic rosary (costochondral beading; small round masses on anterior rib cage)
    - Delayed fontanelle closure
    - Bossing of the skull
    - Kyphoscoliosis
    - Bow-legs and knock-knees
      Bone changes appear first at the lower ends of the radius and ulna.

11. **Which vitamin is given to all newborns?**

    Vitamin K is given as prophylaxis against hemorrhagic disease of the newborn.

12. **Which clotting factors are affected by vitamin K? What is the interaction of vitamin K and the liver?**

    Vitamin K is needed for hepatic synthesis of factors II, VII, IX, and X as well as proteins C and S. Chronic liver disease (e.g., cirrhosis) can cause prolongation of the prothrombin time and international normalized ratio because of the liver's inability to synthesize clotting factors even in the presence of adequate vitamin K levels. This problem should be corrected with fresh frozen plasma; vitamin K is ineffective in the setting of severe liver disease.

13. **Describe the relationship between vitamin K and broad-spectrum antibiotics.**

    Prolonged therapy with broad-spectrum antibiotics is a potential cause of vitamin K deficiency. These medications can eliminate the normal gut bacteria that synthesize much of the vitamin K required daily.

14. **What is the classic Step 2 description of a vitamin C-deficient patient?**

    An elderly person with a diet of "hot dogs and soda" or "tea and toast" who presents with bleeding gums and bone pain.

INDEX

Note: Page numbers in boldface type indicate complete chapters. Page numbers followed by *t* indicate tables; *f* indicate figures; *b* indicate boxes.